CARDIOLOGY

International Journal of Cardiovascular Medicine, Surgery, Pathology and Pharmacology

Founded 1937 as 'Cardiologia' by Bruno Kisch and Wilhelm Löffler, continued by R. Hegglin (1962–1969), I. Mahaim (1962–1965), P. Moret (1966–1969), P.M. Galletti (1966–1979), Jan J. Kellermann (1980–1990) and Joseph S. Alpert (1990–2005)

Incorporating Heart Drug (published 2001–2005)

(Continued on next page)

KARGER

Printed in Switzerland on acid-free and non-aging paper (ISO 9706) by Reinhardt Druck, Basel

Appears monthly: 3 volumes per year (12 issues)

KARGER

Guidelines for Authors

CARDIOLOGY

Submission

'Cardiology' publishes original reports in research and observations pertaining to cardiovascular physiology, epidemiology, pharmacology, disease and therapy. Only original papers written in English are considered. The articles should be readily comprehensible to a reader who is fluent in English. Therefore, all manuscripts originating from non-English-speaking authors must be edited prior to submission to assure that standard English grammar and usage are observed. This may require help from a colleague or other editorial assistant. It must be evident from the covering letter that this has been done. Submissions that are not edited in this way will not be considered for publication until such editing has been achieved. Manuscripts should be submitted using the online submission website:

www.karger.com/crd

If any problems with submission, please contact:

S. Karger AG
Editorial Office 'Cardiology'
P.O. Box
CH-4009 Basel (Switzerland)
Tel. +41 61 306 1357
Fax +41 61 306 1434
E-Mail crd@karger.ch

All manuscripts must be accompanied by a covering letter signed by all authors. Assurance should be given that the manuscript is not under simultaneous consideration by any other publication and that there are no conflicts of interest, see below. The preferred word processing package is Word for Windows®. Presentation of manuscripts should conform with the Uniform Requirements for Manuscripts Submitted to Biomedical Journals (see N Engl J Med 1997;336:309–315).

Main Sections

1. *Original Research*
2. *Original Research – Clinical Trial Design*
   Submissions will be accepted reporting the study design protocols of planned clinical trials that have been appropriately registered with regulatory authorities. These submissions will be limited to 4500 words and 35 references.
3. *Review*
4. *Letter to the Editor*
5. *Novel Insights from Clinical Experience*
   We invite contributions to this section that provide novel insight into a clinical problem. We recognise the value of case reports and thus submissions can be based on a single case or a number of similar cases. While a case report can describe an entirely novel clinical condition, we recognise that it is unlikely that most case reports will provide such information. In the more common setting of a description of a well-recognized condition, the *most important* aspect of the presentation, on which editorial judgments will be based, is the description of the new perspective(s) on the phenotype, pathophysiology, clinical presentation, evaluation strategy and/or management that can be drawn from the case findings. This category replaces the previous case report section.
   We require that a highlighted box containing one or two bullet points on **'Established facts'** and **'Novel insights'** should be placed on the first page of the report. These should be selected to reinforce the novelty of the clinical observation.
   The manuscript should be presented with an abstract (up to 200 words), brief introduction, case or case series description and results, followed by a discussion. Case reports should be no more than 2,500 words (including statements in the highlighted box) and should contain no more than 20 references.
6. *Short Communications*
   These manuscripts should not contain more than 2,000 words, including key words, essential references (not more than 15) and not more than 3 tables or figures. Such communications should represent complete, original studies and should be arranged in the same way as full length manuscripts.

Conditions

All manuscripts are subject to editorial review. Manuscripts are received with the explicit understanding that they are not under simultaneous consideration by any other publication. Submission of an article for publication implies the transfer of the copyright from the author to the publisher upon acceptance. Accepted papers become the permanent property of 'Cardiology' and may not be reproduced by any means, in whole or in part, without the written consent of the publisher. It is the author's responsibility to obtain permission to reproduce illustrations, tables, etc. from other publications.

Conflict of Interest in Cardiovascular Publications

Declaration of potential conflict of interest should be part of each publication or presentation and be designated as one or more of four categories: (1) No relationship. (2) Relationship with a For Profit Organization. (3) Research relationship with a For Profit or Not For Profit Organization, which should be named. (4) Employee of a For Profit or Not For Profit Organization. For legal reasons, all authors are required during submission of their manuscript to complete and sign a **Copyright Transfer & Conflicts of Interest Statement.** The corresponding author must ensure that all authors have been asked to sign this form and to disclose any conflicts of interest.

Ethics

Published research must comply with the guidelines for human studies and animal welfare regulations. Authors should state that subjects have given their informed consent and that the study protocol has been approved by the institute's committee on human research. Further, they should also state that animal experiments conform to institutional standards.

Arrangement

Title page: The first page of each paper should indicate the title, the authors' names, the institute where the work was conducted, and a short title for use as running head.
NB: Authors wishing to preserve the phonetic meaning of diacritics (PubMed reduces diacritics to their root characters) must spell their names accordingly when submitting manuscripts (e.g. Müller should be Mueller).

Full address: The exact postal address of the corresponding author complete with postal code must be given at the bottom of the title page. Please also supply phone and fax numbers, as well as e-mail address.

Key words: For indexing purposes, a list of 3–10 key words in English is essential.

For submissions to Main Sections 1, 2 and 3:

Abstract: The abstract is an essential and most read part of the paper. It should be printed on a separate page, up to 200 words, factual, free of abbreviations (except as specifically defined within the abstract text at first use) and should be structured as follows:
Objectives: Should describe the purpose of the study and the problem addressed; should include at least one sentence providing the rationale or justification for the study.
Methods: Should explain how the study was performed (samples and/or population, procedures, analytical methods).
Results: Should describe the main findings with specific data and their statistical significance, if possible.
Conclusions: Should contain a succinct interpretation of the inferences to be drawn from results.

Footnotes: Avoid footnotes. When essential, they are numbered consecutively and typed at the foot of the appropriate page.

Tables and illustrations: Tables and illustrations (both numbered in Arabic numerals) should be prepared on separate sheets. Tables require a heading and figures a legend, also prepared on a separate sheet. Due to technical reasons, figures with a screen background should not be submitted. When possible, group several illustrations in one block for reproduction (max. size 180 × 223 mm) or provide crop marks. Each illustration must be labelled with its number and the first author's name. b/w half-tone and color illustrations must have a final resolution of 300 dpi after scaling, line drawings one of 800–1,200 dpi. Figure files must not be embedded in a document file but submitted separately (see detailed instructions at http://www.karger.com/crd/).

Color illustrations
Online edition: Color illustrations are reproduced free of charge. In the print version, the illustrations are reproduced in black and white. Please avoid referring to the colors in the text and figure legends.
Print edition: Up to 6 color illustrations per page can be integrated within the text at CHF 760.– per page.

References: In the text identify references by Arabic numerals [in square brackets]. Material submitted for publication but not yet accepted should be noted as 'unpublished data' and not be included in the reference list. The list of references should include only those publications which are cited in the text. Do not alphabetize; number references in the order in which they are first mentioned in the text. The surnames of the authors followed by initials should be given. There should be no punctuation other than a comma to separate the authors. Preferably, please cite all authors. Abbreviate journal names according to the Index Medicus system. (Also see International Committee of Medical Journal Editors: Uniform requirements for manuscripts submitted to biomedical journals. N Engl J Med 1997;336:309–315.)

Examples
(a) Papers published in periodicals: Sun J, Koto H, Chung KF: Interaction of ozone and allergen challenges on bronchial responsiveness and inflammation in sensitised guinea pigs. Int Arch Allergy Immunol 1997;112:191–195.
(b) Papers published only with DOI numbers: Theoharides TC, Boucher W, Spear K: Serum interleukin-6 reflects disease severity and osteoporosis in mastocytosis patients. Int Arch Allergy Immunol DOI: 10.1159/000063858.
(c) Monographs: Matthews DE, Farewell VT: Using and Understanding Medical Statistics, ed 3, revised. Basel, Karger, 1996.
(d) Edited books: Parren PWHI, Burton DR: Antibodies against HIV-1 from phage display libraries: Mapping of an immune response and progress towards antiviral immunotherapy; in Capra JD (ed): Antibody Engineering. Chem Immunol. Basel, Karger, 1997, vol 65, pp 18–56.

Reference Management Software: Use of EndNote is recommended for easy management and formatting of citations and reference lists.

Digital Object Identifier (DOI)

S. Karger Publishers supports DOIs as unique identifiers for articles. A DOI number will be printed on the title page of each article. DOIs can be useful in the future for identifying and citing articles published online without volume or issue information. More information can be found at www.doi.org.

Author's Choice™

With this option the author can choose to make his article freely available online against a one-time fee of CHF 2750.–. This fee is independent of any standard charges for supplementary pages, color images etc. which may apply. More information can be found at www.karger.com/authors_choice.

Page Charges

There are no page charges for papers of 6 or fewer printed pages (including tables, illustrations and references). Each additional complete or partial page is charged to the author at CHF 310.–. The allotted size of a paper is equal to approx. 18 manuscript pages (including tables, illustrations and references).

Proofs

Unless indicated otherwise, proofs are sent to the first-named author and should be returned with the least possible delay. Alterations made in proofs, other than the correction of printer's errors, are charged to the author. No page proofs are supplied.

Reprints

Order forms and a price list are sent with the proofs. Orders submitted after the issue is printed are subject to considerably higher prices.

KARGER

Fax +41 61 306 12 34
E-Mail karger@karger.ch
www.karger.com

The Guidelines for Authors are available at:
www.karger.com/crd_Guidelines

CARDIOLOGY

General Information

ISSN Print Edition: 0008–6312
ISSN Online Edition: 1421–9751

Journal Homepage: www.karger.com/crd

Publication Data: 'Cardiology' is published 12 times a year. Volumes 112–114, each with 4 issues, appear in 2009.

Subscription Rates: Subscriptions run for a full calendar year. Prices are given per year.

Personal subscription:

Print or Online	**Print+Online combined**
CHF 593.55	CHF 728.55
EUR 423.90	EUR 519.90
USD 565.20	USD 694.20

postage and handling (added to print and print+online)
CHF 75.60 Europe, CHF 113.40 Overseas
EUR 54.–
USD 107.40

Institutional subscription:

Print or Online	**Print+Online combined**
CHF 3957.–	CHF 4353.–
EUR 2826.–	EUR 3108.–
USD 3768.00	USD 4146.00

postage and handling (added to print and print+online)
CHF 94.80 Europe, CHF 141.60 Overseas
EUR 67.20
USD 134.40

Airmail surcharge: CHF 96.– / USD 91.20

Back Volumes and Single Issues: Information on availability and prices of single print issues and print or electronic back volumes can be obtained from Customer Service at *service@karger.ch.*

Bibliographic Indices: This journal is regularly listed in bibliographic services, including *Current Contents®* and PubMed/MEDLINE.

Photocopying: This journal has been registered with the Copyright Clearance Center (CCC), as indicated by the code appearing on the first page of each article. For readers in the US, this code signals consent for copying of articles for personal or internal use, or for the personal or internal use of specific clients, provided that the stated fee is paid per copy directly to
Copyright Clearance Center Inc.
222 Rosewood Drive
Danvers, MA 01923 (USA)
A copy of the first page of the article must accompany payment. Consent does not extend to copying for general distribution, for promotion, for creating new works, or for resale. In these cases, specific written permission must be obtained from the copyright owner,
S. Karger AG, P.O. Box
CH–4009 Basel (Switzerland).

Subscription Orders:
Orders can be placed at agencies, bookstores, directly with the Publisher or further Karger offices or representatives:

S. Karger AG
Medical and Scientific Publishers
P.O. Box
CH–4009 Basel
Switzerland
(for courier services only:
Allschwilerstrasse 10
CH–4055 Basel)
Tel. +41 61 306 11 11
Fax +41 61 306 12 34
E-Mail karger@karger.ch
www.karger.com

France:
Librairie Medi-Sciences Sarl
36, bd de Latour-Maubourg
75007 Paris
France
Tél. +33 (0) 1 45 51 42 58
Fax +33 (0) 1 45 56 07 80
E-Mail librairie@medi-sciences.fr
www.medi-sciences.fr

Germany:
S. Karger GmbH
Postfach
79095 Freiburg
Deutschland
(Hausadresse: Lörracher Strasse 16A
79115 Freiburg)
Tel. +49 761 45 20 70
Fax +49 761 45 20 714
E-Post information@karger.de
www.karger.de

India, Bangladesh, Sri Lanka:
Panther Publishers Private Ltd.
33, First Main
Koramangala First Block
Bangalore 560 034
India
Tel. +91 80 25505 836
Tel. +91 80 25505 837
Fax +91 80 25505 981
E-Mail panther_publishers@vsnl.com
www.pantherpublishers.com

Japan:
Karger Japan, Inc.
Yushima S Bld. 3F
4-2-3, Yushima, Bunkyo-ku
Tokyo 113-0034
Japan
Tel. +81 3 3815 1800
Fax +81 3 3815 1802
E-Mail publisher@karger.jp

China, Taiwan and Malaysia:
Karger China
Suite 409, Apollo Building
1440 Central Yan An Road
Shanghai 200040
China
Tel. +86-21-6133 1861
Fax +86-21-6133 1862
E-Mail karger.ray@gmail.com

South America and Central America:
Cranbury International LLC
7 Clarendon Ave., Suite 2
Montpelier, VT 05602
USA
Tel. +1 802 223 6565
Fax +1 802 223 6824
E-Mail
eatkin@cranburyinternational.com
www.cranburyinternational.com

United Kingdom, Ireland:
S. Karger AG
c/o London Liaison Office
4 Rickett Street
London SW6 1RU
United Kingdom
Tel. +44 (0) 20 7386 0500
Fax +44 (0) 20 7610 3337
E-Mail uk@karger.ch

USA:
S. Karger Publishers, Inc.
26 West Avon Road
P.O. Box 529
Unionville, CT 06085
USA
Toll free: +1 800 828 5479
Tel. +1 860 675-7834
Fax +1 860 675-7302
E-Mail karger@snet.net

Change of Address:
Both old and new address should be sent to the subscription source.

KARGER

Fax +41 61 306 12 34
E-Mail karger@karger.ch
www.karger.com

The Journal Home Page is available at:
www.karger.com/crd

CARDIOLOGY

Abstracts
International Heart Forum

Beijing, China, September 11–13, 2009

Guest Editor
Shengshou Hu, Beijing, China

KARGER

Basel · Freiburg · Paris · London · New York · Bangalore ·
Bangkok · Shanghai · Singapore · Tokyo · Sydney

S. Karger
Medical and Scientific Publishers
Basel • Freiburg • Paris • London •
New York • Bangalore • Bangkok •
Shanghai • Singapore • Tokyo • Sydney

Printed in China
ISBN 978–3–8055–9259–8
e-ISBN 978–3–8055–9260–4

KARGER

Fax +41 61 306 12 34
E-Mail karger@karger.ch
www.karger.com

Cardiovascular Intervention

1

Persistent Inhibition of Neointimal Hyperplasia after Firebird2 Sirolimus-Eluting Stent Implantation Long-Term (Up to 3 Years) Clinical Follow-Up a Single Center Experience

Qian J, Xu B, Chen JL, Yang YJ, Qiao SB, Li JJ, Qin XW, Yao M, Liu HB, Wu YJ, Yuan JQ, Chen J, You SJ, Dai J, Gao RL
Cardiovascular Institute & Fu Wai Hospital, Chinese Academy of Medical Science & Peking Union Medical College, Beijing 100037, China

Objective To investigate the late outcomes of Firebird2 sirolimus-eluting stent implantation in patients with coronary artery disease.
Methods The study population consisted of 36 patients who had undergone coronary Firebird2 stent implantation (First in Man). Patients were eligible for enrollment if there was symptomatic coronary artery disease or positive exercise testing, and angiographic evidence of single or multivessel disease with a target lesion stenosis of > or = 70% in a > or = 2.5 mm vessel. Follow-up coronary angiography and intravascular ultrasound was performed 6 months after stent deployment. Patients were clinically followed-up for a mean of 36.1 ± 1.1 months.
Results All patients survived after stent implantation, no patients experienced any kinds of myocardial infarction. Recurrent angina pectoris and Re-PCI was observed in 6 (13.8%) patients, but none of them because of in-stent or in-segment restenosis. IVUS verified late malaposition was found in 3 patients (6.9%), but no MACE was reported so far.
Conclusions The results of the present study indicate that Firebird2 sirolimus-eluting stents showed persistent inhibition of neointimal hyperplasia for up to 3 years of follow-up.

2

Percutaneous Coronary Intervention for Native Coronary Arteries of Post-CABG Subjects with Grafts Occlusion

Wang G, Han YL, Li Y, Jing QM, Wang SL, Ma YY, Wang B, Wang XZ
General Hospital of Shenyang Military, Region Shenyang Cultural Shenhe Road, No. 83

Objective To evaluate the feasibility and efficacy of PCI for native coronary artery lesions in patients with bypass graft occlusion.
Methods The clinical data of 135 post-CABG patients with bypass graft occlusion presenting angina pectoris between June 2003 and June 2007 were analyzed. The mean interval from CABG to index angiography was 33.8 ± 23.5 months. There were 318 grafts, including 128 LIMA (22.7% occluded) and 188 saphenous vein grafts (77.3% occluded). A total of 146 native coronary vessels with 158 target lesions were treated with PCI. All target lesions were B2/C type lesions, including 29.7% (47/158) of chronic total occlusions.
Results All native target lesions were treated with drug eluting stents. Overall success rate of PCI procedure was 96.3% (130/135), and lesion success rate was 96.8% (153/158). No major clinical complications were occurred during peri-operative period. All patients were relieved from myocardial ischemic symptoms. Angiographic follow-up was obtained in 89 patients (91 lesions). The angiographic binary restenosis rate was 5.5% (5/91). All patients underwent successful PCI were followed at 12 month. The rates of major adverse cardiac events and

target vessel revascularization were 6.2% (8/130) and 3.8% (5/130), respectively.

Conclusions This study demonstrates that PCI for native coronary arteries in post-CABG patients with graft occlusion is feasible with a high procedure success rate and favorable long-term clinical and angiographic outcomes. A randomized comparison of this strategy with PCI for bypass graft is needed to confirm those findings.

3

Comparison between Drug-Eluting Stents and Coronary Artery Bypass Surgery for the Treatment of Unprotected Left Main Coronary Artery Stenosis

Wang HZ, Zhao Q, Liu J
The Department of Cardiac Surgery, RuiJin Hospital Affiliated to JiaoTong University, Shanghai, China

Objective To evaluate the clinical outcomes of patients treated with coronary artery bypass grafting surgery or percutaneous coronary intervention with drug-eluting stents for unprotected left main disease and find out the better choice of revascularization for such kind of patients.

Methods This study was a retrospective cohort study. From August 2004 to March 2006, a total of 115 patients with unprotected left main disease received revascularization in Zhongshan Hospital, Fudan University. Sixty-six of them underwent CABG (CABG group) and forty-nine received drug-eluting stents (PCI group). Baseline features, angiographic characteristics and operation data were recorded at entry point. The clinical end point was MACCE (major adverse cardiac and cerebrovascular event), including death of all causes, myocardial infarction, stroke and target vessel revascularization. All analysis was performed using the SPSS 17.0. Survival curves were computed by the Kaplan-Meier method and compared with the Log-rank test. Cox regression was used for multivariate analysis of prognostic factors.

Results 1. Patients in the CABG group were older and had more diabetes mellitus, hypertension, myocardial infarction and heart failure than that in the PCI group. The average Euroscore of the CABG group was higher than that of the PCI group. More patients in the CABG group had distal LMCA stenosis and coupled 3-vessel disease. 2. The combination of death, myocardial infarction, stroke, and target vessel revascularization (MACCEs) at 30 days occurred in 9.09% of the patients in the CABG group, but there was none MACCE in the PCI group. 3. There were more target vessel revascularization events in the PCI group than in the CABG group at 1 year (22.9% vs. 3.6%; $P = 0.006$), although MACCE-free rate was similar (84.2% CABG vs. 77.6% DES, $P = 0.483$). Moreover, there were no significant differences of survival rate (87.1% CABG vs. 92.2% DES, $P = 0.441$) or MACCE-free rate (69.9% CABG vs. 58.0% DES, $P = 0.155$) at a long-term follow-up, but the TVR-free rate was still lower in the DES group (62.8% DES vs. 94.5% CABG, $P < 0.001$). 4. Cox regression analysis indicated that CABG had a better outcome in patients with low-risk (Euroscore < 6) and distal LMCA stenosis. The hazard ratio was 0.320 (95% CI 0.135-0.758, $P = 0.01$) in patients with low risk and 0.373 (95% CI 0.165-0.843, $P = 0.018$) in patients with distal LMCA stenosis.

Conclusions Despite a higher percentage of high-risk patients in the CABG group, the long-term follow-up showed no difference in the rate of death, myocardial infarction, stroke and MACCE between PCI with DES and CABG for the treatment of unprotected left main coronary artery stenosis. However, the rate of target vessel revascularization was higher in the PCI group than that in the CABG group. In patients with low-risk and distal LMCA stenosis, CABG is a better choice.

4

Selection of Heart Valve Substitute in the Young Adult Population

Loisance D
Membre de l'Academie Nationale de Medecine

The selection of the optimal valve substitute in the young adult is a real challenge. Two major changes are leading to reconsider the strategy in the young adult patient: a) life prolongation is not any more the only objective for the valve replacement. The life style of the patient now plays a role in the decision at least as important than the prolongation of life; b) the recent progress in the development of truly non invasive techniques for valve replacement (using trans catheter valves and a true per cutaneous technique) rapidly leads to a new therapeutic approach: the repetition of the non invasive procedures making acceptable a limited longevity of the valve substitute.

Historical data do not help much in the decision in the young adult: the longevity after valve replacement is identical in the group of patients receiving a mechanical valve when compared to the patients receiving a tissue valve. The only difference is the nature of the complications: the mechanical valves are exposing the patient to the risk of thrombo embolism and/or hemorrhagic complications, as the tissue valves may fail. The difference in the vital risk is quite significant: the first ones, often acute, are more frequently lethal than the second one, usually progressive and treatable by a low risk re operation.

Little progress in mechanical valves has been made over the past 20 years. The noise made by the mechanical valve impairs the quality of life. Reduction of bleeding and thrombo-embolism remains a daily challenge. The real progress are still under evaluation: the low anticoagulation regimen, the self monitoring of the anticoagulation, the new anti thrombotic agents and mainly the oral anti thrombin agents (Megabatran), the surface treatment (ForceField) permitting to decrease the level of required anticoagulation.

In another hand, major progress has been made in the field of the tissue valve. The main one is the better understanding of the evolution of tissue materials after implantation. This has permitted new procedures in the manufacturing of the tissue valves (harvesting modalities, rapid fixation, zero pressure fixation, new fixation agents, anti-calcification agents) which finally permit to preserve the tissue structure, the mechanical properties and to decrease the risk of calcification. The analysis of the effect of the stress distribution on the leaflets has permitted to develop two new concepts: the flexible stent and the stentless valve. Both are improving the durability of the tissue valves. The most significant evolution is the transcatheter valve, implantable through a percutaneous approach, which will impact dramatically the strategy in valve replacement in the young adult.

Finally, a priority has to be given to the patients requirements, making quite important the dialogue.

5

Clinical Evaluation of Ventricular Assist Device Implantation (VAD) in 1280 Patients with End-stage Heart Failure (ESHF) in German Heart Institute (Berlin)

Weng YG, Hetzer R

Deutsches Herzzentrum Berlin

Objective Heart failure treatment guidelines recommended utilizing of VAD for ESHF. The implantation of VAD in 1280 patients with ESHF in German Heart Institute (Berlin) has been evaluated.

Methods Between July 1987 and March 2009, 1377 VADs were implanted in 1280 patients. Mean age was 43.43 years (range 3 days-81 years). 1042 (81.4%) were male. 106 were children (< 18 years). Left ventricular assist device (LVAD) were implanted in 703 (54.9%) patients, right ventricular assist device (RVAD) in 29, biventricular assist device (BVAD) in 548 (42.8%) patients, 49 of them total artificial heart. There were a variety of devices used Excor, Novacor, HeartMate I, De Bakey VAD, Incor, HeartMate II, Javik 2000, LionHeart, Abiomed BVS5000, Levitronix, DuraHeart, VentrAsist, CorAid and so on. Patients were divided into 3 groups for survival analyses. Group I as saving lives, a total of 191 cases had severe ESHF postcardiotomy, donor failure underwent heart transplantation (HTX) or already using extracorporeal membrane oxygenation. The most of patients were younger than 60 years old and not known for the survival prognosis. All Patients require immediately VAD for circulatory support. Group II as a bridge to HTX or to recovery, 1011 cases due to various causes of ESHF underwent emergency VAD implantation in profound cardiogenic shock (defined as presence of ongoing multiorgan failure requiring VAD support in next 24 hours). Group III as a destination therapy, a total of 78 patients over the age of 65 ESHF, for various reasons precluding HTX. Anticoagulation therapy (INR maintained at 3.0 ± 0.25) in all cases.

Results The mean duration of support was 134 days and maximal duration 1876 days (5 years). Of 731 cases VAD supporting more than 30 days, 224 supporting 1 year, 78 supporting 2 years, 24 supporting 3 years, 9 supporting 4 years, 2 support 5 years. LVAD was implanted in 519 (71%) patients, BVAD in 208 (28.5%) patients, RVAD only in 4 cases. More than 30-days VAD supporting as a survival is 40.3% (n = 77) in group I, of them recovery of cardiac function in 25, HTX in 15, switch from a short-term to longer-term VAD in 37. Group II had 57.7% (n = 583) 30-days survival, HTX in 316 patients (HTX in DHZB between 1987 and March 2009 in 1630 patients). There no significant differences in long-term survival after HTX among patients with and without previous VAD. Removal of VAD in 81 cases due to cardiac function recovery, follow-up 2 years 7 of them died a non-cardiac diseases, infection and bleeding, 23 further deterioration of cardiac function which had 14 cases of HTX, 3 re-implantation of LVAD, 6 still under medical treatment. Other 47 cases had the average follow-up time 7.5 ± 5.5 years, an average of echocardiography left ventricular ejection fraction (45 ± 3%), left ventricular end-diastolic diameter (50 ± 5 than 58 ± 7 mm, p value = 0.007). Up to March 2009 were still 96 patients with VAD support, including 51 cases of discharge. In group 3 for the permanent treatment there were 71 (91%) cases of success VAD supporting, 24 of them support for more than 3 years, up to 5 years, the eldest patient is now 82 years old. 549 cases of early death, cause of death in 379 cases of multiple organ failure (69%), 135 cases of brain death (25%), other event such as bleeding, infection in 35, no mechanical problems. Late complications had thromboemblism in 241 cases, caused 195 cases of cerebral infarction, VAD thrombosis due to low cardiac output leading to even stop switch for device 45 cases, over the insurance period of VAD, the replacement of VAD in 1 case.

Conclusions VAD implantation can save lives of patients with postcardiotomy heart failure, as a bridge to HTX or to recovery in patients with severe cardiogenic shock, as a destination therapy for patients with ESHF precluding HTX.

6

Perioperative Haemostsis and vWF in Cardiovascular Surgery

Ao HS
Beijing Cardiovascular Institute & Fu Wai Hospital, China

Hemorrhagic disorders must be excluded prior to any operation or other invasive procedure that has the potential to involve serious bleeding, especially in open-heart surgery. Excessive bleeding after cardiopulmonary bypass (CPB) may lead to increased mortality, morbidity, transfusion requirements and re-intervention. Less than 50% of patients undergoing re-intervention exhibit surgical sources of bleeding. Excessive perioperative and postoperative bleeding continue to comnlicate cardiovascular surgery. When assessing the individual risk of bleeding, screening tests of homeostasis must be combined with the patient's clinical history and symptoms, and any history of bleeding must be explored under direct medical supervision using a standardized questionnaire. Screening tests that have been found to be useful include platelet count, activated partial thrombo plastin time (aPTT), prothrombin time (PT) and clottable fibrinogen. No reliable, sensitive and specific screening test is available today to screen for platelet dysfunction or von willebrand disease (vWF). vWF plays an important role in primary homeostasis by contributing to platelet adhesion and aggregation as well as in secondary homeostasis by contributing to in vivo survival of coagulation factor Ⅷ. Patients with very mild hemophilia A, with factor VIII generally in the 20-30% range, may not manifest any serious bleeding, however, it may induce serious bleeding if patients undergoing CPB. It is important to investigate the vWF in CPB patients. This article will evaluation of few factors in bleeding diathesis in cardiac perioperative setting and the treatment will be discussed.

7

Aortic Valve Sparing Operation for Aortic Root Aneurysm in Patients with Marfan Syndrome

Chang Q, Qian XY, Yu CT
Department of Aortic Surgery, Cardiovascular Institute and Fu Wai Hospital, Chinese Academy of Medical Science and Peking Union Medical College, Beijing, China

Objective We report our experiences in patients with Marfan syndrome operated on exclusively with the aortic valve sparing operation for aortic root aneurysm.

Methods Between August 2003 and July 2007, we used aortic valve sparing technique in 43 patients with aortic root aneurysm, 20 had Marfan syndrome. Their mean age was 28 ± 10 years (range, 10 to 57 years), and 9 were female, 11 were male. Reimplantation technique in 9 patients, remodeling technique in 8 patients, patch technique in 3 patients. Additional procedures were total aorta replacement in 1 patient, aortic arch replacement + stent-elephant trunk in 2 patients. The mean follow-up was 46 ± 16 months (range, 17 to 64 months).

Results No in-hospital and late death occurred, there was one reexploration for bleeding one day postoperative. No valve-related complication occurred during the follow-up. At the end of follow up, trivial or no aortic regurgitation was demonstrate in 14, mild in 4, moderate in one and severe in one. 2 patients with moderate and severe aortic regurgitation need reoperation.

Conclusions The early and mid-term results of valve sparing operations were favorable, and durability of the preserved valve should encourage use of this technique in patients with Marfan syndrome. But the long term follow-up is necessary.

8

Comparison of Treatment of Simple Abdominal Aortic Aneurysm by Open Surgery and Endovascular Stent

Chang Q, Wei YZ, Yu CT, Sun XG, Meng YH
Vascular disease center, Fu Wai hospital, Chinese Academy of Medical Sciences

Objective Covered stents have been widely utilized since Parieli treated an abdominal aortic aneurysm with a stent-graft in 1991. This article analyzed the result of different treatment of simple abdominal aneurysm and explored the advantage and disadvantage of both methods.

Methods From April, 2003 to June 2009, 53 patients received endovascular strent-graft repair for abdominal aortic aneurysm, during the same period, 66 patients received open surgery of artificial graft replacement. In stent-graft group, there are 47 male patients and 6 female patients and mean age is 69.63 ± 10.21 years old. Mean body weight of stent-graft group is 71.20 ± 12.77 kg. There are 17 patients with hypertension in this group (32.1%). In open surgery group, there are 55 male patients and 11 female patients and mean age is 58.15 ± 12.41 years old. Mean body weight of open surgery group is 68.55 ± 11.70 kg. There are 24 patients with hypertension in this group (36.3%). 46 patients in stent-graft group used local anesthesia and 7 patients in this group used general anesthesia. While all patients in open surgery group used general anesthesia and two patients also used cardiopulmonary bypass.

Results All patients in stent-graft group were successfully implanted with stent-grafts and angiogram at the time of intervention confirmed there were no endoleak and stent movement. One patient had sudden cerebral infarction 15 days after operation and the mortality of this group is 1.88%. All patients of open surgery group had successful operation. One patient had sudden cerebral infarction 5 days after operation and the mortality of this group is 1.52%. Patient's age of stent-graft group is obviously older than that of open surgery group, ($p < 0.05$). There was no statistical difference in body weight between two groups. There was one case of re-operation for bleeding in each group and there were no statistical difference. There were 7/53 (13.2%) patients in stent-graft group with coronary artery disease while there were 10/66 (15.15%) in open surgery group. There was no statistical difference. The ICU stay and hospital stay time of stent-graft group is significantly shorter than open surgery group ($p < 0.05$). The consumption of blood product of stent-graft group is also significantly reduced than open surgery group ($p < 0.05$), although the total cost of medical expenditure is higher for stent-graft group than open surgery group ($p < 0.05$).

Conclusions For simple abdominal aortic aneurysm, both endovascular stent-graft repair and open surgery is safe and reliable. Both treatments have very good short term result. Endovascular stent-graft repair has the advantage of minimally invasive, quick recovery and low consumption of blood product. Open surgery has the advantage of direct vision, convenient for combined surgery and reliability. Endovascular stent-graft repair has advantage in patients with complex morphology of aneurysm and atherosclerosis and stenosis of iliac or femoral artery. Open surgery has disadvantage for elder patients and patients with comorbidity. Long term result of both treatments is yet to be followed.

9

Transcatheter Closure of Secondum Atrial Septal Defect with Severe Pulmonary Hypertension Using Fenestrated Amplatzer Septal Occluders

Chen HY, Zhu XY, Hou CJ, Deng DG, Han XM, Sheng XT, Zhang DZ, Cui CS, Wang QG
Department of Congenital Heart Disease; General Hospital of Shenyang Military Region, Shenyang 110016, China

Objective To evaluate the effects of using fenestrated Amplatzer septal occluders (ASO) closure secundum atrial septal defect (ASD) with severe pulmonary hypertension (SPH).

Methods 9 patients with ASD combined SPH, 1 male and 8 female, aged from 18 to 54 years (mean 39.29 ± 14.04), were treated with fenestrated ASD occulder device. The diameter of ASD was 25-34 (mean 25.71 ± 5.02) mm by using TTE. Systolic pulmonary artery pressure (sPAP) 83-107 (92.71 ± 9.69) mmHg, mean pulmonary artery pressure (mPAP) 46-62 (56.43 ± 5.13) mmHg were measured by cardiac catheterization before the occlusion.

Results The diameter of fenestrated ASO was 32-42 (36.57 ± 4.86) mm. sPAP 37-99 (71.14 ± 20.84) mmHg and mPAP 31-51 (43.71 ± 8.64) mmHg were measured post-occlusion and femoral arterial oxygen saturation (SatO2) more than 93%. Heart function improved obviously and the sPAP deceased in certain degree, left heart insufficiency disappear in the follow-up. As yet, the longest tern follow-up exceeds 5 years.

Conclusions To closure ASD with SPH was a high risk. The long-term effects of a prolonged left-to-right atrial shunt promotes pulmonary vascular changes, the aging right ventricle was doubly beset by pressure and volume overload, left ventricle filling volume decrease owing to the dilated right ventricle crushing, all having degraded stroke volume that may induced heart failure. Interatrial pressure delivered through the hole, left ventricle capacity increase moderately, can improve left heart function and prevent left heart insufficiency. If sPAP decrease incompletely, the right ventricle pressure relieve effectively through the remain hole. We consider the indication that can implant the fenestrated ASO include Qp/Qs≥1.4, SO2≥90%, sPAP decrease less than 20% after occlusion, and without symptom. Percutaneous occlusion device provide a strategy to be safe and useful for ASD with SPH patients using fenestrated ASOs. However, lesser operated patient, the long-term effect demands to observe further.

10

Two-Year Clinical Outcome after Successful Implantation of Drug-Eluting and Bare Metal Stents in Diabetic Patients: Results from a Real-World Single Center Registry

Dou KF, Xu B, Yang YJ, Qiao SB, Gao RL
Cardiovascular Institute and Fu Wai Hospital, CAMS and PUMC, Beijing 100037, China

Background Drug-eluting stents (DES) have revolutionized the field of interventional cardiology by dramatically improving the clinical and angiographic outcomes. The patients with diabetes mellitus (DM) are associated with increased risk of adverse clinical outcome after PCI. The available information on efficacy and safety of DES and BMS in diabetic patients remains scarce.

Methods From April 2004 to October 2006, 1565 consecutive patients with diabetes, who underwent successful elective stenting at Fu Wai Hospital in Beijing, China, were prospectively enrolled in this study. All enrolled patients were divided into drug eluting stent group and bare metal stent group. We obtained follow-up data, including death, myocardial infarction (MI), thrombus, target lesion revascularization (TLR) and target vessel revascularization (TVR) defined by Academic Research Consortium (ARC) definition, at 30 days and 12 and 24 months. We calculated and compared all the unadjusted cumulative frequencies of the various adverse events in the two groups. Cox's proportional-hazards models adjusted with the propensity score were used to assess relative risks of all the outcome measures at 24 months

11

Comparison of Long-Term Clinical Outcome after Successful Implantation of Firebird and those after Cypher Sirolimus-Eluting Stents in Daily Clinical Practice: Analysis of a Large Single Center Registry

Dou KF, Xu B, Yang YJ, Qiao SB, Gao RL
Cardiovascular Institute and Fu Wai Hospital, CAMS and PUMC, Beijing 100037, China

Background Recent data has shown that sirolimus-eluting stents (SES) reduced not only the incidences of restenosis but also of target vessel revascularization (TVR) and myocardial infarction (MI). CYPHER and FIREBIRD stents are both widely used SES in China. However, comparative data concerning differences in long-term safety and efficacy regarding CYPHER and FIREBIRD stents in the Chinese population are still not available.

Methods From April 2004 to October 2006, 3, 979 consecutive patients who underwent successful SES (FIREBIRD 2274; CYPHER 1705) implantation were prospectively enrolled into this study. All enrolled patients were divided into two groups based upon stent type. We obtained 24-month follow-up data, including death, MI, thrombosis, target lesion revascularization (TLR), TVR, and major adverse cardiac events (MACE, the composite of death, MI, and TVR). Cox's proportional-hazards models were used to assess relative risks of all the outcome measures between the two groups before and after propensity match.

Results Unadjusted clinical outcomes demonstrated higher TVR (HR 1.78, 95% CI 1.26-2.50) and MACE (HR 1.40, 95% CI 1.08-1.82) for patients treated with FIREBIRD SES. After propensity match, however, no significant differences were found for all events at 24 months between FIREBIRD and CYPHER groups. All thrombosis rates by ARC definition were comparable between the two groups, except for higher very late thrombosis in the CYPHER group (0.3% vs. 1.3%, $p = 0.007$).

Conclusions In this large, real-world population, use of China's domestic FIREBIRD SES was associated with same safety and efficacy as the imported CYPHER SES.

12

Experience of 200 Cases of Robotic Cardiac Surgery

Gao CQ, Yang M, Wang G, Wang JL, Xiao CS, Wu Y, Li LX, Zhao Y
Department of Cardiovascular Surgery, PLA General Hospital, Beijing 100853, China

Objective To summarize the experience of the robotic heart surgery with da Vinci S system in China.
Methods Two hundred patients underwent robotic cardiac surgery form January 2007 to July 2009 in the Department of Cardiovascular Surgery in PLA General Hospital. All the patients were divided into 2 groups according to the approach of ports. The procedures included group I: totally endoscopic coronary artery bypass graft on beating heart (TECAB, 20 cases), Endoscopic atraumatic coronary bypass graft (63 cases), and hybrid robotic coronary artery bypass graft (10 cases), and group II: totally robotic mitral valve repaired or replacement (30cases), totally robotic myxoma excision (15 cases), totally endoscopic atrial septal defect closure (59 cases), tricuspid valve repair (8 cases) and totally robotic repair of partial anomalous pulmonary veins connection with pulmonary stenosis (1 case). In group I, 96 patients were operated on via left lateral approach, the mean age was 58. 8 ± 9. 4 years old (33 to 77 years old), the mean weight was 61. 8 ± 12. 0 kg (40 to 86 kg) and the mean height was 168. 9 ± 6. 4 cm (150 to 181 cm). Via 3 port incisions in the left chest and 1 port in the left subcostal area of xiphoid process for endostabilizer, beating-heart TECAB were completed with the da Vinci S robot, and the others were completed via left minithoracotomy after IMA was taken down robotically. In group II, 104 patients were done via right lateral approach, the mean age was 38. 6 ± 14. 8 years old (11 to 70 years old), the mean weight was 61. 8 ± 12. 0 kilogram (31 to 91 kg) and the mean height was 164. 2 ± 8. 4 cm (144 to 181 cm). Via 3 port incisions in the right chest and a 1. 5 cm working port, all the procedures were completed with the da Vinci S robot.
Results All patients had successful operations. There were no operative deaths or other complications. One patient was reexplored for bleeding in the trocar site, 1 patient had hemolysis. There were no intraoperative conversion to alternative approach, and there were no da Vinci system-related adverse events. All the cases were followed up.
Conclusions Our study shows that robotic cardiac surgery is feasible and safe and the surgical results are excellent for selected patients.

13

Totally Endoscopic Robotic Coronary Artery Bypass Grafting on Beating Heart

Gao CQ, Yang M, Wu Y, Wang G, Xiao CS
Minimally Invasive and Robotic Cardiac Surgery Center, Department of Cardiovascular Surgery, PLA General Hospital, Institute of Cardiac Surgery, Beijing 100853, China

Objective The ultimate goal of minimally invasive coronary artery bypass grafting is to perform the entire anastomosis in a closed chest. Robotic technology has been proven safe and efficacious in the performance of some cardiac surgeries. However, reports on totally endoscopic coronary artery bypass grafting on beating heart (TECAB-BH) are very limited. This study describes our experience of TECAB-BH in order to address procedural feasibility, safety and efficacy.
Methods From April 2007 to July 2009, a total of 83 patients underwent selective robotic CABG on the beating heart with da Vinci Surgical System, of which 63 patients underwent off-pump coronary artery bypass graft surgery through small lateral thoracotomy using robotic assistance for harvesting of left internal mammary artery (LIMA); 20 patients underwent TECAB-BH. In TECAB-BH cases, through 3 ports about 1 cm in the left thorax and an endostabilizer inserted via the 4th port in the xiphoid area under endoscopic vision, all the procedures were completed with the da Vinci S robot. Patients underwent postoperative angiography or CTA and were followed up to now.
Results TECAB with single-vessel LAD revascularization was successfully completed with da Vinci S robotic system in 20 cases. There were no operative deaths and no incisional conversion. The mean LIMA flow was 63. 2 ± 26. 7 ml/min. The patency of graft was checked by CTA (n = 10) or coronary angiography (n = 10) after operation, and the patency rate was 100%. The cosmetic results were excellent.
Conclusions Our study shows that TECAB on beating heart for LIMA-LAD is a feasible and safe procedure in selected patients, and clinical results are excellent. Further follow-up for graft patency is necessary. Use of robotics is now extended to achieve complete revascularization by

harvesting both internal mammary arteries and making a small thoracotomy for direct anastomosis.

14

Long Term Follow-Up of Dual Drug Eluting Stents Strategy for True Coronary Artery Bifurcation Lesions

Gao Z, Yang YJ, Xu B, Qiao SB, Gao RL
Cardiovascular Institute and Fu Wai Hospital, CAMS 100037, China

Objective True bifurcation lesions still are big challenge to percutaneous coronary intervention, it is still a controversy of dual drug eluting stent (DES) strategy for this kind of lesions.

Methods From April 2004 to April 2008, 506 consecutive patients (420 male, 57.7 ± 11.5 years old) with true bifurcation lesions in our center underwent DES implantation were analyzed. The double stents technique included Crush (62.8%), T (23.9%), Kissing stents (7.5%), T and protruding (4.3%) and Culotte technique (1.4%).

Results Mean clinical follow up duration was 537 ± 340 days, combination of ASA and plavix antiplatelet time was 256 ± 96 days. Major adverse cardiac events rate was 11.66%, including cardiac death (0.98%), no fatal myocardial infarction (3.16%) and target vessel revascularization (7.51%). Stent thrombosis (definite and probable) rate was 2.57%, including early (1.58%), late (0.59%) and very late (0.39%) thrombosis. 7 months Angiographic follow-up rate was 26.5%. Restenosis rate was 11.94% in main vessel and 14.93% in side branch.

Conclusions Long term follow-up indicated that DES strategy for true bifurcation lesions was comparatively safe and efficient.

15

Long Term Follow-Up of Crush versus No Crush Technique for Coronary Artery Bifurcation Lesions

Gao Z, Yang YJ, Xu B, Qiao SB, Gao RL
Cardiovascular Institute and Fu Wai Hospital, CAMS 100037, China

Objective Lesions at coronary bifurcations always are a big challenge for interventionists even with the advent of drug eluting stent (DES). Even with more and more clinical tails were published, operators still can not confirm one more efficient strategy than others, given these highly selected patients with short term follow-up.

Methods From April 2004 to April 2008, 505 consecutive Chinese patients underwent DES implantation for true bifurcation lesions including 258 crush strategy (213 male, 56.7 ± 10.8 years old) and 247 No Crush strategy (206 male, 58.1 ± 10.1 years old) were analyzed.

Results The follow-up period ranged from 237 to 1223 days [(537 ± 340) days for Crush group and (538 ± 351) days for No Crush group]. There was no significant difference of MACE rate in Crush and No Crush group (10.1% vs. 12.1%; $p = 0.481$), and so were cardiac death, nonfatal MI and TVR (0.4% vs. 1.6%; $p = 0.207$, 2.7% vs. 2.8; $p = 1.000$ and 7.0% vs. 7.7%; $p = 0.865$). Stent thrombosis rate was similar in two groups (1.6% vs. 2.0%; $p = 0.409$), late and very late stent thrombosis in both groups were very low (0.4% vs. 0.4%; $p = 1.000$). 7 months Angiographic follow-up showed no difference of restenosis rate in both groups (11.0% vs. 13.5%; $p = 0.786$). During follow-up, cardiac death, nonfatal MI, TVR and ST free survival rate showed no significant difference in both groups. The only variant identified as predictor of MACE was PCI by first two years, which accounted for 47% patients of all four years' cases.

Conclusions Crush technique showed similar long term clinical effect compared with other two DES techniques for coronary bifurcation lesions, operators' skills are very important improving clinical outcome.

16

Angioplasty of Stenosis Adjacent to Coronary Artery Ectasia: Long Term Follow-Up of Drug Eluting Stent versus Bare Metal Stent

Gao Z, Yang YJ, Xu B, Qiao SB, Gao RL
Cardiovascular Institute and Fu Wai Hospital, CAMS 100037, China

Objective Malaposition and coronary aneurysm after coronary stenting especially for drug eluting stent (DES) implantation are big concerns for interventionists, so the outcomes for stenting at stenotic lesions with adjacent ectasia need to be identifed.
Methods From April 2004 to October 2008, 136 consecutive Chinese patients underwent stent implantation for stenotic lesions with adjacent ectasia including 53 bare metal stent (BMS) and 83 DES were analyzed.
Results The follow-up period ranged from 132 to 1056 days [(566 ± 234) days for BMS group and (478 ± 251) days for DES group]. There was only 2 cardiac death (cardiogenic shock one day after acute myocardial infarction) in BMS group and 1 non fatal myocardial infarction 378 days after percutaneous coronary intervention (PCI) and 1 target vessel revascularization (TVR) in DES group (no significant difference of any of cardiac events). Except for 1 very late probable stent thrombosis in DES group (1.2%), no other stent thrombosis episodes were found. 19 patients (6 in BMS group and 13 in DES group) experienced 7 month coronary angiogram follow up, none of them suffered restenosis, stent malaposition or aneurysm, and original ectasias did not changed.
Conclusions From this long term follow up results, PCI for stenotic lesions with adjacent ectasia including DES was safe and efficient.

17

The One-Year Follow-Up of Bioabsorbable Polymer versus Durable Polymer Sirolimus-Eluting Stents in Real World

Gan Z, Yang YJ, Xu B, Qiao SB, Gao RL
Cardiovascular Institute and Fu Wai Hospital, CAMS 100037, China

Objective To compare the comparative effect of the bioabsorbable polymer sirolimus-eluting Stent (Excel) and the durable polymer sirolimus-eluting stent (Cypher) for daily practice in Chinese patients.
Methods From May 2006 to November 2006, 591 consecutive Patients implanted Excel (E group: n = 350, 58.1 ± 10.9 years old) or Cypher (C group: n = 241, 56.4 ± 10.7 years old) in our center were analyzed. 1 year clinical and 7 months angiographic follow-up were performed.
Results Baseline characteristics indicated that, compared with C group there were older myocardial infarction and triple vessel disease and less left main in E group, and there were larger reference vessel diameter, stent diameter and minimal diameter in stent and less rate of post-dilation in E group. 1 year follow-up results showed no difference of major adverse cardiac event (MACE) rate in E and C group (8.3% vs. 7.1%; P = 0.641), and no difference of cardiac death rate, non fatal myocardial infarction and target vessel revascularization (TVR) (0.9% vs. 0%; P = 0.274, 2.0% vs. 1.2%; P = 0.747and 5.4% vs. 5.8%; P = 0.857 respectively). There was no difference of total stent thrombosis or its components in both groups (total: 0.9% vs. 0.4%; P = 0.649, early: 0.6% vs. 0%; P = 0.516 and late: 0.3% vs. 0.4%; P = 1.000) according to Academic Research Consortium (ARC) standard definitions (definite + probable). 7 months angiographic follow-up indicated that there were no difference of in-stent and in-segment restenosis rate between two groups (4.7% vs. 3.2%; P = 0.725 and 5.6% vs. 3.2%; P = 0.505), but in-stent and in-segment late loss were significantly smaller in E group (0.18 ± 0.07 mm vs. 0.21 ± 0.08 mm; P = 0.000 and 0.21 ± 0.09 mm vs. 0.23 ± 0.11 mm; P = 0.003).
Conclusions Results from this, single-center study showed that both of the Excel and Cypher Sirolimus-eluting stent had similar effects on reducing the incidence of MACE and the risk of restenosis (both in-stent and in-segment binary restenosis) after PCI in 1 years follow-up.

18

Comparative Study of Long Term Follow-Up of Drug Eluting Stents for In-Stent Restenosis

Gao Z, Yang YJ, Xu B, Qiao SB, Gao RL
Cardiovascular Institute and Fu Wai Hospital, CAMS 100037, China

Objective To compare the long-term effect of three different drug-eluting stents (DES) for in-stent restenotic lesions.

Methods From April 2004 to June 2006, 390 consecutive patients with in-stent restenotic lesions underwent DES implantation including 187 Cypher (group C), 89 Taxus (group T) and 114 Firebird (group F) were analyzed. Mean 2 years clinical and 7 months angiographic follow-up were performed.

Results Baseline characteristics indicated there were more unstable angina in T group and less left main disease and more triple vessel disease in F group. Mean 2 years follow-up results showed no difference of major adverse cardiac events (MACE) rate in three groups (23.0% vs. 22.5% vs. 13.2%; P = 0.081), and no difference of cardiac death, no-fatal myocardial infarction (MI) and target vessel revascularization rate (1.1% vs. 4.5% vs. 1.8%; P = 0.210, 5.9% vs. 2.2% vs. 2.6%; P = 0.226 and 2.9% vs. 2.2% vs. 0.9%; P = 0.509). There was no difference of total stent thrombosis or its components in three groups (total: 4.8% vs. 3.4% vs. 2.6%; P = 0.605, early: 0.5% vs. 0% vs. 0.9%; P = 0.560, late: 1.6% vs. 1.1% vs. 0.9%; P = 0.849 and very late: 2.9% vs. 2.2% vs. 0.9%; P = 0.509) according to Academic Research Consortium (ARC) standard definitions (definite + probable). 7 months angiographic follow-up indicated that there were lower rate of both in-stent and in-segment restenosis in C and F groups (17.9% vs. 29.4% vs. 13.6%; P = 0.214 and 21.8% vs. 35.3% vs. 15.9%; P = 0.132), and in-stent and in-segment late loss were significantly smaller in C and F groups (0.31 ± 0.12 mm vs. 0.75 ± 0.24 mm vs. 0.31 ± 0.13 mm; P = 0.000 and 0.33 ± 0.18 mm vs. 0.61 ± 0.23 mm vs. 0.31 ± 0.14 mm; P = 0.001).

Conclusions Results from this 2 years follow-up, single-center study showed comparable effectiveness and safety of Cypher, Taxus and Firebird DES for in-stent restnotic lesions, but Cypher and Firebird tended to reduce restensis more.

19

Comparison of Zotarolimus-Eluting and Sirolimus-Eluting Stents in Elderly Patients with Coronary Artery Disease

Gao Z, Yang YJ, Xu B, Qiao SB, Gao RL
Cardiovascular Institute and Fu Wai Hospital, CAMS 100037

Objective To compare the comparative effect of the zotarolimus-eluting (Endeavor) with sirolimus-eluting Stent (Cypher) for daily practice in Chinese elderly patients.

Methods From October 2006 to May 2007, 635 consecutive patients (≥60 years old) implanted Endeavor (E group, n = 334, male: 75.7%) or Cypher (C group, n = 301, male: 81.4%) were analyzed. 7 months clinical and angiographic follow-up were performed.

Results Baseline characteristics indicated there were more hyperlipidemia, restenosis lesion and left main disease in C group, and there were longer stent length, stent deployed pressure and more rate of post-dilation in C group. 7 months follow-up results showed no difference of major adverse cardiac event (MACE) rate in E and C group (4.5% vs. 4.3%; P = 1.000), and no difference of rate of cardiac death, non-fatal myocardial infarction and target vessel revascularization (TVR) (0.6% vs. 0%; P = 0.501, 0.6% vs. 2.0%; P = 0.159 and 3.3% vs. 2.3%; P = 0.485 respectively). There was no difference of total stent thrombosis or its components in both groups (total: 0.3% vs. 0.7%; P = 0.606, early: 0.3% vs. 0.3%; P = 1.000 and late: 0% vs. 0.3%; P = 0.474) according to Academic Research Consortium (ARC) standard definitions (definite + probable). 7 months angiographic follow-up indicated that there were no difference of in-stent and in-segment restenosis rate between two groups (5.9% vs. 3.5%; P = 0.700 and 7.4% vs. 4.7%; P = 0.509), but in-stent and in-segment late loss were significantly larger in E group (0.48 ± 0.12 mm vs. 0.24 ± 0.09 mm; P < 0.001 and 0.21 ± 0.09 mm vs. 0.23 ± 0.11 mm; P = 0.003).

Conclusions Results from this 7 months follow-up, single-center study showed that both Endeavor and Cypher sirolimus-eluting stent had similar effects on reducing the incidence of MACE and restenosis rate (both in-stent and in-segment binary restenosis) for elderly patients in daily practice.

20

Long-Term Outcomes of Percutaneous Coronary Intervention for Unprotected Left Main Coronary Artery Disease: Comparison of Transradial Versus Transfemoral Approach

Gao Z, Yang YJ, Xu B, Qiao SB, Gao RL
Cardiovascular Institute and Fu Wai Hospital, CAMS 100037, China

Background The efficacy and safety of percutaneous coronary intervention (PCI) for unprotected left main coronary artery (LMCA) disease by transradial approach need to be established in comparison with tranfemoral approach.
Methods From April 2004 to November 2008, 874 consecutive Chinese patients underwent PCI for LMCA disease including 373 by transradial approach and 501 by transfemoral approach were analyzed.
Results Compared with the transfemoral group, the transradial group had more left main bifurcation disease and underwent more bifurcation stenting. There were no significant difference in terms of major adverse cardiac events (MACE) and its ingredients including cardiac death, no fatal myocardial infarction (MI) and target vessel revascularization (TVR) during mean 17 months follow-up in transradial group compared with transfemoral group (12.6% vs. 9.6%, $p = 0.187$; 2.1% vs. 3.2%, $p = 0.262$; 3.8% vs. 2.2%, $p = 0.218$ and 6.7% vs. 4.2%, $p = 0.125$). And there were also no significant difference of stent thrombosis and restenosis rate between two groups (1.6% vs. 2.8%, $p = 0.361$ and 9% vs. 14%, $p = 0.221$). During follow-up, cardiac death, no fatal MI and TVR free survival rate showed no significant difference in both groups. Cox regression results indicated that transradial approach was not a predictor of cardiac death, no fatal MI and TVR.
Conclusions Transradial approach showed similar long term clinical effect compared with transfemoral approach for LMCA disease, transradial approach is feasible for LMCA disease.

21

Endovascular Stent-grafting via the Aortic Arch for Type B Dissection Involving Distal Aortic Arch

Guo HW, Yu CT, Chang Q, Sun XG, Qian XY, He D, Wu YB, Feng J
Department of Surgery, Cardiovascular Institute and Fu Wai Hospital, Chinese Academy of Medical Sciences and Peking Union Medical College, Beijing 100037, China

Objective To evaluate effectiveness of endovascular stent-grafting via the aortic arch for type B dissection involving distal aortic arch and short-term results.
Methods Between January 2008 and March 2009, 7 patients with type B dissection involving distal aortic arch underwent endovascular stent-grafting via the aortic arch. A stent graft was implanted through aortotomy under circulatory arrest and selective cerebral perfusion. The proximal end of graft was sutured to the aortic arch. Concomitant surgery was underwent in 6 patients, including bypass from ascending aorta to brachiocephalic artery in six, and coronary artery bypass grafting (CABG) in one.
Results There was no operative death. One patient wasn't able to wean from cardiopulmonary bypass (CPB) due to myocardial ischemia, after CABG the patient was weaned from CPB successfully. One patient showed left upper limb venous return disturbance due to compression of innominate vein 3 days after operation, the patient recovered unevenfully after release the compression. One patient underwent pericardial window drainage procedure due to large pericardial effusion in 12 days after discharge. The other patients recovered and discharged uneventfully. CT examination showed one patient had an endoleak. The endoleak disappeared in 3 months of CT examination. Follow up ranged from 2 to 16 months, mean (12.75 ± 6.26) months. Symptoms of chest and back pain disappeared or released.
Conclusions Endovascular stent-grafting via the aortic arch is a safe, effective and economic way for type B dissection involving distal aortic arch. Short-term results were satisfied, and Long-term results need to be followed up.

22

Long-term Outcomes of Percutaneous Coronary Intervention for Patients with Distal Left Main Coronary Artery Disease

Han YL, Li Y, Wang SL, Jing QM, Ma YY, Wang G, Luan B, Wang B
Cardiovascular Research Institute and Department of Cardiology, Shenyang Northen Hospital, Shenyang 110016, China

Objective Distal left main (LM) coronary artery disease remains one of the most challenging lesion subsets in percutaneous coronary intervention (PCI). Impacts of different PCI strategies for such lesions on long-term outcomes are uncertain.
Methods Between January 2001 and December 2006, a total of 174 patients having PCI for distal LM diseases either with single vessel stenting (SVS, n = 125) or bifurcation stenting (BS, n = 49) were consecutively registered. The stents being used were paclitaxel eluting stents (PES) or bare metal stents (BMS). All patients were followed 1-year for occurrence of major adverse cardiac events (MACE).
Results Clinical characteristics were comparable between patients received SVS or BS except a higher numbers of diabetes within patients received SVS (29% vs. 14%, p = 0.046). Patient received BS displayed a higher proportion of significant stenosis in ostial or proximal circumflex (82% vs. 43%, p < 0.001). A higher proportion of BS than SVS procedures used PES (88% vs. 68%, p = 0.008). One-year clinical outcomes were not significantly different between the two strategies, either for MACE (15% in SVS vs. 8% in SB, p = 0.22) or target vessel revascularization (8% in SVS vs. 4% in BS, p = 0.36). Kaplan-Meier curves showed that PES implantation, instead of stenting strategies, was associated with favorable MACE-free survival (log rank p < 0.001). Multivariate analysis showed PES implantation (HR 0.16, 95% CI 0.07 ~ 0.41, p < 0.001) and EuroSCORE ≥6 (HR 3.0, 95% CI 1.3 ~ 7.0, p = 0.01) were predictors of MACE.
Conclusions In PCI for distal LM disease, PES implantation is more effective in reducing MACE rate compared with BMS. However, SVS or BS, based on physician's discretion, performs equally in long-term clinical outcomes.

23

Long-Term Safety and Efficacy of A Biodegradable Polymer Coated Sirolimus Eluting Stent: 2-Year Clinical Outcome of the CREATE Registry

Han YL, Jing QM, Yan GL, Wang SL, Ma YY, Wang G, Luan B
Shenyang Northern Hospital, Shenyang 110016, China

Objective Drug eluting stents with biodegradable polymer coatings were developed to overcome the potential adverse effects of durable polymers. However, long-term safety and efficacy of such stents were still unclear. The aim of this study was to assess the 2-year clinical outcomes of a biodegradable polymer coated sirolimus eluting stent (ExcelTM, JWMS, China) in real world practice.
Methods A total of 2077 patients were enrolled in the prospective, multicenter CREATE registry and were exclusively treated with the Excel stents. 80.5% of discharged patients discontinuated clopidogrel at 6 months after index procedure according to the study protocol. Patients were visited at 30d, 6-month and every 6 months thereafter. The primary outcome was the composite of cardiac death, non-fatal myocardial infarction (MI) and target lesion revascularization (TLR). The safety outcome was the incidence of stent thrombosis.
Results Clinical follow-up was completed in 2043 (98.4%) patients at 2 years post the index procedure. Primary events occurred in 71 patients (3.5%). The incidence of all-cause death, cardiac death, MI and TLR were 2.4%, 1.4%, 0.54% and 2.0%, respectively. At the 2-year follow-up, stent thromboses had developed in 24 patients (1.17%), including 2 (0.1%) acute, 8 (0.39%) subacute, 7 (0.34%) late, and 7 (0.34%) very late stent thrombosis. The occurrence of Academic Research Consortium definite or probable stent thrombosis was 0.73% (15/2043). A landmark analysis showed that the cumulative primary events-free survival rate during 6-to 24-month were not significantly different between patients had clopidogrel treatment ≤6 months and >6 months (96.5% vs. 97.6%, log rank p = 0.259).
Conclusions The 2-year clinical outcomes of the present study indicate the safety and efficacy of Excel stent in real world practice. The 6-month dual antiplatelet treatment seems safe after Excel stent implantation. However, the conclusions require further confirmation by longer follow-up results and head-to-head comparisons.

24

Immediate and Long-term Effects of Transcatheter Closure of Ventricular Septal Defect in Combination with Percutaneous Coronary Intervention in Patients with Ventricular Septal Rupture Complicating Acute Myocardial Infarction

Han YL, Zhu XY, Zhang DZ, Qin YW, Wang P, Liu YF, Xu YW, Jin QM, Li Yi, Wang XZ
Department of Cardiology, Department of Congenital Heart Disease, Northern Hospital of Shenyang, Liaoning 110016, China

Objective Ventricular septal rupture (VSR) complicating acute myocardial infarction (AMI) has been a life-threaten disease. The objective of this study was to assess the immediate and long-term effects of transcatheter closure of ventricular septal defect (VSD) in combination with percutaneous coronary intervention (PCI) in patients with VSD complicating AMI.

Methods Data were prospectively collected for 16 patients (9 females) with a mean (SD) age of 69.0 (5.8) years who underwent attempted trascatheter VSD closure and PCI therapy in 5 Chinese centers between April 2001 and November 2007. All the patients who survived the procedures were followed up clinically and by X-ray, electrocardiogram and echocardiography.

Results Of all patients studied, 8 patients had one-vessel disease, 4 had two-vessel disease, and 4 had three-vessel disease. The mean duration from AMI symptom onset to PCI was 33.8 ± 28.5 days. Successful PCI therapy was performed in all patients without major procedural complications. A mean (SD) of 1.3 (0.5) stents per patient were implanted. All patients but two had a one-orifice defect and the diameter of the defects ranged from 6 mm to 22 mm (10.8 ± 4.6 mm). The post-VSR cardiac function was Killip Class Ⅱ in 4, Class Ⅲ in 4 and Class Ⅳ in 8 patients. Six patients underwent urgent VSD closure in acute phase (within 3 weeks from VSR) while the others underwent elective closure. 14 of 16 patients including two patients with two-orifice defects underwent successful transcatheter VSD closure. The VSD closure device success was 88.9% (16/18) and the procedure success was 87.5% (14/16). Residual shunts were small in 2 patients and moderate in 5 patients immediate after device release. At a mean (SD) of 48 (23) months follow-up period, 13 patients are all alive and only 3 had small residual shunt at the last follow-up. Cardiac function assessed clinically and by echocardiography improved significantly after successful combined interventional therapy compared with that at admission.

Coclusions Combined transcatheter VSD closure and PCI therapy to treat VSR complicating AMI is safe and feasible and is a promising alternative to the surgery in the patients with anatomically suitable VSDs and coronary vessels.

25

Non-calcified Attenuated Plaque and Neointima Hyperplasia after Drug-eluting Stents in Patients with Acute Myocardial Infarction

Han YL, Jing QM, Wang SL, Ma YY, Wang XZ, Zhang J
Department of Cardiology, Shenyang Northern Hospital, Shenyang 110016, China

Background Intravascular ultrasound (IVUS) non-calcified plaque with attenuation is plaque with deep ultrasound attenuation without calcification or very dense fibrous plaque. Natural evolution of attenuated plaques and their affect on vessel responses to stent implantation are not fully understood.

Methods We analyzed 13 month follow-up IVUS in 147 patients with acute myocardial infarction who undergone primary percutaenoues coronary intervention using drug-eluting stents. The neointima hyperplasia in the segments with attenuated plaques was analyzed.

Results At follow-up, there was less neointima in lesions with attenuated plaques ($n = 41$) compared to lesions without ($n = 106$) (mean neointima area: $0.91 \pm 0.41\ mm^2$ vs. $0.51 \pm 0.32\ mm^2$, $p < 0.05$). In the plaques with attenuation, there was more neointima hyperplasia in the arc without attenuation ($n = 106$) than in the arc with ($n = 106$) (mean neointima arc: $23° \pm 12°$ vs. $78° \pm 32°$, $p < 0.05$, figure).

Conclusions Non-calcified attenuated plaques maybe related to late healing after drug-eluting stents implantation in patients with acute myocardial infarction.

26

Clinical Analysis of the Death Cases for Children after Complete Repair of Tetralogy of Fallot

He D, Shen XD, Liu YL
Department of Cardiac Surgery, Cardiovascular Institute and Fu Wai Hospital, CAMS and PUMC, Beijing 100037, China

Objective To analyze the modes of death for children after complete repair of Tetralogy of Fallot and to determine the indication and contraindication of complete repair of Tetralogy of Fallot in the children.
Methods Between August 1999 and February 2007, 1284 children with Tetralogy of Fallot received complete repair procedure with mean age of 2. 4 ±5. 1 (3 months-8. 0) years and body weight of 11. 2 ±8. 5 (4. 0 ~28. 0) kg. Of the 1284 patients, there were 372 infants not elder than six months, and 53 emergency surgeries were included.
Results 49 patients died with mortality 3. 8% (49/1284) and 4 patients died after emergency operation with mortality 7. 5% (4/53). Acute and subacute cardiac failure was the mainly cause of death, 16 patients died of low cardiac output syndrome. Pulmonary insufficiency or edema in 6 patients. 5 patients could not withdraw cardiopulmonary bypass because of anomalous origin of coronary artery, pulmonary artery atresia or complete atrioventricular septal defect and died during the repairs. Severe infection led 5 patients to death. Complete cardiac block, multiple subsystem failure, neurological complication and improperly postoperative management and nursery contributed 4 patients to die equally. One patient died of upper gastric bleeding and DIC.
Conclusions Cardiac catheterization and angiography for children with severe Tetralogy of Fallot is required. Staged repair of Tetralogy of Fallot is necessary for minority patients with severe Tetralogy of Fallot. Appropriate and intensive postoperative care can decrease the mortality.

27

Re-operative Coronary Artery Bypass Grafting in 25 Patients

He D, Xu JP, Sun HS
Department of Cardiac Surgery, Cardiovascular Institute and Fu Wai Hospital, CAMS and PUMC, Beijing 100037, China

Objective To summarizes and analyzes the experience and surgical results of re-operative coronary artery bypass grafting (Re-CABG).
Methods 25 patients who underwent Re-CABG in Fu Wai Hospital between March (1997) and May 2007 were analyzed. There were 22 males and 3 females aged from 50 to 72 (62. 5 ± 8. 1) years old. The average time from the first CABG was 48. 7 ± 35. 2 months (range, 3-109 months).
Results There was no operative death and myocardial infarction happened. The patients were followed up for 38. 7 ± 30. 6 months (range, 8-90 months), no recurrent angina pectoris and no related events occurred.
Conclusions Satisfactory outcome of Re-CABG can be achieved if proper indication was chosen and reasonable management was performed.

28

Comparison of Safety and Effectiveness of Drug-eluting Stents versus Bare Metal Stents in Octogenarians

Hu FH, Yang YJ
Cardiovascular Institute and Fu Wai Hospital, CAMS and PUMC, Beijing 100037, China

Objective To compare the outcomes of Drug-eluting stent (DES) with bare metal stent (BMS) in over 80 years old patients.
Methods From Jan 2005 to December Apr. 2008, 326 consecutive patients who underwent coronary stent implantation, including 196 (118 male, 80-98 years old) and 130 (90male, 80-97 years old) with BMS were analyzed. Incidence of major adverse cardiovascular events (MACE) including death, no-fatal myocardial infarction (MI), and target lesion revascularization (TLR) was evaluated at 30 days and 1 year after percutaneous coronary intervention (PCI).
Results There was no statistical difference between two groups, except for longer stents length and smaller stents diameter (27. 10 ± 14. 23 mm vs. 24. 83 ± 11. 85 mm, P = 0. 038; 3. 01 ± 0. 37 mm vs. 3. 31 ± 0. 53 mm, P = 0. 028) in the DES group. There was no statistical difference

in the MACE rate between the group both at 30 days and 1 year follow-up (DES vs. BMS: 1.5% vs. 3.3%, P = 0.358; 5.8% vs. 12.9%, P = 0.073), and there also no statistical difference in death and MI in the two groups (DES vs. BMS: 2.6% vs. 3.7%, P = 0.43; 2.4% vs. 2.6%, p = 0.47), but TLR was significantly lower in DES group ((0.78% vs. 7.2%, P = 0.013) and the rate of late stent thrombosis was lower in BMS group (0% vs. 1.4%).

Conclusions DES could reduce restenosis compared with BMS in over 80 years old patients, but its late stent thrombosis needed to be considered.

29

Surgical Treatment of Complete Atrioventricular Septal Defect

Hu XP, Li SJ, Shen XD, Liu YL, Xu JP
Cardiovascular Institute and Fu Wai Hospital, CAMS and PUMC, Beijing 100037, China

Objective To summarize the experience of surgical treatment of complete atrioventricular septal defect (CAVSD) in 130 patients.

Methods One hundred and thirty patients with CAVSD underwent surgical therapy from 2003 to 2008. Patients with complex anomalies such as tetralogy of Fallot, or double-outlet right ventricle were excluded. Mean age was 3.6 ± 6.4 years (range, 3 months to 46 years. Twenty-two patients underwent repair before 6 months of age, 73 patients between 6 months and 3. years and 35 patients after 3 years of age. CAVSD were repaired by two-patch technique in 85 patients, single-patch technique in 12 patients and modified single-patch technique in 33 patients.

Results There were 14 hospital deaths (10.8%). patients less than 6 months had the mortality of 9.1%, compared with 15.1% in 6 months to 3 years group and 2.9% in older than 3 years group. The in-hospital mortality of two-patch group, single-patch group and modified single-patch group was 8.3%, 9.4% and 15.2% respectively. Ten patients died of pulmonary hypertensive crises and acute respiratory distress syndrome, 3 died of septic shock and one died of intractable ventricular fibrillation. Fifteen patients had moderate mitral regurgitation and 7 had a 2 mm residual ventricular septal defect at discharge. Follow-up was completed in 92 patients, with duration of 9.4 months (range, 1 month to 64 months). Moderate to large degree mitral valve regurgitation was observed in 5 patients.

Conclusions Postoperative pulmonary hypertensive crises and acute respiratory distress syndrome were the main cause of deaths for correction of CAVSD. Early correction of CAVSD before 6 months of age might prevent the development of pulmonary vascular obstructive disease and decrease the operative mortality. The modified single-patch technique was used commonly in recent years because of its simplicity. It produced results comparable with the two-patch technique in patients with shallow ventricular septal defects.

30

Surgical Repair of Ascending Aortic Pseudoaneurysm with Previous Cardiac Operation

Hu XP, Xu JP, Yu CT, Chang Q
Cardiovascular Institute and Fu Wai Hospital, CAMS and PUMC, Beijing 100037, China

Objective Ascending aortic pseudoaneurysm are a rare complication of cardiac surgery. It can occur several months to years after the initial operation. We reviewed 15 cases of ascending aortic pseudoaneurysm with previous cardiac operation to summarize the clinical presentation, surgical technique and outcomes of the disease.

Methods From 1999 to 2009, fifteen patients with previous cardiac surgery underwent 18 times repair of ascending aortic pseudoaneurysm. One patient had pseudoaneurysm repair twice and one patient had three times. Mean age was 44 ± 14 years. Intervals between operations varied from 1 month to five years. The cannulation site was femoral-femoral in 83% (n = 15), with deep hypothermic circulatory arrest in 67% (n = 12).

Results Principal etiology of ascending aorta pseudoaneurysm with previous cardiac surgery was infection (n = 9). Of these, five patients had deep sternal wound infection. Staphylococcus aureus was the most prevalent microorganism. Intrinsic aortic wall diseases (Marfan syndrome, Behcet's disease and Takayasu's arteritis) account for four patients' pseudoaneurysm. Six patients had moderate or severe aortic valve periprosthetic leakage. The pseudoaneurysm was resected and the aorta replaced in 8 operations; the pseudoaneurysm repaired with or without patch in 10 operations. Hospital mortality was 20% (n = 3). During mean follow-up of 3.6 ± 2.3 years, 3 additional patients died.

Conclusions Ascending aortic pseudoaneurysm with previous cardiac operation often have an infectious etiology and carry a high mortality and morbidity rate. Other risk factors include Marfan syndrome, Takayasu's arteritis and Behcet's disease. Ascending aortic pseudoaneurysm can be safely approached using femorofemoral cardiopulmonary bypass and deep hypothermic circulatory arrest.

31

Radial versus Femoral Approach for Percutaneous Coronary Interventional Procedures in the Aged

Huang WG, Wu TG, Wei JR
Department of Cardiology, Guangzhou Red Cross Hospital, Guangzhou 510220, China

Objective To evaluate the safety and effect of transradial approach for coronary intervention in the elderly patients.
Methods There were 314 cases >60 years old with coronary artery disease in hospital from Mar 2007 to May 2009 who accepted coronary intervention. They were divided into Transradial group (TRA, n = 157) and Transfemoral group (TRF, n = 157). The success rate and time of puncture, x-ray exposure time, procedure duration, complication in puncture site and pulmonary embolism were observed in the two groups.
Results 149 out of 157 cases success in TRA group and 155 cases in TRF group. The success rate was not different. The success rate of puncture, x-ray exposure time and procedure duration had no difference between the two groups. But the complication in puncture site and pulmonary embolism were more in TRF group than in TRA group.
Conclusions Percutaneous transradial artery approach is secure and effective for coronary intervention treatment in the aged and has few vascular complications.

32

Interventional Treatment of Congenital Heart Disease- Current Status and Perspective in China

Jiang SL
Cardiac Catheterization Laboratory, Department of Radiology, Cardiovascular Institute and Fu Wai Hospital, CAMS and PUMC, & Peking Union Medical College, Beijing 100037, China

About 150 000 infants were born with congenital heart disease every year and 2 millions with congenital heart disease in Mainland China. The application of intervention in treatment of congenital heart disease develops rapidly. On the basis of clinical practice the first Chinese guidelines of interventional treatment of congenital heart disease were issued in 2004. Now about 120 medical centers performed more than 13 000 cases of congenital heart disease intervention in a year in Mainland China. Of them, only 4 centers performed more than 500 cases with congenital heart disease every year, but in quite a lot of centers the number of the cases performed annually are still less than 70 cases.
The data of retrospective study were analyzed by 18 centers. Pediatric cardiac intervention in China was started in 1985 when the first balloon valvuloplasty for pulmonary valve stenosis was successful. Up to March 2008, 36 068 patients with congenital heart disease were performed by interventional therapy, including 10580 patients with patent ductus arteriosus, 10059 with atrial septal defect, 9660 with ventricular septal defect, 4 886 with pulmonary valve stenosis, 134 with coronary fistula, 121 with coarctation of aorta, 103 with congenital valvular aortic stenosis, other interventions in 525 patients. Homemade devices were used in most of them. The technical successful rate was 92.3% ~99.6%. The complication rate was 1.97% ~4.45%. The mortality was ≤0.11%.
The first hybrid cardiac catheterization laboratory in Asia was built in Beijing Fu Wai hospital in 2006. We have performed some hybrid interventions for treating complex congenital heart disease.
Percutaneous aortic and pulmonary valve replacement on animal study was made in few centers, but has not been tried on study of human.
Interventional treatment of congenital heart disease is an effective and safe nonsurgical method in selected cases. It has been become a routine treatment for common congenital heart disease in majority of medical centers. More patients with congenital heart disease will benefit from this effective treatment. Long-term follow-up study is important to clarify the long-term prognosis in pediatric through adults.
The great progress of Interventional treatment of congenital heart disease has been achieved in China, especially recent years. But the number of cases we accomplished so far is still too little to satisfy the need of patients with congenital heart disease. The development of the interventional technique is unbalanced in different areas. Technique training and academic exchanges are still very important, especially young special-

ists. We also need to develop interventional devices and technique. The first Chinese guidelines of interventional treatment of congenital heart disease will be revised Some regulation of administration and supervision of interventions of cardiovascular disease were drew up by Ministry of Health of the People' s Republic of China in 2007. We believe that the interventional treatment of congenital heart disease in China will get great development continuously.

33

The Effects of Intracoronary Tirofiban in Acute ST-segment Elevation Myocardial Infarction Patients with No Reflow and Slow Flow Phenomenon During Primary Percutaneous Coronary Intervention

Li CS, Wei YL, Pan JS
Department of Cardiology, 152 Central Hospital of PLA, Pingdingshan, Henan 467000, China

Objective To observe the effects of intracoronary tirofiban on infarct-related artery (IRA) thrombolysis in acute myocardial infarction (TIMI) flow during primary percutaneous coronary intervention (PCI) in acute ST-segment elevation myocardial infarction (STEMI) patients, analyze the effects of intracoronary tirofiban with no reflow and slow flow phenomenon after PCI, evaluate its clinic therapeutic effect and safety.
Methods 108 cases with acute STEMI were randomized to divided into treatment group ($n = 56$, male35, female21, age 68.5 ± 5.8) and control group ($n = 52$, male30, female 22, age 62.3 ± 4.6) of hospitalization in department of Cardiology from March 2007 to March 2009. Two group cases were received PCI therapy within 12 hours. The treatment group cases were received 3 minutes intracoronary tirofiban injection by the 10 ug/kg^{-1} concentration after be attenuated to 20 milliliters with Sodium Chloride during PCI and were to last to venous pump 36 hours by the 0.15 $ug/kg^{-1} \cdot min^{-1}$ concentration after PCI. The control group cases were received intracoronary 200 ug glycerol trinitrate injection and were to be rechecked coronary angiography 20 minutes later, evaluated the IRA TIMI flow. Both the two group cases were intracoronary heparin 8000-10000U during PCI, took orally clopidogrel 300 mg and aspirin 300 mg before PCI, took orally clopidogrel 75 mg and aspirin 100 mg per day after PCI. Both the two group cases were observed the IRA TIMI flow before and after PCI, the complication and major adverse cardiac event three months after PCI.
Results Compared with the control group cases, both the incidence rates of no reflow or slow flow phenomenon with intracoronary tirofiban and the incidence rates of major adverse cardic events three months after PCI in treatment group cases were found significantly decreased ($P < 0.05$), but the incidence rates of complication were not found significantly increased ($P > 0.05$).
Conclusions Intracoronary tirofiban treatment in patients with STEMI during. Primary PCI can improve the IRA TIMI flow, decrease the incidence rates of no reflow or slow flow phenomenon immediately after PCI and major adverse cardic events three months after PCI, but not increase the incidence rates of complication. It is safe and effective.

34

Terapeutic Strategies of Coronary Heart Disease Patients with Diabetes Mellitus in Era of Drug-eluting Stent

Wu YJ, Zheng Z, Yang YJ, Hu SS, Song GY, Li W, Wang Y, Gao RL
Center of Coronary Heart Disease, Center of Interventional Therapy, Department of Cardiovascular Surgery, Department of Biostatistics, Cardiovascular Institute & Fu Wai Hospital, Peking Union Medical College and Chinese Academy of Medical Sciences, Beijing 100037, China

Objective In the era of drug-eluting stent (DES), to explore the change of therapeutic strategies in patients with coronary heart disease and diabetes mellitus; and also to compare the prognosis of percutaneous coronary intervention (PCI) with coronary artery bypass graft surgery (CABG).
Methods Therapeutic strategies of patients with coronary heart disease and diabetes mellitus from January 1, 1999 to December 31, 2003 (Era of bare metal stent, BMS) and from January 1, 2004 to July 2, 2009 (Era of DES) were analyzed. And we identified 2669 consecutive patients with coronary heart disease and diabetes mellitus who underwent isolated CABG surgery or received PCI between April 1, 2004, and December 31, 2006, and we compared safety (cardiac mortality, acute myocardial infarction) and efficacy (any revascularization) during a 1-year and 2-year follow-up, The 2 primary databases used in the study were our institutional CABG registry and PCI registry.

Results In the era of BMS, there were 4062 patients with coronary heart disease and diabetes mellitus, in which 820 (20.2%) were treated with PCI, another 919 (22.6%) were treated with CABG, and the other 2323 (57.2%) received medication only. Whereas in the era of DES, there were 10989 patients with coronary heart disease and diabetes mellitus, in which 4815 (43.8%) were treated with PCI, another 2427 (22.1%) were treated with CABG surgery, and the other 3747 (34.1%) medication only. From April 1, 2004, to December 31, 2006, Patients with coronary heart disease and diabetes mellitus receiving PCI (1761) had considerably higher rates of acute myocardial infarction (2.1% vs. 0.3%, $P < 0.001$ and 2.2% vs. 0.9%, $P < 0.05$) and any revascularization (8.2% vs. 1.0%, $P < 0.001$ and 9.9% vs. 1.7%, $P < 0.001$) compared with those treated with CABG (908) during 1-year and 2-year follow-up. However, there was no difference in cardiac death (1.0% vs. 0.8%, P = NS and 1.4% vs. 2.4%, P = NS) between both groups during this era.

Conclusions In the era of DES, PCI treatment for patients with coronary heart disease and diabetes mellitus were sharply increased. And during the 1-year and 2 year follow-up, PCI and CABG therapy for the treatment of coronary heart disease patients with diabetes mellitus was both safe; however PCI treatment was associated with higher rates of acute myocardial infarction and any revascularization than CABG.

35

Long-Term Results of Transcatheter Device Closure of Perimembranous Ventricular Septal Defectsxi Jing Experience

Yang J, Zuo J, Yi DH
General Hospital of Shenyang Military Region, Shenyang City Cultural Shenhe Road, No 83

Objective The most common congenital heart disease is perimembranous ventricular septal defect (pmVSD). Transcatheter closure of pmVSD is a newly appeared technique and its long-term follow-up results are limited. The purpose of the study was to evaluate the safety and efficacy of transcatheter closure of pmVSD and its long-term prognostic results.

Methods Between June 2002 and June 2008, 865 patients with pmVSD were enrolled in our institution and were treated with transcatheter closure using different types of pmVSD occluders. All patients were followed up for an average of 37 months until Dec 2008. Clinical examination, electrocardiography, chest roentgenogram, and transthoracic echocardiography (TTE) were performed at 1, 6, and 12 months after the procedure and yearly thereafter. This trial is registered with ClinicalTrials. gov, number NCT00890799.

36

Clinical Outcomes of Stent Revascularization as Treatment for Atherosclerotic Renal Artery Stenosis

Yang Q, Jiang XJ
Dept. of Cardiology, Cardiovascular Institute and Fu Wai Hospital, PUMC and CAMS, Beijing 100037, China

Objective To evaluate the safety and clinical efficacy of stent revascularization as treatment for atherosclerotic renal artery stenosis, and to analyse the predictors for clinical efficacy.

Methods In the prospective non-randomized cohort study in our hospital from January 2003 to October 2008, 238 consecutive patients with severe atherosclerotic renal artery stenosis (ARAS) (diameter stenosis ≥60%) underwent percutaneous transluminal renal angioplasty and stenting (PTRAS) for severe hypertension and reserving renal function. They were followed up for 6-72 months and the effects of the procedure on renal function, blood pressure and cardiovascular events were observed. The predictors for blood pressure control, renal function reservation and cardiovascular events were analyzed.

Results The success rate of stent revascularization was 99%. During 6-72 months of follow-up, both systolic and diastolic blood pressure significantly decreased ($P < 0.05$), with less antihypertensive medication was taken ($P < 0.05$). Serum creatinine decreased significantly at 6-48 months ($P < 0.05$) and did not change significantly at 54-72 months ($P > 0.05$). Blood urea nitrogen decreased significantly at 6-24 months ($P < 0.05$) and did not change significantly at 30-72 months ($P > 0.05$). Complications related with the procedure occurred in 13 cases. 23 patients failed to follow up. Cardiovascular events occurred in 24 patients, including 5 cases of renal events, 4 cases of myocardial infarction, 4 cases of stroke and 11 cases of cardiovascular deaths during follow-up. The survival rates of free-of-events at year 1, 2, 3, 4, 5 and 6 were 92.7%, 92.4%, 82.9%, 81.1%, 66.7% and 42.3%, respectively. The survival rates at year 1, 2, 3, 4, 5 and 6 were 95.0%, 92.4%,

88.3%, 81.1%, 66.7% and 42.3%, respectively. Higher baseline systolic blood pressure and more number of antihypertensive drugs taken before the procedure were independent predictors of improved blood pressure. Higher baseline serum creatinine was independent predictor of improved renal function. Both improved blood pressure and improved renal function at 12 months were independent predictors of decreased mortality and decreased all cardiovascular events.

Conclusions Renal artery stenting as treatment for ARAS has a beneficial effect on blood pressure control and on renal function during mid-term and long-term follow-up. The treatment may be helpful in reduction of cardiovascular events and mortality, which should be investigated further.

37

Acute Total Occlusion of Left Main Coronary Artery in Acute Myocardial Infarction: Successful Treatment with Percutaneous Coronary Intervention

Yang SL, Liu HL, Zhang H, Qiu XM, Luo JP
Department of Cardiology, the General Hospital of Chinese People's Armed Police Forces, Beijing 100039, China

Objective Acute myocardial infarction (AMI) due to acute total occlusion of left main coronary artery (ATOLM) is a rare but life-threatening situation. Most patients die suddenly or go into cardiogenic shock (CS). In patients with AMI due to ATOLM identified by coronary angiography (CA), percutaneous coronary intervention (PCI) performed in left main coronary artery as diagnostic CA is the fastest option to complete revascularization. However, no prospective studies regarding the outcome of such procedures have been published so far.

Methods In this prospective single-center study, between October 2004 and March 2008, consecutive patients with acute coronary syndrome (ACS) were evaluated for ATOLM by means of emergent CA. When diagnosed with ATOLM, PCI of the left main coronary artery was performed. Clinical data were obtained at baseline, discharge, after 6 months, and after 1 year.

Results Out of 526 patients with ACS, 447 patients (85.0%) suffered an AMI. In 16 patients CA revealed an ATOLM. PCI was performed in 13 patients. Two patient died in-hospital due to cardiac shock and ventricular fibrillation before PCI. One patient died in-hospital due to early in-stent thrombosis after PCI. At 6-month follow-up and at 1-year follow-up, 13 patients were alive.

Conclusions In spite of the complex interventions, PCI patients had low in-hospital mortality and good clinical results at 6-month follow-up and 1-year follow-up. Our observations are important in the clinical decision-making process of AMI due to ATOLM.

38

Clinical and Procedural Predictors of No-Reflow Phenomenon after Primary Percutaneous Coronary Interventions: Experience at a Single Center

Yang SL, Liu HL, Zhang H, Qiu XM, Luo JP
Department of Cardiology, the General Hospital of Chinese People's Armed Police Forces, Beijing 100039, China

Objective The aim of the study was to identify clinical factors, angiographic findings, and procedural features that predict no-reflow phenomenon (Thrombolysis In Myocardial Infarction (TIMI) flow grade < or = 2) in patients with acute myocardial infarction (AMI) who underwent primary percutaneous coronary intervention (PCI).

Methods A series of 286 consecutive patients with AMI underwent primary PCI within 12 h of symptom onset. Patients who had continuing ischemic symptoms for more than 12 h were also included. Clinical, angiographic and procedural data were collected for each subject.

Results Fifty-two (18.1%) of the patients developed no-reflow phenomenon, and their findings were compared with those of the reflow group. Univariate analysis showed that advanced age (>60 years), delayed reperfusion (> or = 4 h), low (< or = 1) TIMI flow prior to PCI, cut-off type total occlusion, high thrombus burden on baseline angiography, long target lesion (>15.2 mm) and large vessel diameter all correlated with no-reflow ($p < 0.05$ for all). Multiple logistic regression analysis identified that advanced age (odds ratio (OR) 1.13, $p < 0.01$), delayed reperfusion (OR 1.38, $p < 0.01$), low TIMI flow before primary PCI (OR 1.23, $p < 0.01$), target lesion length (OR 4.8, $p < 0.01$) and high thrombus burden (OR 4.6, $p < 0.01$) on angiography as independent predictors of no-reflow phenomenon.

Conclusions The occurrence of no-reflow phenomenon after primary PCI can be predicted using simple clinical, angiographic and procedural features. In this selected group of patients, adjunctive pharmacotherapy and/or distal protection device may be of value.

39

Clinical Significance and the Characteristics of Coronary Angiography of Coronary Artery Disease in Patients with Complete Left Bundle Branch Block

Yuan JQ, Jin C, Xu B, Wang Y, Gao LJ, Qin XW, Yao M, Liu HB, Wu YJ, Chen J, Dai J, Wu Y, You SJ, Qian J, Zhang P, Hu FH, Yang WX, Dou KF, Li JJ, Qiao SB, Yang YJ, Chen JL, Gao RL, Chen ZJ
Coronary Heart disease Division, Cardiovascular Institute and Fu Wai Hospital, CAMS and PUMC, Beijing 100037, China

Objective To analyze the characteristics of coronary angiography of coronary artery disease (CAD) in patients with complete left bundle branch block.
Methods 285 patients with electrocardiographic findings of Left bundle branch block (LBBB) had been subjected to coronary angiographic study. The age range was 33 to 86 years old (mean 60 ±9 years). There were 165 male and 120 female. The diagnosis of LBBB was based upon electrocardiography. Patients underwent selective coronary angiography and left ventriculography by use of the Judkins technique. Statistical analysis was performed using SAS software methods for small samples.
Results Of the 285 patients, 61% had CAD, Compared with the patients without CAD, the patients with CAD were older; more likely to be men; more likely to have previous myocardial infarction, diabetes mellitus and hypertension. Coronary angiogram revealed that single vessel disease, two vessels disease and three vessels disease were 32%, 20% and 46% respectively. Of the cases had LAD lesion was most. In multivariable analysis the independent predictors are male gender, advanced age, diabetes mellitus and hypertension.
Conclusions The most subjects with LBBB and concomitant CAD are likely to have certain clinical characteristics, the patients with CAD were older; more likely to be men; more likely to have previous myocardial infarction, diabetes mellitus and hypertension. In patients who have left bundle branch block came to the hospital with chest pain of uncertain etiology, or unexplained electrocardiographic abnormality, coronary angiogram was helpful to identify the etiology.

40

Treatment of Mild-moderate Calcified Coronary Lesions with Sirolimus-Eluting Stent: A Real World Data from a Single Center

Yuan JQ, Li JJ, Qin XW, Xu B, Yang YJ, Chen JL, Qiao SB, Ma WH, Yao M, Liu HB, Wu YJ, Chen J, You SJ, Dai J, Xia R, Gao RL
Department of Cardiology, Fu Wai Hospital, Chinese Academy of Medical Sciences, Peking Union Medical College, Beijing 100037, People's Republic of China.

Objective Calcified coronary lesions have commonly been considered as a challenge for interventional cardiologists, and few previous studies of sirolimus-eluting stent (SES) for calcified lesion have been limited by small sample size. Therefore, we evaluated the effectiveness of SES implantation for the treatment of calcified lesions in a large Chinese cohort of real world practice.
Methods A total of 956 consecutive patients who successfully received SES placement were enrolled in this study, and were divided into the two groups according to whether the mild-moderate calcified lesion treated with SES exists or not: non-calcified groups ($n = 637$) and calcified group ($n = 319$). Lesions treated with SES were subjected to quantitative coronary angiography at immediately and 8 months following stenting.
Results Baseline characteristics including clinical, demographic or angiographic data were well balanced between the non-calcified and calcified group. Angiographic follow-up at 8 months, the in-stent restenosis (ISR) and in-segment restenosis rate were similar in both groups. (ISR: 3.8% vs. 4.0%; $p > 0.05$; in-segment restenosis: 8.5% vs. 9.7%, $p > 0.05$). The target lesion revascularization was no difference between the two groups (5.2% vs. 6.8%; $p > 0.05$). In addition, the in-stent late loss and overall thrombosis rate were also similar in both groups (0.17 ±0.41 mm vs. 0.18 ±0.35 mm and 1.8% vs. 1.8%, $p > 0.05$ respectively).
Conclusions Although calcified lesion was hard to stenting, successful treatment with SES for mild-moderate calcified lesions was conferred to similar favorable results compared with non-calcified lesions in patients with coronary artery disease.

41

Transcatheter Closure of Congenital Coronary Artery Fistulae: Immediate and Long-term Follow-up Results

Duan ZZ, Zhu XY, Han XM, Cui CS, Sheng XT, Wang QG
Department of Congenital Heart Disease, General Hospital of Shenyang Military Region, Shenyang 110016, China

Background Coronary artery fistulae (CAF), the anomalous communications between a major subepicardial coronary artery and a cardiac chamber or thoracic vessel, are rare congenital anomalies. Although most patients with such anomalies are asymptomatic, early treatment is recommended to prevent complications such as congestive heart failure, pulmonary hypertension, myocardial ischemia or infarction, fistula rupture with cardiac tamponade and infective endocarditis. Transcatheter closure of CAF has emerged as an alternative to surgery, but the long-term outcome is lacking.
Objective We report immediate and long-term results in 24 patients after transcatheter closure of congenital CAF.
Methods Between November 1998 and August 2008, 24 patients (14 females) with symptomatic CAF and coronary dilation (maximal coronary artery diameter > 5 mm) underwent transcatheter fistula closure using various devices. Device deployment was performed either anterogradely or retrogradely. The immediate closure results and clinical follow-up were reviewed.
Results At the time of procedure, the patient's mean age was 18.0 ± 13.1 years and the body weight were 43.4 ± 21.2 kg. Most of the CAF originated from the right coronary arteries, draining into the right heart. Two patients had multiple fistulae, both of which originated from left anterior descending coronary artery and right coronary artery and drained into pulmonary artery through multiple orifices. Of the 24 patients, 20 (83.3%) underwent successful transcatheter closure using various devices. Devices were deployed from transvenous approach in 8 (40%) and from transarterial approach in 12 patients. The mean diameter of the fistulae closed by using one device was 5.4 ± 1.7 mm and the mean size of the devices was 11.3 ± 0.7 mm. The angiogram right after device deployment revealed complete occlusion in 15 patients (75.0%) and trivial to mild residual flow in 5 (25.0%). Three patients (15.0%) had transient ST-T wave changes after procedure. The left ventricular end-diastolic volume decreased from 165 ± 31.4 mm^3 to 128.6 ± 24.4 mm^3 ($P = 0.012$) 24 hours after procedure, and the cardiothoracic ratio from 0.57 ± 0.02 to 0.53 ± 0.01 ($P = 0.003$). Follow-up was 100% complete and ranged from 3 months to 10 years. There were no early and late deaths. All patients were in asymptomatic with complete closure of CAF except one (5.0%) who had recurrence of shunt which was re-closed by percutaneous technique.
Conclusions Transcatheter closure of CAF is feasible and safe in the anatomically suitable vessels and is a promising alternative to the surgery in most patients.

42

Long-term Outcomes of Drug-eluting Stent Implantation in Patients with Multivessel Chronic Total Coronary Artery Occlusions

Han YL, Zhang J, Jing QM
Department of Cardiology, General Hospital of Shenyang Military Command, Shenyang 110016, China

Objective There are limited data on the efficacy of drug-eluting stents (DES) for treatment of multivessel chronic total occlusions (CTO). The aim of the study was to evaluate the long-term clinical outcomes of DES implantation for multivessel CTO compared with bare-metal stent (BMS) implantation.
Methods We analyzed 137 patients who underwent interventional revascularization in their multivessel CTO lesions with DES from January 2003 to December 2005 (DES group). A control group was composed of 97 consecutive patients with multivessel CTO lesions treated with BMS from January 2001 to December 2003 (BMS group). All patients were followed up for up to 3 years for occurrence of major adverse cardiac events (MACE). Long-term survival rates were estimated with the Kaplan-Meier method.
Results Baseline clinical and angiographic characteristics were comparable between the two groups except that there was higher target vessel numbers (64.7% vs. 51.2%, $P < 0.05$), mean stent numbers (1.47 ± 0.86 vs. 1.29 ± 0.80) and mean stent length (41.5 ± 11.8 mm vs.

22.7 ±9.2 mm) of patients in the DES group ($P < 0.001$). Average follow-up periods were (3.5 ±0.7) and (3.3 ±1.1) years for the BMS and DES groups, respectively. At 3-year follow-up, the 3-year target vessel revascularization (TVR)-free survival rate in the DES group was significantly higher than that in the BMS group (78.1% vs. 71.3%, log rank $P < 0.05$). The cumulative MACE-free survival in the DES group was also significant higher than that in the BMS group (81.0% vs. 72.3%, log-rank $P < 0.05$). The rates of re-admission caused by cardiovascular disease (29.2% vs. 38.3%, $P < 0.05$) and the need for bypass surgery were significantly lower in the DES group (2.2% vs. 7.4%, $P < 0.05$).

Conclusions This study demonstrates the long-term (up to 3 years) efficacy of DES for treatment of multi-vessel CTO, which is superior to BMS implantation in reducing the rates of TVR and MACE, as well as the need of re-admission and bypass surgery.

43

Comparison on Long-term Effects of Atorvastatin or Provastatin Combined with Clopidogrel for Patients Undergoing Coronary Stenting

Zhang Y, Cheng WP

PUMC & CAMS, Department of Anesthesiology, Cardiovascular Institute and Fu Wai Hospital, Beijing 100037, China

Capital University of Medical Sciences, Department of Anesthesiology, An Zhen Hospital, Beijing 100029, China (CHENG Wei-ping)

Objective This prospective, randomized controlled study aimed at evaluating the effects of drug-drug interaction between statins (atorvastatin or pravastatin) and clopidogrel on platelet activation and aggregation function in patients with ACS undergoing coronary stenting.

Methods A total of 1275 hospitalized patients undergoing coronary stenting were randomly given atorvastatin 20 mg/d (638patients) or provastatin 20 mg/d (637 patients). Inclusion criteria included age 20-80, of unstable angina pectoris, acute myocardial infarction or old myocardial infarction, emergency or elective PCI. All patients received standard antiplatelet treatment including aspirin 300 mg/d and a 300 mg clopidogrel loading dose for 30 days, then aspirin 100 mg/d for lifetime, clopidogrel followed by a maintenance dose of 75 mg/d for 12 months. The primary end point was cardiovasculate and cerebral ischemic events at 12 months, defined as the composite of cardiac death, non-fatal myocardial infarction (MI), stroke. The second end point were major adverse cardiac and cerebral events (MACCE) at 12 months, defined as the composite of cardiac death, non-fatal myocardial infarction (MI), stroke or target vessel revascularization (TVR), stent thrombosis events and TIMI hemorrhagic events.

Results The baseline clinical characteristics, angiographic and PCI result were comparable in there the two groups. At 12 months clinical follow-up, no significant difference existed in cardiac and cerebral ischemic events (4.70% vs. 5.49%, $P > 0.05$). Also no significant difference existed in cardiac death rate (1.88% vs. 2.51%), non-fatal MI (0.47% vs. 0.31%), stroke (2.35% vs. 2.67%) and TVR (7.68% vs. 5.49%, $P > 0.05$). No significant difference existed in the composite of MACCE (12.38% vs. 11.00%, $P = 0.447$), the rate of stent thrombosis events (2.04% vs. 2.51%, $P = 0.828$) and hemorrhagic events (13.0% vs. 12.2%, $P = 0.927$) between the two groups. Kaplan-Meier survival analysis showed the cumulative hazard rate for the cardiac and cerebral ischemic events and MACCE was similar ($P = 0.525$, $P = 0.240$).

Conclusions 12-months therapeutic effects of atorvastatin 20 mg/d combined with clopidogrel for the patients undergoing coronary stenting is similar to that of provastatin combined with clopidogrel. Longer-term therapeutic efficiency and safety of the two strategies need to be further investigated.

44

Successful Transcatheter Closure of Congenital Coronary Artery Fistula Complicated with A Giant Coronary Artery Aneurysm by Utilization of Double Chinese home-made PDA Occluders: Report of Two Cases

Zheng H, Lan T, Liu M
Department of Radiology, Cardiovascular Institute and Fu Wai Hospital, CAMS and PUMC, Beijing 100037, China

Objective We have described our experience with transcatheter occlusion of congenital coronary arterial fistulas complicated with a giant coronary artery aneurysm by utilization of double Chinese home-made PDA occluders.
Methods and Results Two symptomatic patients, one man aged 36 and one woman aged 56 years old underwent transcatheter occlusion of both fistulas and giant coronary artery aneurysm at same procedures by utilization of double Chinese home-made PDA occluders. All two patients had chest distress and dyspnea on exertion. The fistula originated from the left circumflex artery (LCX) to coronary sinus in man patient was closed by operation 20 years ago but it was showed reopened and complicated with a giant coronary artery aneurysm nearby remote end (the diameter of aneurysm was 36 mm) this time. The fistula in woman was drained into right atrium from LCX with a giant coronary artery aneurysm of diameter 45 mm. Two Chinese home-made PDA occluders, which were two of the type of 22/20 mm in man and two of the type of 20/18 and 18/16 mm in woman, were deployed into the coronary arteries to occlude the opening of the aneurysm and the end of the fistulas one after another in both patients through a 14F and 12F deliver sheath, respectively. The procedures were uncomplicated and successful. Two patients were followed up after 3 and 25 months and underwent examination of UCG and Chest film to show that the left to right shunt were disappeared and cardiothoracic ratio was smaller. The chest distress and dyspneas of these two patients have also resolved or improved after the procedure.
Conclusions Transcatheter closure of congenital coronary fistulas complicated with a giant coronary artery aneurysm by utilization of double Chinese home-made PDA occluders are safe and effective, and can be regarded as an acceptable alternative to surgery, especially for the patient complicated with remains of shunt after operation.

45

Coronary Intervention in Patients ≥75 years old with ST-elevation Myocardial Infarction: in-hospital and 6 Months Clinical Outcome

Zheng X, Yuan JQ, Li JJ, Qin XW, Guo YL, Mu CW, Hua YH, Yang YJ, Chen JL, Xu B, Qiao SB, Wu YJ, Yao M, Liu HB, Chen J, You SJ, Dai J, Xia R, Gao RL
Department of Cardiology, Fu Wai Hospital, Chinese Academy of Medical Sciences, Peking Union Medical College, Beijing 100037, China.

Background Elderly acute myocardial infraction (AMI) patients present specific clinical characteristics which differ from younger patients. However, the efficacy and safety of percutaneous coronary intervention (PCI) in elderly patients (≥75 years) with ST-segment elevation myocardial infarction (STEMI) has not yet been definitely established.
Objective To investigate outcomes including clinical characteristics and in-hospital and 6 months results of PCI in elderly patients with STEMI.
Methods The study population included 522 consecutive STEMI patients undergoing PCI within 12 hours from symptoms onset. Clinical characteristics and in-hospital and 6 months outcome of 66 elderly patients (≥75 years, group A) were compared to that of 456 younger patients (< 75 years, group B).
Results Compared to younger patients, elderly patients were more frequently female (42.4% vs. 17.8%, $p<0.005$), and a history of cerebral vascular events (7.6% vs. 0.9%, $p<0.05$). In elderly patients, smokers were lesser (28.8% vs. 45.4%, $p<0.05$) but had worse left dysfunction (Killip I class: 69.7% vs. 85.7%, $p<0.05$). In elderly patients, less frequently DES was implanted and TIMI flow 3 was restored following PCI (33.3 vs. 47.1 and 84.8 vs. 94.7%, $p<0.05$ respectively). In addition, both in-hospital mortality and myocardial infarction rate were much higher in elderly patients (16.7% vs. 1.5%, and 7.6% vs. 2.6%, $p<0.05$ respectively), which was also observed until 6-month follow up (25.8% vs. 15.6%, and 13.6% vs. 2.6%, $p<0.05$ respectively). In multivariable logistic regression analysis, the data suggested that plasma creatinine (Cr) level on admission ($p=0.03$), history of hypertension ($p=0.025$) and Killip class ($p=0.007$) were independent predictors of mortality at 6-month follow up in elderly patients.

Conclusions Primary PCI in elderly patients with STEMI is safe, efficacious, and with a low rate of PCI failure. However, it is still associated with a worse outcome than that seen in young group.

46

Transcatheter Closure of Patent Ductus Arteriosus in Middle-aged and Old Patients

Zhu XY, Chen HY, Zhang DZ, Han XM, Sheng XT, Cui CS, Zhang P, Wang QG
Department of Congenital Heart Disease, General Hospital of Shenyang Military Region, Shenyang 110016, China

Objective To evaluate the clinical feature of patients with patent ductus arteriosus (PDA) and the safety of transcatheter closure of PDA in Middle-aged and Old patients.

Methods Between January 2001 and April 2009, 139 patients (22 male) aged from 40 to 74 (49.8 ± 6.8) years underwent attempted transcatheter PDA closure. The cardiac function was NYHA class I in 64, class II in 53, class III in 16 and class IV in 6 patients before procedure, respectively. The pre-and post-closure clinical feature, pulmonary artery pressure (PAP) and cardiac function were evaluated.

Results In 139 patients, 107 (77.0%) were complicated with pulmonary arterial hypertension (PAH) and 3 were unsuitable for closure because of severe PAH. The remaining 136 patients (97.8%) underwent successful PDA closure without major complications. Check cardiac angiography after device deployment showed trace residual shunt in 14, small residual shunt in 2 and moderate shunt in 1. The cardiac function ameliorated and PAP decreased significantly after PDA closure. The systolic PAP decreased from 47.3 ± 23.9 mmHg to 28.1 ± 12.3 mmHg and mean PAP from 31.7 ± 17.4 mmHg to 17.9 ± 8.8 mmHg.

Conclusions PDA in middle-aged and old patients is commonly associated with PAH and cardiac insufficiency. Transcatheter PDA closure is safe in such patients as their PAP can be monitored before and after device closure.

47

Right Coronary Angiographic Characteristics in Patients with Acute Inferior, Posterior and Right Ventricular Myocardial Infarction

He CH, Yuan JQ, Gao RL
Coronary Heart disease Division, Cardiovascular Institute and Fu Wai Hospital, CAMS and PUMC, Beijing 100037

Objective To analyse the right coronary artery angiographic characteristics in patients with acute inferior, posterior and right ventricular myocardial infarction.

Methods Sixty patients with acute inferior, posterior and right ventricular myocardial infarction were subjected to coronary angiographic and intervention study. The age range was 31 to 80 years old (mean 57 ± 11 years). There were 50 men and 10 women. Statistical analysis was performed using SAS software methods for small samples.

Results (1) Clinical characteristics: Among 60 patients, males comprised 83.3%. The risk of acute myocardial infarction was significantly higher in males than in females ($p < 0.0001$). (2) Electrocardiographic characteristics: In 60 patients with acute inferior myocardial infarction or posterior myocardial infarction which final diagnosed by electrocardiogram, 55 patients (91.7%) combined with right ventricular infarction. (3) Coronary angiography characteristics: In 60 patients, 55 are dominating RCAs. The culprit lesions mainly happened in proximal portion and midprotion (76.4%). 33 patients are total occlusion (60%). (4) Left ventricular function: the mean left ventricular ejection fraction was normal (60% ± 13%).

Conclusions Right coronary artery as culprit artery mainly happened in patients with acute inferior, posterior and right ventricular myocardial infarction. The most of the culprit lesions were severe stenosis or total occlusion of proximal and midprotion.

48

Minimally Invasive Perventricular Device Closure of Ventricular Septal Defect without Cardiopulmonary Bypass: Multi-center Experience and Mid-term Results

Xing QS, Pan SL, Wu Q
The Heart Center of Qingdao Children's Hospital, Qingdao 266011, China.

Bacground Significant drawbacks exist in open heart repair with cardiopulmonary bypass (CPB) and transcatheter intervention of ventricular septal defect (VSD). Lately developing perventricular device closure of VSD under transesophageal echocardiography (TEE) guidance was widely used in China.

Objective To summary the clinical experiences and short and mid-term follow-up results of perventricular closure of ventricular septal defect (VSD) without cardiopulmonary bypass under TEE guidance.

Methods A total of 408 cases, 5 months to 15 yeas (3.1 ± 1.7years), underwent minimally invasive perventricular device closure under guidance of transesophageal echocardiography (TEE), with a bodyweight of 4.5 to 26 kg (13.6 ±5.5) kg. 57 VSDs close to aortic valve. Diameters of VSD ranged from 3 to 12 mm (5.1 ±2.6) mm. An inferior sternal incision of 3 to 5 cm was made and incision was made in the third left intercostal space for a small number of children. A single per-right ventricular "U" like suture was established and a guidewire was inserted from right ventricular wall through VSD to the left ventricle after puncturing under TEE guidance. Proper devices were delivered and released under real-time TEE monitoring if no significant aortic regurgitation, abnormal atrioventricular valvular motion or residual interventricular shunt was indicated.

Results 393 cases of this group were successfully closed (96.3%) and the other 15 cases (3.7%) converted to traditional open heart repair. 213 (54.2%) of the perventricular closed 408 cases were implanted a symmetrical device and 180 (45.8%) were closed with asymmetrical ones. 387 cases (96.5) received no transfusion. New tiny or mild tricuspid regurgitation (TR) was found in 13 cases (3.3%), but no worsening regurgitation in those with existed TR. Incomplete atrioventricular right bundle block from ECG happened in 11 cases (2.8%). No obvious residual shunt or aortic regurgitation was detected. Total process was no more than 90 min, and time for device implantation was 5 to 60 min (17.8 ±8.7 min). All were extubated two hours after operation, and most discharged 3 to 5 days after operation. Complete atrioventricular block (AVB) was observed in another 3 cases and recovered to sinus rhythm after therapy. All cases were follow-upped for 3 months to 2 years, but no related complications were found. 9 of the 13 newly-happened TR decreased. 6 of 11 incomplete atrioventricular right bundle block diminished. No residue shunt, new or aggravating aortic regurgitation, obstruction of left or right outflow tract and device dislocation were detected. No thrombosis or hemolysis happened.

Conclusions Minimally invasive perventricular device closure of VSD off CPB, is a simple, effective and safe intervention under guidance of TEE. It is agreeable to considerable VSD clients and clinically valuable to be promoted. Long-term follow-up is necessary.

Pacing and Electrophysiology

1

Clinical Investigation of Ibutilide-induced Cardioversion of Persistent Atrial Fibrillation in the Cardiac Catheterization Laboratory

Hou H, Li XF, Liu J, Cao DF, Hu JQ, Fang PH
The center of arrhythmia diagnosis and treatment, Fu Wai Hospital, Chinese Academy of Medical Sciences & Peking Union Medical College, Beijing 100037, People's Republic of China.

Objective Ibutilide is a type III antiarrhythmic agent approved for the pharmacologic conversion of atrial fibrillation (AF) and atrial flutter (AFl). The purpose of this study was to investigate the efficacy and safety of ibutilide in terminating persistent or permenent atrial fibrillation (AF) post-radiofrequency ablation.
Methods Of 36 consecutive patients (27men, mean age 51.7 ±7.4 years) with persistent or permanent AF who underwent circumferential pulmonary vein ablation (CPVA) plus linear ablation along roof of LA and endocardium of mitral annulus between October 2008 and June 2009. If AF was not terminated, the CAF potential was ablationed. Finally 30 patients who did not convert to sinus rhythm after RFCA received a infusion of ibutilide 1 mg in 10-minute. Successful conversion was defined as restoration of sinus rhythm within 30 minutes after administration. Continuous electrocardiographic monitoring was performed, and 12-lead electrocardiograms were recorded during administration of the drug. The AF cycle length (CL) was measured and averaged by atrial-atrial (A-A) interval recorded in coronary sinus lead.
Results Eighteen of 30 patients with PAF were converted to sinus rhythm (conversion rate = 60%). The mean time between infusion of drug and arrhythmia termination was 10.17 ±5.18 minutes. There was statistical significant difference between converted and not-converted group on duration of Persistent AF (4.25 ±2.86 years vs. 9.38 ±4.34 years, $P < 0.041$). No differences were found regarding gender, age, body mass index, left ventricular function, left atrial diameter between two groups. Ibutilide prolonged atrial CL (171.85 ±29.53 ms vs. 242.00 ± 40.06 ms, $P < 0.001$). The mean QTc interval was significantly decreased at 1 hour after administration of ibutilide compared with those after successful conversion immediately (441.00 ±37.40 ms vs. 421.50 ±24.76 ms, $P < 0.05$), which suggested that QT interval tended to restoring to normal after 1 hour. There were no significant changes in blood pressure or the QRS intervals. No significant complications occurred.
Conclusions Ibutilide is a reasonable therapy choice for PAF patients post-radiofrequency ablation in the cardiac catheterization laboratory.

2

Study on Clinical Application of a Portable Remote Real-time Electrocardiogram Monitoring System

Sun XL, Guan J, Wang L, Wang GG
Department of Cardiology, Fu Wai Hospital, CAMS&PUMC, Beijing 100037, China
The company of ZHONGWEILAIKANG

Objective A remote real-time wireless electrocardiography monitoring system based on GPRS was tested in order to contrast the accuracy and stability of electrocardiosignal with the 12 leads electrocardiogram (ECG), and then evaluated this device's clinical practice value, security and validity.

Methods The data were collected from in-patient with from April 2008 to December 2008 in Fu Wai hospital. All subjects were received the portable remote real-time ECG monitoring and the 12 leads ECG, and these patients were divided into two groups. The aspects of ECGs were compared between 2 systems including the general waves, clinical diagnosis, time and voltage parameters.

Results The electrocardiographic evaluation of the mobile ECG demonstrated three characteristics: Reliability, 1006 lines (93.8%); Interference, 51 lines (4.8%); Unsharpness, 15 lines (1.4%). The baseline stability of precordial leads is better than limb leads. The mobile ECG identified 266 cases of arrhythmia, including 135 cases of tachyarrhythmia and 131 cases of bradyarrhythmia. The mobile ECG was the same as the 12 leads ECG in the general waves and clinical diagnosis of ECGs. The electrocardiographic parameter of the two groups, such as the heart rate, swing and time of the ECGs, has no statistical difference ($P > 0.05$), and was significant correlation ($P < 0.01$).

Conclusions The accuracy and stability of the portable remote real-time ECG monitoring system is in accordance with the standard ECG instrument. The portable remote real-time electrocardiogram monitoring system may be a helpful tool in assisting physicians in the diagnosis of common arrhythmia and malignant ventricular arrhythmia disorders, and showed high safety in data transmission.

3

Changes of QRS Duration after Optimization of VV Intervals by Cardiac Resynchronization Therapy

Li DF, Wang DM, Zang HY, Yu HB, Han YL
Department of Cardiology, General Hospital of Shenyang Command of Chinese PLA, Shenyang 110016, China

Objective To investigate the changes of QRS duration after different optimization of VV intervals by echocardiogram in patients with Cardiac Resynchronization Therapy (CRT).

Methods 54 patients after CRT treatment due to congestive heart failure (CHF) in our hospital were enrolled in this study, of which 43 cases with the QRS duration of surface electrocardiogram > 120 ms and 11 cases with QRS duration ≤120 ms (Tissue Doppler ultrasound showed the existence of ventricular asynchrony), all patients were appropriate for CRT or CRT-D implantation with type I or IIa indication.

The aortic velocity time integral (VTI) was measured by echocardiography after CRT implantation, and we defined the VV intervals with the highest VTI as the "best VV interval", meanwhile, QRS duration of surface electrocardiogram was recorded. The changes of the QRS duration before CRT, after CRT and "at the best VV interval" were assessed.

Results QRS duration of the 54 patients before CRT was 148.89 ± 36.11 ms, the instant QRS duration after CRT was 124.82 ± 28.53 ms, thus, QRS duration after CRT was quite narrower than that before CRT. And QRS duration at the "best VV intervals" was 135.00 ± 20.35 ms. QRS duration at the "best VV intervals" was much narrower than before CRT, but it was wider than the instant moment after CRT (VV has not been optimized).

Conclusions QRS duration after CRT was much narrower than it before CRT, but the QRS duration at the "best VV intervals" which was optimized by echocardiography was not the narrower, so it was inaccurate for assessing the best VV interval merely by the width of QRS wave, and we'd better to optimize VV intervals with the help of echocardiography.

4

Ventricular Repolarization Turbulence, a New Risk Stratification Factor for Patients after AMI

Li D, Wang HY
Department of cardiology, The Second Hospital of ShanXi Medical University, TaiYuan 030001, China.

Objective We investigated a new factor termed VRT and explored its value for risk stratification.
Methods We segmented ventricular-repolarization interval J-T into five sections, separately researched the fluctuations of their length after a single VPC recorded in Holter, characterized the fluctuations (termed ventricular repolarization turbulence, VRT) by a series of numerical parameters and compared them among groups. 104 patients and 100 controls were chosen.
Results 1, VRT in AMI patients are obviously attenuated: JTe-TS, Tbp-TS, Tpe-TS are lower; JTp-TT, JTe-TO, Tpe-TO, JTb-TOc, JTp-TOc, JTe-TOc are higher ($p < 0.05$). 2, In subsets of AMI group, VRT of high risk patients are more weaker: JTe-TS ($p < 0.01$) in group combined heart failure and JTp-TS, JTe-TS ($p < 0.05$, $p < 0.01$) in group combined malignant ventricular arrhythmia are obviously lower. 3, After following-up, VRT in patients who recurred heart event also attenuated more: JTe-TS in AMI patients recurred myocardial infarction or stenocardia are lower ($p < 0.01$); JTp-TS, JTe-TS, Tpe-TS in AMI patients with cardiac death or malignant arrhythmia are lower ($p < 0.05$); AMI patients who suffered endpoint events of following-up are older, RR-TS, JTp-TS, Tpe-TS, JTe-TS are lower too ($p < 0.05$). 4, VRT-TS was not correlated with age, HRT-TS and HR, but correlated with SDNN ($p < 0.05$). 5, Statistical analyzing with Kaplan-Meier, the stratification critical values of JTp-TS, JTe-TS, Tpe-TS are 4.80, 5.68, 6.00 (ms/RRI). 6, In Cox analysis, JTe-TS have the best predicted worth ($RR = 2.82$) than other traditional predictors.
Conclusions VRT could serve as a potent and independent risk stratification factor of AMI patients.

5

Comparative Study on Diagnostic Value of Electrocardiogram and Coronary Angiography in the Coronary Artery Disease

Li F, Guo JH, Zhang P
Beijing Public Security Hospital

Objective The present study was conducted to investigate the diagnostic value of electrocardiogram and coronary angiography in the coronary artery disease.
Methods Totally 94 suspicious cases of coronary artery disease was evaluated by silent electrocardiogram, Holter or exercise test orderly: 66 positive cases (70.2%) was defined as A group and 28 negative (29.8%) as B group and then all were conducted coronary angiography. There were 55 cases (83.3%) showed coronary artery diameter stenosis ≥50% and 11 cases (16.7%) showed that <50% in group A. There were 19 cases (67.9%) diagnosed as coronary artery diameter stenosis ≥50% and 9 cases (32.1%) diagnosed as that <50% in group B. The change of electrocardiogram in myocardial infarction, coronary artery diameter stenosis ≥50% and coronary artery diameter stenosis <50% in group A were compared. The coronary angiography evaluation results were compared in group A and group B. Electrocardiogram was conducted again after coronary angiography and intracoronary stent placement.
Results There was significant difference in the acute myocardial infarction between group A and group B. There was significant difference between the elevation of ST segment and temporal change of T wave, permanent Q wave, ST-T segment change in the leaders (II III avF, V_{1-3}) of group A. There was significant difference in the coronary stenosis and TMI 3 flow between group A and group B in coronary artery angiography. 3 cases had new ST-T segment changes after coronary artery angiography in group B.
Conclusions Electrocardiogram test is still one of the important diagnostic methods for coronary artery disease although there is no complete concordance between electrocardiogram and coronary angiography.

6

Comparisons of Electrocardiogram Characteristics between Pre-and post-Transcatheter Closure of Atrial Septal Defect in Patients over 40 Years

Li X, Zhu XY, Wang QG
Department of Congenital Heart Disease, Shenyang Northern Hospital, Shenyang 110016

Objective To evaluate characteristics of the electrocardiographic (ECG) before and after transcatheter closure of atrial septal defect (ASD) in patients over 40 years.
Methods Twelve leads ECG were recorded before and 24 hours after closure procedure one time per patient, nineteen patients were evaluated cardiac dysrhythmias with 24-hour ambulatory ECG monitoring. Observing and analyzing the features of ECG.
Results The QRS axis declined from 79.1 ± 36.1 to 76.4 ± 36.8 ($P < 0.05$); The incidence of normal ECG increased and right bundle branch block signi cantly decreased after transcatheter closure; The number of right heart dilatation decreased but has no difference ($P > 0.05$); The incidence of sinus bradycardia increased signi cantly ($P < 0.05$), it has irrelevance with age, diameter of defect and size of closure ($P > 0.05$); There was no signi cant change in other arrhythmias ($P > 0.05$); Seven patients developed new atrial brillation, age, diameter of defect and size of closure has significant difference ($P < 0.01$) between patients with atrial brillation and without atrial brillation.
Conclusions Volume load of right ventricle is decreased after transcatheter closure of atrial septal defect in patients over middle age, It may protect against the subsequent complications; New arrhythmias may occur while some persist arrhythmias remained for short time after transcatheter closure.

7

Effect of Serum Creatinine on Mortality and Response to Cardiac Resynchronization Therapy

Wang DM, Han YL, Zang HY, Yu HB, Zhang DH, Wang SL, Wang ZL, Jin QM
Department of Cardiology, General Hospital of Shenyang Command of Chinese PLA, Shenyang 110016, China

Objective We aimed to assess the influence of the level of serum creatinine (SCr) before implantation on the prognosis of patients with cardiac resynchronization therapy (CRT).
Methods 91 patients with heart failure were divided into three groups (Group I: SCr ≤ 1.0 mg/dl, n = 33; Group II: 1.1 mg/dl < SCr ≤ 1.5 mg/dl, n = 35; Group III: SCr > 1.5 mg/dl, n = 23).
Results There were 6 patients (18.18%) died in Group I and 7 (20%) died in Group II and 8 (34.78%) died in Group III. The heart function improved significantly after 6 and 12 months of operation in 3 groups ($P < 0.01$). 6-minute hall-walking test increased significantly in Group I and Group II ($P < 0.01$) and did not increase significantly in Group III ($P > 0.05$) at 6-12 months of postoperation. Left ventricular end-diastolic dimension diminished significantly at the 6-12 month follow-up in Group I ($P < 0.05$-0.01) and did not decrease obviously in Group II and III ($P > 0.05$). Left ventricular ejection fraction increased significantly in 3 Groups ($P < 0.05$-0.01). There was significantly statistical different in 3 Groups.
Conclusions The higher level SCr (> 1.5 mg/dl) before implantation predicts the worse reversing LV remodeling and the increase of patients' mortality from heart failure aggravation after CRT implantation.

8

Effect of Pulmonary Hypertension to the Prognosis of Patients with Cardiac Resynchronization Therapy

Wang DM, Han YL, Zang HY, Yu HB, Zhang DH, Wang SL, Wang ZL, Jin QM
Department of Cardiology, General Hospital of Shenyang Command of Chinese PLA, Shenyang 110016, China

Objective To investigate the effect of pulmonary artery systolic pressure (PASP) to the response of patients with CRT.
Methods Ninety-three patients (76 male, mean ages: 61.23 ± 15.56) with heart failure involved in our study. According to the level of preoperative PASP, they were divided into three groups (Group I: PASP ≥50 mmHg, n = 29; Group II: 30 mmHg < PASP < 50 mmHg, n = 17; Group III: PASP≤30 mmHg, n = 47). New York Heart Association (NYHA) class, 6-minute hall-walking test (6-MWT), left ventricular end-diastolic dimension (LVEDD), left ventricular ejection fraction (LVEF) and mortality (cardiac and noncardiac) were followed by 3 to 6 months after implantation.
Results 1, eight patients died in Group I (28%), sudden death in two, r acute myocardial infarction in one and heart failure in five. One patient died of sudden death in Group II (6%). Eight patients died (17%) in Group III, 1 for aggravation of heart function, 4 for sudden death and 3 for other noncardiac diseases. The total mortality (28% vs. 6% vs. 17%) and the proportion of death for heart function aggravation (62.5% vs. 0 vs. 12.5%) were highest in Group I. 2, The NYHA class improved obviously in three groups after the implantation ($P < 0.01$), but which in Group III was improved more significantly than in Group I ($P < 0.01$). 3, The 6-MWT increased at 3-6 months after operation in three groups ($P < 0.05$-0.01), especially in Group III which had increased by 130 m over the preoperation and by 70 m over Group I ($P < 0.05$-0.01). 4, LVEDD in Group III diminished significantly from 71 mm to 66 mm at 3-6 months ($P < 0.05$), but which had no significant change in Group I (from 71 mm to 68 mm, $P > 0.05$) and Group II (from 69 mm to 66 mm, $P > 0.05$). 5, LVEF increased averagely by 31-38% ($P < 0.01$) in Group III at 3-6 months, But in Group I and II which had not obvious increased at 3 months ($P > 0.05$) and had increased by 17% (Group I, $P < 0.05$) and 26% (Group II, ($P < 0.01$) at 6 months. LVEF in Group III had increased more than that in Group I and Group II ($P < 0.05$-0.01).
Conclusions Clinical outcome post-CRT was assessed based on elevated PASP. PASP≥50 mmHg had an increased risk for an adverse outcome and a higher Mortality for aggravation of heart function.

9

The Long-Term Effects of Pacemakers Upgraded into Biventricular Pacing in Patients with Heart Failure

Wang DM, Han YL, Zang HY, Yu HB, Zhang DH, Wang SL, Wang ZL, Jin QM
Department of Cardiology, General Hospital of Shenyang Command of Chinese PLA, Shenyang 110016, China

Objective Long-term right ventricular apex pacing had potential harm to the heart function in bradyarrhythmia patients. This study was to observe the long-term effects of pacemakers upgraded intobiventricular pacing in patients with heart failure.
Methods Thirteen patients (11 men, mean ages: 63.46 ± 14.13) with left ventricular end-diastolic dimension (LVEDD) > 55 mm and left ventricular ejection fraction (LVEF) < 40% had indication of pacemaker implantation. There were 2 patients with NYHA heart function Class II, 7 with Class III, 4 with Class IV and 10 patients with the QRS duration≥130 ms, 3 with < 120 ms. The dual-chamber pacemakers had been implanted in 2 patients before implanting CRT. CRTs were implanted directly in 11 patients. NYHA class, 6-minute hall-walking test (6-MWT), LVEDD, LVEF and mortality were followed from 3 months to 5 years (mean months: 31.77 ± 20.67).
Results 1, 3 patients died (23.08%) in follow-up. Among them, 1 patient with heart function Class II died for sudden cardiac death, 1 with Class III-IV for ventricular fibrillation-and 1 for cancer with Class II. 2, the heart function improved significantly from 3 months to 36 months after CRT implantation ($P < 0.05$-0.01), the mean improvement was more than 1 grade. The 6-MWT increased meanly by 84-165 m at 3 months, 12 months and 36 months after implantation ($P < 0.05$-0.01). LVEDD diminished obviously at 3 months and 36 months ($P < 0.05$) after CRT. The mean decreasing diameter was 6-9 mm. LVEF showed significant improvement from 3 m to 36 months after CRT implantation and averagely increased by 24-36% ($P < 0.05$-0.01).
Conclusions The heart function was improved significantly after CRT implantation and Mortality due to aggravation of heart function decreased after pacemakers upgraded into CRT in patients with heart failure and depending on ventricular pacing.

10

Left Ventricular Pacing Lead Placement and Anatomy of Coronary Vein System

Wang DM, Han YL, Zang HY, Yu HB, Wang SL, Jin QM, Wang ZL, Geng JC
Department of Cardiology, General Hospital of Shenyang Command of Chinese PLA, Shenyang 110016, China

Objective The purpose of this study was to analyze coronary venogram in 123 patients, focusing on the relationship between the abnormality of lateral vein and the placement of LV pacing lead.

Methods The coronary sinus venogram in 123 patients was obtained during occlusion using a balloon catheter in both the anteroposterior and the left anterior oblique (LAO) projections. The lateral marginal veins and postero-lateral veins were analyzed.

Results Transvenous LV pacing leads were successfully placed in optimal coronary vein in 118 cases (95.93%), among which 44 were in lateral marginal vein (37.29%), 47 were in postero-lateral vein (39.83%), 24 cases were in middle cardiac vein (20.34%), 3 cases were in great cardiac vein (2.54%). There was at least one or more vessel abnormality (thinness, stenosis, tortuousity, lack of lateral marginal vein or postero-lateral vein) in 98 of 123 cases (79.67%). The incidence of thinner lateral marginal vein was more frequent than that of postero-lateral vein ($p < 0.01$). Lack of large vein was more frequent in male than that in female (37.00% vs. 13.04%, $p < 0.05$). The incidence of thin lateral marginal vein in female was more frequent than that in male ($p < 0.05$). Total number of lateral marginal vein and postero-lateral vessel variability was markedly more frequent in non-ischemic heart disease than in ischemic heart disease (96.59% vs. 74.29, $P < 0.01$). Coronary sinus myocardial bridges all occurred in non ischemic cardiomyopathy (10.23%).

Conclusions The anatomic variations of coronary vein system are great and occur often. These anatomic variations are not associated with gender. The ratio of vessel abnormality is higher in patients with non-ischemia heart disease than that in patients with ischemic heart diseases. Many patients had a lateral marginal vein or postero-lateral vein using LV pacing lead, therefore CRT implantation success rate can not be affected.

11

The Characteristic of the Prevalence of J Wave in Apparently Healthy Subjects in China

Tang YH, Chen K, Huang CX, Wang X, Bao MW, Deng HH, Zhu GY
Cardiology Department of Renming Hospital of Wuhan University, Wuhan 430060, China.

Background J wave can be observed in idiopathic ventricular fibrillation, Brugada syndrome that is closely connected with sudden death. But the characteristic its in healthy subjects is unknown.

Objective To observe the characteristic of the incidence of J wave in apparently healthy subjects.

Methods The study subjects comprised of apparently healthy 1817 subjects. One thousand one hundred and thirty one subjects were males, was averaged in 46.38 ± 15.81 years old; six hundred eighty six subjects were females, was averaged in 42.77 ± 14.15 years old. Routine medical examinations, including ECG were performed. J wave was defined as a wave followed QRS complexes with amplitude of at least 0.05 mV and 0.03 ms.

Results The incidence of J wave in all subjects was 7.6%. The incidence of J wave in males was significantly higher than that in female (10.53% vs. 1.87%, $p < 0.01$). The incidence of J wave in inferior wall (II, III, avF), right wall (V1-V3) and left wall (V4-V6) was 4.57%, 0.50%, and 2.20% respectively. J wave located in inferior wall was more than in left and right wall (both $p < 0.05$). The incidence of J wave was positive correlation with age. With the age increasing, the incidence of J wave increased ($r = 0.78$, $p < 0.01$).

Conclusions J wave is more frequently observed in male, elderly people and is more frequently occurred in inferior wall than in left and right wall.

12

Electroanatomic Mapping and Catheter Ablation of Sustained Atrial Tachycardia Originated from Right Atrial Appendage

Chen YL, Xu J, Lu FM, Fu NK, Xin TW
Department of cardiology, Tianjin Chest Hospital, Tianjin 300051, China

Objective The study was to evaluate the use of the electro-anatomic mapping system in four patients with sustained atrial tachycardia originated from right atrial appendage. Furthermore, to characterize the electrocardiographic and electrophysiologic features of this kind of arrhythmia.
Methods Electroanatomical mapping of right atrial activation was performed in four patients with sustained atrial tachycardia to identify the earliest local activation for radiofrequency catheter ablation. ECG pattern was analyzed carefully.
Results The 3D mapping allowed a rapid demonstration of focal mechanism and the earliest action wave front originated from the right atrial appendage. Atrial tachycardia in two patients were terminated successfully in right atrial appendage without complication. Long-term success was achieved in four of the four patients over a mean follow-up of nearly 6 months. ECG pattern was identified, consisting of positive P wave in lead II, III, aVF and V1, and a transition to positivity in the rest of the precordial leads.
Conclusions Visualization of atrial activation in a 3D construction of the right atrial appendage using electroanatomic mapping system facilitates the analysis and the ablation of tachycardia originated from right atrial appendage. There is consistent P-wave morphology and endocardial activation associated with this type of atrial tachycardia.

13

The Initial Experience of Low Energy Mapping for Treating Ventricular Tachyarrhythmia without Premature Ventricular Contraction

Jia YH, Wang J, Mao KX, Wei W, Zhao YJ, Zhang S, Chu JM
Clinical Electrophysiologic laboratory and arrhythmia center of Fu Wai Hospital, Chinese Academy of Medical Sciences, Peking Union Medical College, Beijing 100037, China.

Objective This study reported initial experience of a new mapping method for treating syncope-caused ventricular tarchycardia (VT) without combining frequent premature ventricular contractions (PVCs).
Methods All 11 recruited patients were female, mean age 39.9 ± 13.7 years. They had experienced at least 1 syncope episode and been treated with 2 or more antiarryhthmic agents (atenolol, propafenone, mexiletine and amiodarone) in the last 1 to 3 years.
Results 1. Clinical arrhythmia characteristic analysis: Five patients can be induced PVC or VT on right ventricular outflow tract (RVOT) by programed stimuli without intravenous injection of isoproterenol, which suggested micro-reentrent could be the possible mechanism. In these patients, holter monitoring recorded more PVCs (mean 3678 beats/24 hour) with ventricular bigeminy or trigeminy, but less VT (mean 5.8 episodes/24 hours). These patients suffered more temporarily amaurosis (or presyncope attacks) than syncope except one older woman combining hypertension; The other 6 patients could not be induced VT with programmed stimuli unless isoproterenol been administrated; these patients all suffered syncope in their medical history, their holter monitoring recorded more VT (mean 15.5 episodes/24 hour) less PVC (mean 1208 beats/24 hour) with few ventricular bigeminy or trigeminy. Trigger activity may be the possible mechanism of VT in these 6 patients. It suggested exertion or emotional activity would induce pulseless VT and syncope in those patients. 2. Electrophysiologic mapping and catheter ablation: Induced PVC or VT were fixed on monitor screen as reference, based on this reference PVC/VT morphologic characteristic combine previously ablation experience, ablation catheter was positioned on expected area of RVOT, pace mapping was performed firstly and low radiofrequency (RF) energy (15-20 J) was delivered at sites where paced VT morphology is identical to reference VT in all 12 leads of ECG, once the sites was found that VT morphology induced by thermo effects was identical to reference VT in all 12 leads of ECG, this site would be view as final target and origin of VT/PVC, the radiofrequency energy would be increased to 35-50 J (50-55℃) until VT was eliminated. Then enlarge ablation area to about 1 cm^2 around this site. No VT/PVC were induced through program stimuli or intravenous isoproteronol repeatly after ablation was considered as successful end point. All patients were induced identical VT during low radiofrequency energy and these VTs also were eliminated by high RF energy. 3. Ten out of eleven patients reached the end of ablation in the procedure, 9 targets located at septal or

posterior wall in RVOT, 1 at base of right coronary sinus. The only failure one could be induced few PVC by isoproterenol before ablation, activating mapping finding the earliest activation site located in inferior of left coronary sinus, and identical VT also could be induced by RF delivery, however, PVC couldn't be eliminated, which suggested the target locating the epicardial layer and then the ablation was aborted. 4. No syncope or amaurosis were observed in following 3-14 months out-patient follow-up.

Discussion Radiofrequency catheter ablation is a mature method for treating VT/PVC arise from ventricle out-flow tract. Activating mapping sometime combined with pacing mapping are primary methods. Those two methods both need enough PVCs showed in the EPS, even 8000 PVCs/24 hour or more. However, relative number of patients who suffer from frequent syncope due to VT have few PVCs, it is hard to map using above mapping methods in the EPS, implantation of implantable cardiac defibrillator (ICD) will be a big psychologic and economic burden for those patients. In this study whatever mechanisms of VT/PVC, although induced VT/PVC was few not enough to activate mapping, enough to be frozen on monitor screen as reference, and enough to low energy mapping the successful target site that thermo-induced VT/PVC identical to reference in all 12 leads of ECG. Follow-up results confirm that this new mapping method have high success rate for determining final ablation target. We concluded low energy ablation mapping will be a potential mapping method, as well as activity mapping, pacing mapping, and P potential, especially for the syncope caused VT but less PVCs.

14

A Rapid Electrocardiographic Algorithm to Differentiate Repetitive Monomorphic Ventricular Tachycardia between Right Outflow Tract and Left Side Origin

Jia YH, Ma J, Li X, Yao Y, Zhang KJ, Fang PH, Zhang S, Chu JM

Clinical Electrophysiologic laboratory and arrhythmia Center and Epidemiology Department of Fu Wai Cardiovascular Disease Hospital, Chinese Academy of Medical Sciences, Peking Union Medical College, Beijing 100037, China.

Objective This study aim to establish a rapid surface ECG algorithm on RMVT differentiating right outflow tract from left outflow tract origin, and determining catheter approaches before ablation procedure. Study population: sixty-six consecutive patients, refractory to 2-3 antiarrhythmic agents (30 male, 36 female, mean age 36.9 ± 13.9 years), with spontaneously or induced symptomatic idiopathic ventricular tachycardia (VTs) and/or frequent monomorphic ventricular premature contraction (VPCs) during Radiofrequency Catheter Ablation (RFCA) procedure were enrolled.

Methods successful ablation site and corresponding arrhythmic ECG characteristics including 1) lead Ⅰ, avR, avL, Ⅱ Ⅲ avF, V1; 2) Duration of R wave in lead V1; 3) the ratio of R wave width to QRS complex duration in lead V1; 4) the R/S transition zones (first precordial lead with R/S ratio > 1) in the precordial leads were analyzed.

Results Successful RF ablation was performed in right side in 32 patients (48.5%), and in left side in 34 patients (51.5%). The surface ECG morphologic characteristics of lead, avR, avL, Ⅱ, Ⅲ, avF, V1 and duration of R wave in lead V1 have been founded no predictive value in location the origin of VTs or VPCs through SPSS 10.0 software analysis, However, the R/S transition zones in the precordial leads and the ratio of R wave width to QRS complex duration in lead V1 (D_r/D_{QRS}) show excellent predictive ability to locate the right side or left side origin of VTs or VPCs. In this study, the R/S transition after leads V3 (no including lead V3) were found in 0 of 34 patients (0/34) whose successful RF target were left side including either 17 left ventricular origin or 17 left coronary cusps origin. while 12 of 32 patients (12/32, 37.5%) whose successful target were right ventricular were found the R/S transition after leads V_3; therefore, Although the sensitivity of the R/S transition after leads V_3 predict successful ablation in right side was low (37.5%), the specificity to predict outside right side (left side) was 100%. Thus positive and negative predictive values of the R/S transition after leads V_3 (leads V_4 to V_6) for successful ablation in right side was 100% (12/12) and 63% (34/54). The other 54 patients whose the R/S transition before V_3 (including V_3) were further analyzed. There were 19 patients and 35 patients who presented with $D_r/D_{QRS} < 0.5$ and $D_r/D_{QRS} \geq 0.5$, respectively. $D_r/D_{QRS} < 0.5$ predict right ventricular origin were 90% (18/20) sensitivity and 97.1% (33/34) specificity, Its positive and negative predictive value were 94.7% (18/19) and 94.3% (33/35), respectively. $D_r/D_{QRS} \geq 0.5$ predict left ventricular origin were 97.1% (33/34) sensitivity and 90% (18/20) specificity, Its positive and negative predictive value were 94.3% (33/35) and 94.7% (18/19), respectively.

Conclusions Sequence analysis of two surface ECG morphologic characteristics of R/S transition zones in the precordial leads and ratio of R wave width to QRS complex duration in lead V1 (D_r/D_{QRS}) can excellent predict the origins of VTs or VPCs Prior to RFCA.

15

Aminoglycosides Restore Nonsense Mutation Herg Channels

Yan Y, Si YT, Ning L, Pu JL
Cardiovascular Institute and Fu Wai Hospital, Beijing 100037

Background Pharmacological restoration of the trafficking defect of HERG missense mutations has been documented. However, whether it is possible to correct HERG nonsense mutations remains unknown.
Objective To investigate the effect of aminoglycosides on the expression of nonsense mutants.
Methods Herg channel and mutant currents were recorded by whole-cell patch clamp techniques. Pharmacological rescue was applied by culturing the cells in 400 μg/mL G-418 or gentamicin for 24 hours.
Results Current densities were significantly reduced in cells expressing R1014X and W927X mutants compared to those of cells expressing wild type (WT) HERG. R863X and E698X mutants failed to generate any typical HERG currents. The mean peak tail current density of R1014X mutant was significantly lower than that of WT (3.9 ± 1.4 pA/pF, $n = 8$ vs. 47.8 ± 6.3 pA/pF, $n = 12$, $p < 0.05$), and it increased to 12.7 ± 3.3 pA/pF ($n = 7$, $p < 0.05$) and 18.3 ± 3.7 pA/pF ($n = 8$, $p < 0.05$) after G-418 and gentamicin treatment. The voltage dependence of activation of R1014X was also restored after drug treatment. Furthermore, the expression of full-length proteins for R1014X induced by drugs was detected by western blot and confocal imaging. Similar results were observed on W927X. For R863X and E698X, however, gentamicin treatment had no effect. In the cells co-transfected with WT/R1014X, gentamicin and G-418 demonstrated different results: gentamicin, but not G-418, increased the current density by 2.2-fold ($n = 12$, $p < 0.05$).
Conclusions These findings provide proof of principle that interventions designed to read through premature stop mutations may at least partially reverse the LQT2 phenotype in vitro.

16

The Comparison between the Active-fixation Leads and Passive-fixation Leads in Right Ventricular Pacing

Yu HB, Wang DM, Zang HY, Tian Y, Zhang DH, Han YL
Department of Cardiology, General Hospital of Shenyang Command of Chinese PLA, Shenyang 110016, China

Objective To compare the pacing parameters of active-fixation leads and passive-fixation leads in right ventricular pacing in 6 months after operation.
Methods There were 91 patients implanted with single or dual chamber pacemaker involved in this study from January 2008 to December 2008 followed by 6 months after operation. In these patients 55 with active-fixation lead (Group I) and 36 with passive-fixation lead (Group II) implanted in right ventricle, the average age was 66.91 ± 12.95 years old, 31 patients with single chamber pacemaker and 60 with dual chamber pacemaker.
Results 1. Comparison of pacing parameters between the Group I and Group II: The stimulation thresholds of Group I were higher than that of Group II at postoperative moment, 1 month after operation, 3 months and 6 months respectively ($P < 0.05$); The pacing impedances at postoperative moment of Group I were similar to Group II ($P > 0.05$), but those were separately lower than Group II after 1 month, 3 months and 6 months ($P < 0.05$). 2. Comparison of pacing parameters inside the Group I and Group II separately: There were no obvious changes for stimulation thresholds in Group I at postoperative moment, 1 month, 3 months, and 6 months. In Group II the thresholds were higher at postoperative moment than those after 1 month ($P < 0.05$). The pacing impedances inside Group I or II at postoperative moment were higher than that after 1 month, 3 months and 6 months respectively ($P < 0.05$) 3. Severe stimulation thresholds changes: There were 2 of 91 patients with higher pacing thresholds after operation so severely as we had to adjust the ventricular lead again. The two patients both implanted with active-fixation lead, the incidence rate of severe thresholds increase in Group I was 3.6% (2/55). No patients with severely higher pacing thresholds in Group II.
Conclusions It was possible that the stimulation thresholds were individually higher in patients with active-fixation leads than those with passive-fixation leads (3.6% vs. 0%). The long-term changes of parameter were still observed.

17

J Wave and J Wave Syndromes

Yan GX
Main Line Health Heart Center

The J point denotes the junction of QRS complex and ST segment on the ECG and it marks the end of depolarization and beginning of repolarization. The J wave is a deflection with a dome or hump morphology in the same direction of the R wave immediately following the QRS complex. Animal studies have demonstrated that the J wave is the consequence of a transmural voltage gradient resulting from an Ito-mediated action potential notch (spike and dome) in epicardium but not endocardium. Ito-mediated spike and dome morphology predisposes loss or depression of the dome in epicardium, leading to ST segment elevation. ST segment elevation associated with J wave in a structurally normal heart is observed in the early repolarization syndrome (ERS), idiopathic ventricular fibrillation (IVF) and the Brugada syndrome. Because these three clinical syndromes share common molecular, ionic and cellular basis as well as many ECG features, they are now named as J wave syndromes. However, their clinical consequences are different. The ERS based on previous classification is considered as a benign ECG finding characterized by a distinct J wave and ST segment in left precordial leads V4-V6 although early repolarization per se with ST elevation is the common ECG feature of these three syndromes. In contrast, IVF and the Brugada syndrome, characterized by a J wave and ST segment elevation in the inferior and right precordial leads respectively, are the leading cause for sudden cardiac death in young Southeast Asian males who have structurally normal heart. The underlying mechanism for such a difference in clinical consequences among J wave syndromes is due to a difference in Ito density and Ito-mediated epicardial spike and dome. When Ito is prominent, complete loss of the dome may occur due to either a decrease in inward currents or an increase in outward currents secondary to gene mutation or acquired pathological factors, leading to phase 2 reentry (local reexcitation at action potential phase 2) capable of initiating ventricular fibrillation as in IVF and the Brugada syndrome. When Ito is relatively small as in the ERS, partial depression of the dome occurs with a significantly smaller risk in the development of phase 2 reentry.

Cardiovascular Surgery

1

A Comparison of Long-term Outcome of Radial Artery with Saphenous Vein Graft in CABG

Zhu YP, Zhao Q, Chen AQ
Department of Cardiac Surgery, Ruijin Hospital, Shanghai Jiao Tong University, Shanghai 200025

Objective The left internal mammary artery (LIMA) has been shown to improve the outcome of coronary artery bypass grafting (CABG) and become the gold standard graft. However the benefit of the radial artery (RA) has not been determined. The aim of this retrospective study was to compare the long-term outcome of the radial artery with the saphenous vein graft in CABG.

Methods Between January 2004 and December 2005, 324 patients who were underwent isolated OPCAB composed this study. There were 79 patients received the radial artery graft (the RA group), of which 59 patients had total arterial grafts (LIMA and RA), 20 patients had standard procedure (LIMA to LAD, SVG to other target vessels) with RA (LIMA, SVG and RA). The other 245 patients who underwent CABG without RA (LIMA and SVG) composed the SVG group. A complete follow-up was obtained for 254 patients from 36 to 60 months after the operation (mean 41.6 months). Coronary artery CT or angiography were performed in 63 cases after the operation, including 18 cases with angina symptoms. Thus 63 LIMA, 29 RA and 142 SVG were followed up from 3 to 52 months (mean 32.1 months). Outcomes were evaluated by univariate analysis and survival analysis.

Results Clinic outcomes: The mean age of the RA group was younger. The clinic characters showed a significant higher prevalence of female, severe angina (CCS) and smoke in the RA group. The mean number of conduits in the RA group was fewer (RA 3.28 ± 0.88, SVG 3.62 ± 0.70; $p = 0.004$). The prevalence of taking exercise post-operatively was higher in the RA group (RA 58/67, 86.6%; SVG 118/170, 69.0%; $p = 0.006$). The actuarial survival, freedom from MACE (major adverse cardiac event) and angina at 12 months or 36 months were similar. The total survival curve showed significant benefit in the RA group ($p = 0.01$). The MACE-free survival curve also showed significant benefit in the RA group ($p = 0.044$). The angina-free survival curve showed no significant difference. As a subgroup analysis (age 60-70), there was no significant difference of the total survival curve, the MACE-free survival curve and the angina-free survival curve between two groups. Image study outcomes: Results of the LIMA grafts were all excellent. The overall patency of the RA graft was higher than the SVG (RA 27/29, 93.1%; SVG 103/142, 72.5%; $p = 0.018$). The rate of TVR (target vessel revascularization) of the RA graft was less (RA 0/29, 0%; SVG 24/142, 16.9%; $p = 0.036$). There was no difference in the patency rate at 12 months. The patency rate of the RA graft at 24 and 36 months were superior (RA 21/21, 100%; SVG 102/128, 79.7% at 24 months; $p = 0.049$; RA 17/18, 94.4%; SVG 79/115, 68.7% at 36 months; $p = 0.023$). The Long-term patency curve showed significant benefit in the RA group ($p = 0.032$).

Conclusions The RA graft improved survival and reduced MACE after CABG. The RA graft had superior patency. The long-term outcome of the RA was better than SVG.

2

The Recall Alloresponse in Retransplantation is more Intensive than That in Memory-transfer Setting

Liang H, Liao CX, Shan ZG, Zhao YX, Lin Z
Zhongshan Hospital of Xiamen University

Objective The presence of alloreactive memory T cells in recipient is a critical handicap to achieving transplantation tolerance. To establish a mouse model which can as closely as possible mimic the presensitized transplant patient is important for research in this subject. Thus, we developed a novel retransplant model and compared the alloresponse in this model with that in the memory T cells-transfer model (transfer control).

Methods Mean survival time of allograft was compared between 3 groups including blank transplant control, memory transfer control and retransplant groups. Cellular rejection activity in allografts was evaluated via HE staining of cardiac graft section. Proliferation and differentiation of the alloreactive effector T cells were assayedin vitro by mixed lymphocyte reaction and flow cytometry respectively. Real-time quantitive RT-PCR was used to assess gene expression of cytokines and surum IFN-γ was measured via ELISA.

Results It showed that the median survival time of allograft in retransplant recipients was significantly shortened compared with that of transfer control, and it was the same in rejection score of graft. Moreover, proliferation and differentiation of the alloreactive effector T cells were more intensive in retransplant recipients than that in transfer control, which was confirmed in vitro by mixed lymphocyte reaction and by flow cytometry of the splenocytes for detecting $CD44^{high}$CD62L-memory/effector phenotype cells. Furthermore, activation of $CD4^{+}$ memory T cells was reflected by high level of surum IFN-γ and the intensive gene expression of IFN-γ and IL-2 in cardiac allograft in retransplant recipients.

Conclusions Collectively, the recall alloresponse in retransplantation is more intensive than that in memory-transfer setting and this retransplant model is more close to the clinic situation than the memory-transfer model in rodents.

3

Comparative Proteome Analysis between the Sera of Anterior and Posterior Cardiopulmonary Bypass Procedure in Open Heart Surgery Patients

Liu JX, Wu YH, Jin LY
The 3rd Xiangya Hospital of Central South Univesity, Changsha, Hunan, China

Objective In this study, serum proteomics technique was used to screen the differential proteins from the sera of anterior and posterior CPB procedure in open heart surgery patients.

Methods For each patient, blood samples were taken approximately 30 min before initiation of CPB (time point 1), 1 h postweaning from CPB (time point 2), and 24 h postweaning from CPB (time point 3). Serum proteins were isolated using two dimensional gel electrophoresis (2-DE). The protein spots were analyzed by the PDQuest image analysis software and the differential protein spots were identified by matrix-assisted laser desorption/ionization-time of flight-mass spectrometry (MALDI-TOF-MS). Then, enzyme linked immunosorbent assay (ELISA) was used to determine the expression level of serum amyloid A protein (SAA) in the serum of healthy people and at three different time points (30 min before initiation of CPB, 1 h postweaning from CPB, and 24 h postweaning from CPB) of open heart surgery patients. The prospects of clinical application of SAA were further discussed.

Results Through 2-DE combinated with MALDI-TOF-MS, 3 proteins altered in expression were identified, including Haptoglobin (HPT), Leucine-rich alpha-2-glycoprotein (A2GL), Serum amyloid A protein (SAA). ELISA analysis showed that compared with the time point of 30 min before initiation of CPB, SAA levels rise rose three times at the time point of 1 h postweaning from CPB and rise rose nineteen times at the time point of 24 h postweaning from CPB. But levels of SAA in the serum of healthy peopledid not show significant deviation compared with the time point of 30 min before initiation of CPB.

Conclusions This pilot study illustrate HPT, A2GL and SAA may be related with haemolysis, tissue damage, inflammation, and so on following CPB procedures. HPT can be used in judging the degree of haemolysis in open heart surgery patients. SAA is a subservient and sensitive biochemical indicator of the acute-phase response following CPB.

4

Effects of Nicardipine and Diltiazem on Hypertension in the Early Postoperative Period after Coronary Artery Bypass Grafting

Liu P, Du J, Zhao KL, Lu TY

Department of Cardiovascular Surgery ICU, Cardiovascular Institute and Fu Wai Hospital, CAMS and PUMC, Beijing 100037

Objective To evaluate the effects of Nicardipine and Diltiazem on hypertension, heart rate and their changes in the early postoperative period after coronary artery bypass grafting (CABG), so as to guide the choice and regimen of calcium-channel blockers during the early postoperative phase after CABG.

Methods Sixty patients were included with a radial arterial systolic pressure (RASP) greater than 150 mmHg in the early postoperative period after CABG. They were divided into groups I, II, III according to their heart rates (HR), and group II was subdivided into II-A and II-B. Nicardipine and Diltiazem were used in Groups I and II-A, and Groups II-B and III, respectively. Observations were made 2. 5 hours after the initial dosage, on radial arterial systolic and diastolic pressures (RADP), HR and their trends respectively at 15 time points. The means of radial arterial pressures and HR at the initiation and termination of therapy were compared among groups I, II and III and between groups II-A and II-B respectively.

Results In Groups I, II-A, II-B and III at the initiation/termination of therapy, the mean RASP was 162. 3 ±5. 2/135. 5 ±4. 8 mmHg, 161. 3 ±7. 6/134. 8 ±6. 3 mmHg, 161. 3 ±7. 0/132. 3 ±6. 6 mmHg, and 161. 2 ±5. 9/133. 4 ±6. 9 mmHg, respectively, the mean HR was 63. 2 ± 5. 7/78. 6 ±5. 7 beats per minute (bpm), 86. 9 ±8. 0/92. 7 ±5. 9 bpm, 85. 7 ± 11. 4/76. 3 ± 12. 8 bpm, 110. 7 ±5. 5/87. 1 ±5. 0 bpm, respectively. There was no statistical difference of HRs between the initiation and termination of therapy in group II-A ($p = 0.026$), while the RASP, RADP and HR in groups I, II-B and III were significantly different ($p < 0.01$). Between groups II-A and II-B, there was no statistical difference among the three parameters, except the HR at initiation of therapy ($p < 0.01$).

Conclusions Both Nicardipine and Diltiazem could effectively treat the hypertension in the early postoperative period. Nicardipine could increase the HR while Diltiazem could decrease the HR significantly.

5

Middle and Long Term Results of Radical Arterial Switch Operation in Older Patients with Severe Pulmonary Arterial Hypertension: A Challenge to Conventional Surgical Treatment of Congenital Heart Disease with Pulmonary Arterial Hypertension

Liu YL, Huang JB, Kong B, Hu SS, Shen XD, Li SJ, Wang X, Yan J, Wu X

Pediatric Center of Cardiac Surgery, Cardiovascular Institute and Fu Wai Hospital, Chinese Academy of Medical Sciences and Peking Union Medical College, Beijing 100037, China

Objective To analyze the middle and long term results of radical arterial switch operation in older patients with severe pulmonary arterial hypertension.

Methods 86 consecutive patients with transposition of great arteries (TGA) or Taussing-Bing anomaly and severe pulmonary arterial hypertension, aged 7 months to 19 years (24 ±22 months, among 86 patients, 28 patients aged 7-12 mongths、33 patients aged 1-3 years、17 patients aged 4-6 years、4 patients aged 7-12 years、4 patients aged 13-19 years), with mean pulmonary pressure of 50. 0-97. 0 (64. 9 ± 13. 0) mmHg, pulmonary vascular resistance of 46. 0-1261. 9 dyn · s · cm^{-5}, underwent radical arterial switch operation at our institution from May 2000 to October 2008. 80 survived and were discharged. 12 patients were lost (15%, 12/80). The rest 68 patients were followed up by telephone or in out-patient clinic. The pediatric quality of life inventory (PedsQL™) questionnaires were sent to the parents and completed by the parents or patients. Child and parent scores on the PedsQLTM Generic Core Scales were compared to known healthy children or parents.

Results The mean duration of follow-up was 41. 5 ±23 months (range, 9 to 110 months). Follow-up data showed that 2 patients died of sudden death with unknown reason 2 months and 18 months postoperatively respectively, and the other 68 patients survived with pulmonary arterial pressure regressed and significantly improved cardiac function. 97% (66/68) were in NYHA class Ⅰ, and 3% (2/68) were in class Ⅱ. 2 patients were with mild pulmonary artery valve insufficiency, and 1 with mild tricuspid valve insufficiency. There were no other complications and reoperations. Physical and psychosocial developments were normal.

Conclusions Middle and long term results of radical arterial switch operation in older patients with severe pulmonary arterial hypertension are excellent and radical arterial switch operation can be used to treat older vetriculoarterial discordance with severe pulmonary arterial hypertension.

6

Modified Method for Tricuspid Valve Repair with the Cosgrove-Edwards Annuloplasty System: Early Clinical and Echocardiographic Results

Pan SW, Lu ZQ, Guo HW, Liu XJ, Song YH, Hu SS

Department of Surgery, Cardiovascular Institute and Fu Wai Hospital, Chinese Academy of Medical Sciences and Peking Union Medical College, Beijing 100037, China

Objective Flexible rings for tricuspid valve repair are widely used. The purpose of this study was to evaluate the results of modified method for tricuspid valve repair with the Cosgrove-Edwards annuloplasty system.

Methods Between January 2008 and December 2009, 32 consecutive patients with tricuspid valve regurgitation underwent tricuspid valve repair with the Cosgrove-Edwards annuloplasty system, among them, 23 patients developed tricuspid valve regurgitation secondarily to left-sided heart valve diseases; 5 patients secondarily to congenital heart diseases; 2 patients with Ebstein's anomaly and 2 patients with traumatic tricuspid regurgitation. The modification to the classical Cosgrove-Edwards tricuspid valve repair method included: 1. the size of the chosen ring was at least two less than the measured size. 2. In addition to shortening the anterior and posterior annular of tricuspid, two or three stitches were set at the septal region of tricuspid valve to fasten the ring. The diameter of tricuspid valve orifice after repair was 25 mm to 27 mm. 26# Cosgrove-Edwards ring was used in 5 patients, 28# in 9, and 30# in 8.

Results There was no operative death. All patients recovered and were discharged uneventfully. Echocardiograpic tricuspid regurgitation was none or minimum in 17 patients, mild in 15 patients without tricuspid stenosis.

Conclusions The Cosgrove-Edwards annuloplasty system is very effective in the treatment of secondary tricuspid regurgitation.

7

Predictors for the Neo-Aortic Regurgitation after Arterial Switch Operation

Pan XB, Hu SS, Li SJ

Cardiovascular Institute and Fu Wai Hospital, Beijing 100037

Objective The aim of this report was to study the predictors for late insufficiency of the neo-aortic valve in patients with transposition of the great arteries (TGA) and Taussig-Bing malformation undergoing arterial switch operation.

Methods Between February 2001 and December 2007, 185 patients (140 male, 45 female; mean age 13.83 ± 27.76 months) with TGA or Taussig-Bing malformation underwent Switch procedure. All the patients were followed up in out-patient department by ultrasonic cardiogram. Long-term free from aortic regurgitation rates were calculated using the Kaplan-Meier method. Multiple logistic regression analysis was performed to identify the risk factors of the postoperative aortic valvular regurgitation.

Results All patients were followed up. The mean follow-up periods was 34.72 ± 22.49 months, ranging from 3 to 88 months. Aortic regurgitation was presented in 19 patients, including mild regurgitation in 16 patients (8.6%) and moderate regurgitation in 3 patients (1.6%). 90% of patients were Free from regurgitation during the follow-up. The overall actuarial free from regurgitation at 1, 3 and 5 years follow-up resulted to be 95%, 91%, and 83%. Multiple logistic analysis identified associated VSD ($P = 0.0218$), age above 6 months ($P = 0.0083$) and post-operative neo-AV Z-score > 1 ($P < 0.01$) as the risk factors for postoperative aortic regurgitation.

Conclusions ASO remains the procedure of choice for the treatment of various forms of TGA with acceptable long term aortic valve function. Strong predictors for poor insufficiency of the neo-aortic valve are complicating VSD, age > 6 months and postoperative neo-AV Z-score > 1.

8

Surgical Treatment for Prosthetic Heart Valve Dysfunction

Sun HS, Ma WG, Abdurusul A, Gong DX, Wang W, Xu JP, Chang Q, Hu SS
Department of Cardiac Surgery, Cardiovascular Institute and Fu Wai Hospital, Chinese Academy of Medical Sciences, Beijing 100037, China

Objective To review our clinical experience with 44 reoperations for of prosthetic heart valve dysfunction.
Methods Between October 1996 and July 2009, there were 44 reoperations (0.3%) for failed heart valve prostheses among a total of 14546 cases of prosthetic heart valve replacement performed in Fu Wai Hospital. Among them 16 were males and 25 females with an average age of 45.5 ± 11.9 years. At the initial operation, 9 and 35 patients received bioprostheses and mechanical valve prostheses respectively. Initial procedures included mitral valve replacement (MVR) in 25, aortic valve replacement (AVR) in 8, aortic and mitral valve replacement (AVR + MVR) in 9, and mitral and tricuspid valve replacement (MVR + TVR) in 2 patients. Six reoperations were done during the postoperative period with the median time between the 2 operations being 20 hours (1 to 96 hours). The remaining 38 cases occurred after a mean interval of 63 months (1 to 241 months) postoperatively. The median time between the initial procedure and onset of symptoms was 32 months (1 to 189 months). All patients presented with dyspnea on exertion and palpitation and 26 patients suffered from atrial fibrillation. Chest X-Ray showed cardiomegaly (cardiothoracic ratio > 0.55) in 29 cases and 13 patients were in New York Heart Association functional class II, 15 in III and 16 in IV. Diagnosis was established by 2-dimensional echocardiography in all the patients. All patients underwent reoperation under hypothermic cardiopulmonary bypass (CPB), including 41 heart valve replacements, 2 disc rotations and 1 resection of an excessive knot. There were 16 emergency and 28 elective procedures. CPB was set up via the ascending aorta and venae cavae through the initial median sternotomy in 42 cases and via the femoral artery and vein through a left thoracotomy in 1 case. The reasons for mechanical heart valve dysfunction were thrombosis in 16 cases, pannus formation in 8, thrombosis with pannus formation in 8, valve orifice mal-orientation in 2 cases and an excessive knot in 1 case. Degeneration was found in the 9 cases of failed valve bioprostheses. Reoperations included MVR in 25 cases, AVR in 11, MVR + AVR in 3, TVR in 2, disc rotation in 2 cases and resection of knot in 1 case. A total of 37 mechanical valves were used, including 22 in the mitral, 8 in the aortic, 6 in the aortic and mitral, and 1 in the tricuspid position. Bioprosthetic valves were used in 7 cases, including 3 in the mitral, 3 in the aortic and 1 in the tricuspid position.
Results The mean CPB and clamp times were 146.5 ± 56.9 min (58 to 391 min) and 86.2 ± 26.7 min (35 to 133 min) respectively. The median time to extubation was 15.3 hours (5 to 243 hours) and tracheostomy was needed in 5 cases. There were 6 deaths, with a mortality rate of 13.6%. All 6 deaths occurred in emergency cases and patients initially implanted with mechanical valves due to low cardiac output in 3 cases, multiple organ failure in 2 and malignant arrhythmia in 1. No death occurred in patients initially implanted with bioprosthetic valves. Postoperative complications included 1 infective endocarditis, 1 intractable hiccup and 1 incisional infection.
Conclusions Acute failure bioprosthetic and mechanical heart valve is a catastrophic condition which should be treated by emergency reoperation as soon as possible. For chronic prosthetic valve dysfunction, early diagnosis and reoperation are mandatory, especially for mechanical valve prostheses.

9

Pulmonary Flow Study in Choosing Operative Strategy for Cyanotic Congenital Heart Defects

Sun HS, Ma WG, Ma Q, Gong DX, Luo XJ
Department of Cardiac Surgery, Cardiovascular Institute and Fu Wai Hospital, Chinese Academy of Medical Sciences, Beijing 100037, China

Objective To report our experience with intraoperative pulmonary flow study in the choice of surgical strategies for patients with cyanotic congenital heart defects.
Methods Between December 2007 and January 2009, four patients with cyanotic congenital heart defects underwent intraoperative pulmonary flow study before the final operative decision was made. Among them, there are 3 males and 1 female and their ages were 25, 31, 18, and 14 years respectively. The diagnosis was severe tetralogy of Fallot (TOF) in 2 cases, pulmonary atresia with ventricular septal defect and major

aortopulmonary collateral arteries in 1, and single ventricle with malposition of the great arteries and pulmonary stenosis in 1. The diagnosis was made by echocardiography and angiocardiography. The McGoon ratio was 1. 17, 1. 32, 1. 2 and 1. 3, respectively. After induction of general anesthesia and tracheal intubation, the superior and inferior venae cavae and the main pulmonary artery were cannulated and bypass was initiated the right atrium to the pulmonary artery. The flow rate started from 1 L/min and increased by every 0. 5 L/min at a 5-min interval, to the equivalent of at least one indexed cardiac output of 2. 5 L/min/m^2. At each flow rate, the pulmonary arterial (PA) pressures and arterial oxygen saturation were recorded. If anatomic repair was intended, the mean PA pressure should stay consistently below 25 mmHg; otherwise a palliative procedure should be chosen and the intracardiac shunt should be left open. When physiological repair was intended for cases unsuitable for anatomic repair, the mean PA pressure should remain consistently below 16 mmHg. If the PA pressure measurement exceeded 16 mmHg, a palliative procedure should be considered and the intracardiac shunt be left open.

Results The pulmonary flow rate reached 80% of the indexed cardiac output in the first TOF patient and decision was made of complete repair. Postoperatively she had elevated central venous pressure and pleural and pericardial effusion, which dissolved after a surgical atrial septal fenestration of 5 mm. The second TOF patient underwent complete repair and the other two patients received a total cavopulmonary connection. The third patient had moderate left pleural effusion and was cured after drainage.

Conclusions The intraoperative pulmonary flow study we used was a useful criterion in choosing operative strategies for patients with cyanotic congenital heart defects due to three merits. First, it helps in making decisions whether anatomic or physiological repair or palliative procedure should be adopted at the start of the operation. Second, in patients who received a physiological repair, it helps to decide whether the intracardiac shunt should be left open or closed. Finally, it results in a reduction of postoperative complications and the total medical cost.

10

Early Outcome of Hybrid Revascularization in Patients with Concomitant Coronary and Peripheral Artery Disease

Gong DX, Sun HS, Ma WG, Jiang XJ, Luo XJ, Ma Q, Zhang J, Wang XQ, Wang W

Department of Cardiac Surgery and Cardiology, Cardiovascular Institute and Fu Wai Hospital, Chinese Academy of Medical Sciences, Beijing 100037, China

Objective To review our experience with 19 cases of hybrid revascularization combining coronary artery bypass grafting with peripheral artery stenting.

Methods All patients underwent operations in a special hybrid operating room. The femoral artery was cannulated with the use of a 7-or 8-F guiding catheter after general anesthesia. The diseased peripheral arteries were first dilated by balloon angioplasty, followed by stent implantation if the severity of stenosis was more than 80%. After the completion of coronary artery bypass grafting, heparin was antagonized by protamine. Oral clopidogrel of 75 mg/day was administrated daily upon the first day of extubation, and was continued for at least 6 months. Patients also received oral aspirin of 100 mg daily after tracheal extubation.

Results All patients had a LIMA to LAD graft, and the number of grafts was 2 to 5 (mean, 3. 2). Stenting time was 34. 6 ± 3. 6 min (range, 32 to 50) and the CABG time was 185 ± 32. 5 min (range, 145 to 235). A total of 32 stents were implanted, including 20 in the carotid, 8 in renal, and 4 in the left subclavicular arteries. Pleural drainage during the first 24 h was 842 ± 180 ml, the mean ICU stay was 75. 4 ± 25. 2 h, the mean time to tracheal extubation was 24. 2 ± 17. 4 h, the mean length of hospital stay was 9. 8 ± 2. 9 d. Postoperative alanine transarninase (ALT) and aspartate transferase (AST) were 38. 4 ± 6. 9 and 28. 0 ± 8. 2 u/L, respectively and there was no significant change compared to preoperative levels (ALT 36. 6 ± 7. 5 u/L, $t = -0.88$, $p = 0.43$, AST 26. 4 ± 7. 2 u/L, $t = -1.73$, $p = 0.16$). Postoperative blood urea nitrogen and serum creatinine levels did not differ from preoperative levels significantly. All symptoms caused by the coronary and peripheral artery diseases dissolved after this compound procedure. One patient suffered a brain infarction, which was cured by thrombolytic therapy and he was discharged uneventfully. The follow-up time was 2 to 19 months, and no cardiovascular event was observed during the follow-up.

Conclusions For patients with both coronary and peripheral artery disease, hybrid revascularization combining coronary artery bypass grafting with peripheral artery stenting is a safe and effective therapy.

11

Risk Factor of Hypoxemia after Coronary Artery Bypass Grafting

Sun Y, Chi YF, Hou WM, Niu ZZ
Department of Cardiac Surgery, Qingdao Municipal Hospital, Qingdao 266071, China

Objective To analyze the risk factors of hypoxemia in patients after coronary artery bypass grafting.
Methods From January 2006 to January 2009, 318 patients underwent coronary artery bypass grafting and 35 patients suffered from post-operative hypoxemia. The relative-analysis of age, smoking, pulmonary disease, peri-operative LVEF, CPB and CPB time, ACC time, emergency operation and post-operative pneumonia were reviewed.
Results Hypoxemia happened in 35 cases and the incidence of hypoxemia was 11.4%. The risk factors of hypoxemia were exceeding 70 year-old, smoking, pulmonary disease, long CBP time, emergency operation, on lower and post-operative pneumonia.
Conclusions Hypoxemia after coronary artery bypass grafting is proved to occur in patients with advanced-age, smoke, pulmonary disease, long CBP time, emergency operation, post-operative lower-LVEF and post-operative pneumonia.

12

Peri-Operative Usage of Extracorporeal Membrane Oxygenation in Heart Transplantation

Wang W, Liao ZK, Hu SS
Department of Cardiac surgery, Cardiovascular Institute and Fu Wai Hospital, CAMS and PUMC, Beijing 100037, China

Objective To summarize clinical experience in Peri-Operative usage of ECMO in heart transplant patients.
Methods We performed 131 orthotopic heart transplantations from Jun. 2004 to Dec. 2008. Fourteen cases were performed with veno-artery ECMO (Medtronic Ltd) for Peri-Operative mechanical circulatory support in heart transplantation. Active clotting time (ACT) was maintained between 160-200 sec, Mean blood flow was 1.8-3.3 L/min during ECMO assistant period.
Results Twelve survivals were discharged with NYHA I, two patients died of multi-organ failure severe infection and complication of CNS. The ECMO time was 75-824 h and mean time 149 h. After bedside UCG evaluating heart function recovery, ECMO could be weaned off uneventfully after 100 h; Five patients had complication of bleeding and one patient hadcatheter-associated arterial thrombosis of distal limb. All ECMO patients had low-albuminemia and hyperbilirubinemia, eleven patientshad increasing blood creatine. Five patients were treated with CRRT, one patient with pertinacious hyperbilirubinemia was treated with plasma exchange and MARS.
Conclusions ECMO can bridge patients with end-stage heart failure to heart transplant, and extend the use of marginal donors, avoiding irreversible dysfunction of the vital organs and preventing from complication during ECMO, ECMO may decrease mortality of severe patients in the peri-operative period of heart transplantation.

13

One-Stage Repair of the Interrupted Aortic Arch (IAA) Associated with Cardiac Anomaly

Yan J, Cui B, Liu YL
Cardiovascular Institute and Fu Wai Hospital, Beijing 100037

Objective To evaluate the clinical experiences of one-stage repair of the interrupted aortic arch (IAA) associated with cardiac anomaly in neonates and infants.
Methods From July 1996 to October 2008, 48neonates or infants with the interrupted aortic arch (IAA) associated with cardiac anomaly underwent one-stage biventricular repair. male 30, female 18. mean age was 0.08-7.00 (1.97 ± 2.05) years, the mean body weight was 2.70-20.00 (9.28 ± 4.94) kg, 40 patients were IAA type A and 8 patients were type B. combined malformations: double outlet of the right ventricle, aortopulmonary window, ventricular septal defect, mitral valve stenosis, mitral valve insufficiency, tricuspid valve insufficiency, and et al. 42 patients had the middle-severe pulmonary hypertension (PH). the operation was performed through median sternotomy, on the four dif-

ferent CPB: deep hypothermia with circulatory arrest, deep hypothermia with low flow rate, deep hypothermia with low flow rate with low flow rate and circulatory arrest, the patients were operated on the arch anastomosis (30 cases) and arch transplantion (18 cases), the associated cardiac anomalies were completely corrected after IAA operation.

Results The total operative mortality rate was 6. 25% (3/48), the result was the severe pulmonary hypertension crisis, dysfunction of the pulmonary or the serious low cardiac output syndrome. Physical activities of the survivals increased obviously and discharged from hospital uneventfully, follows-up (3 to 144 months) showed survivals with no late complications and death.

Conclusions One-staged repair of IAA with other intracardiac anomalies can be safely applied with good results.

14

Strategy of Expanding Marginal Donor Heart and Clinical Result

Yang KM

Cardiovascular Institute and Fu Wai Hospital, Chinese Academy of Medical Science and Peking Union Medical College, Beijing100037, China

Objective To study the strategy of marginal donor heart application and to analyses the clinical effect on applying marginal donor heart in heart transplantation.

Methods 146 patients were undertaken heart transplantation in Fu Wai Hospital Beijing from June 2004 to February 2009. Marginal donor heart was defined as oversizing by more than 20% body weight, prolonged ischemic time over 6 hours, advanced age up to 40, and blood type ABO mismathched. Blood type exam and PRA test must be taken before operation. The preservative method of donor heart was sequential perfusion using cold St. Thomas and HTK solution. We divided those patients into groups according to different oversizing body weight, ischemic time, and donor age. The purpose of those compare study was to analyse the clinical result after heart transplantation.

Results There were 11 patients died after operation, 3 patients died in 1 month follow up, 7 patients died in 6 months follow up, 9 patients died in 1 year follow up. Ischemic time of donor heart was 262. 1 ± 120. 8 min, and 18 donors ischemic time was over 360 min, the longest one was 605 min. Comparing different groups we concluded there was no significant difference in recipient properties before transplantation, and also there were no different in mortality, heart function, heart rejection, and mainly morbidity after transplantation and follow up.

Conclusions These data support continued aggressive utilization of marginal donor hearts in heart transplantation. Our experience demonstrates that properly expanding marginal cardiac allografts application do not have an increased incidence of mortality and morbidity in recent and midterm results.

15

Reduced-dosed CNI plus Sirolimus for CNI-related Chronic Renal Dysfunction after Heart Transplantation

Yin D, Huang J, Feng L, Liao ZK

Cardiovascular Institute and Fu Wai Hospital, Chinese Academy of Medical Science and Peking Union Medical College, Beijing100037, China

Objective We summarized the preliminary experience of sirolimus-based immunosuppression therapy on 20 heart transplant recipients with renal dysfunction.

Methods From June 2004 to December 2008, 20 cardiac transplant recipients reduced-dose CNI plus sirolimus immunosuppressive regimen due to late CNI-related chronic renal dysfunction laboratory studies and echocardiography were routinely completed during the follow-up period. Endomyocardial biopsies were performed routinely in the first year after transplantation.

Results The mean clinical follow-up was 12. 11 ± 8. 85 months serum creatinine decreased significantly 160. 41 ± 25. 5 umol/l versus 130. 00 ± 27. 3 umol/L ($P = 0.026$). Sirolimus levels averaged 7. 91 ± 4. 28 ng/ml (doses 0. 92 ± 0. 27 mg). Within first year posttransplant, one patient had an episode of acute rejected (ISHLT grade II). Twenty patients were all alive with normal cardiac function by echocardiography. The most common side effect was hyperlipidemia. Cholesterol levels were 4. 68 ± 1. 34 mmol/L at the time of switching and 5. 51 ± 0. 78 mmol/L at the end of follow-up period ($P = 0.021$).

Conclusions In our experience, reduced-dose CNI plus sirolimus and an effective and safe approach to the management of patients with CNI-related chronic renal dysfunction.

16

Anatomic Surgical Repair for Complex Coarctation in Adults

Yu CT, Sun HT, Chang Q

Department of Cardiac Surgery, Cardiovascular Institute and Fu Wai Hospital, CAMS and PUMC, Beijing 100037, China

Objective Treatment of complex coarctation is a surgical challenge. The best approaches are still debatable.

Methods In the past 4 years (2005-2009), anatomic surgical repair was performed in 18 adults for complex coarctation. Age ranged from 16 to 55 years (mean age, 25.8 ± 13 years). Coarctation with hypoplastic aortic arch, n = 5; coarctation with aortic aneurysm, n = 6; coarctation with ventricular septal defect, n = 4; coarctation with aortic dissection, n = 3; coarctation with aortic valve incompetence, n = 2; aortic arch replacement was performed in 4, arch patch enlargenment in 9 and descending thoracic aorta replacement in 5 patients. Midsternotomy in 11 and left thoracotomy in 6 patients, arch reconstruction was performed. A prospective and systematic clinical evaluation of the anatomic surgical repair for complex coarctation was undertaken.

Results There was no hospital mortality and major Morbidity. The median postoperative follow-up was 24 months (range, 6 to 49 months). There were no recoarctation and false aneurysm.

Conclusions On the basis of these results, anatomic surgical repair appears to be a safe alternative in complex coarctation patients. The anatomic repair is the procedure of first choice.

17

The Application of Hybrid Operation in Coronary Heart Disease

Zhang HL, Zhang YF, Xi ZH

Cardiovascular Institute and Fu Wai Hospital, Chinese Academy of Medical Science and Peking Union Medical College, Beijing 100037, China

By reviewing relative literatures and our cases, we analyzed the application of Hybrid operation in coronary heart disease, Our dates showed that the Hybrid Operation combine Bypass surgery and PCI, maybe the best choice for multi-vessel coronary heart disease patient. Currently, PCI and Bypass surgery are two strategies to treat coronary heart disease, Bypass surgery could get the full revascularization but has the heavy operation injury; PCI has the small operation injury but has some limitations, the Hybrid operation combine the advantages of both PCI and Bypass surgery, using LIMA as the bypass artery to improve the prognosis and the quality of life, using PCI for RCA or LCX to avoid the skin injury of taking SVG.

We also analyzed the pre and post operation nursing strategy. For pre-operation care, we focused on psychological care, medical education for the patient on top of the regular care and preparation. For post-operation care, we focused on life style changes, smoking quitting, diet management, and risk factors control on top of the regular care. In conclusions, Hybrid operation seems to be the best choice for the multi-vessel disease, and the nursing program after Hybrid operation is different from the regular care after bypass surgery and PCI, and if need more improvement.

18

Orthotopic Heart Transplantation Report of Four Cases

Zhang XH, Shi BY, Chen X, Li T, Fan LL, Sun SH, Qi YJ, Jin WB, Ma LJ, Cai M
Chinese People's Liberation Army General Hospital, Second Affiliated Hospital Organ Transplant Center of the PLA Cardiothoracic Vascular surgery

Objective To investigate the treatment of orthotopic heart transplantation for end-stage dilated cardiomyopathy of surgical treatment.
Methods In November 1999-2008 year in May, we have four cases of end-stage heart disease in patients with dilated introduced orthotopic heart transplantation, respectively, Stanford University to improve myocardial protective solution and HTK solution Shun irrigation myocardial protection for heart protection; surgery and the use of standard intravenous method of dual-chamber cardiac transplantation. Early postoperative application of methylprednisolone (1000 mg/day) immunosuppressive therapy, and to give the gastrointestinal tract of high nutritional support, after three days of cyclosporine A (or FK506), mycophenolate mofetil, prednisone immune Sanlian suppression therapy. Through the monitoring of CsA blood concentration, T lymphocyte subsets, white blood cell count, enzyme changes, ECG leads of the high peaks of QRS and, echocardiography ventricular systolic and diastolic function, EF values, left ventricular wall thickness and volume and myocardial scintigraphy, etc., to determine whether the occurrence of acute rejection.
Results The results of early postoperative death in 1 case, the other three cases of patients with hemodynamic stability; after early recovery goes well, no hyperacute rejection; no wound infection and lung infection; cardiac function returned to grade I (NYHA).
Conclusions Heart transplantation is end-stage dilated cardiomyopathy only effective method of treatment, perioperative management of patients with heart transplantation is the last long-term effect of the success or failure and a key factor in good or bad.

19

Total Anomalous Pulmonary Venous Drainage of the Surgical Treatment

Zhang XH, Chen X, Wei FL, Ma LJ, Qi YJ, Jin WB, Zheng ML
Chinese People's Liberation Army General Hospital, Second Affiliated Hospital Organ Transplant Center of the PLA Cardiothoracic Vascular surgery

Objective To investigate the total anomalous pulmonary venous drainage surgery and perioperative management experience.
Methods From April 1987 to September 2005, after surgical treatment of total anomalous pulmonary venous drainage in 33 cases of patients. 22 cases of male, female 11 cases; the age of 2 to 32 years of age; supracardiac total anomalous pulmonary venous drainage in 21 cases, cardiac-type total anomalous pulmonary venous drainage in 12 cases; echocardiography confirmed complete supracardiac pulmonary venous drainage in 17 cases, the left vertical vein diameter of 2.6-3.5 cm, atrial septal defect diameter 2.0-3.5 cm, 2 patients with pulmonary valve stenosis. Cardiac-type total anomalous pulmonary venous drainage in 10 cases, atrial septal defect size of 2.8 cm-3.1 cm, of which there are five cases of coronary sinus to expand. Line 12 cases of cardiac catheterization, pulmonary artery pressure of patients for the 1.8-1.2kp (13-84 mmHg), of which 2 cases of pulmonary resistance >8wood units. Surgery in general anesthesia under hypothermic cardiopulmonary bypass. Of supracardiac total anomalous pulmonary venous connection patients, the right atrium-atrial septal defect in the posterior wall of left atrial incision and the common pulmonary vein to 4-0 prolene line will cut the right side wall of the left atrium and the common position of the corresponding vein incision traction suture cooperation, continue to cut the posterior wall of the left atrium and the common vein to vertical vein incision length plus the diameter of 2 cm, with 4-0 prolene line to the left atrium and the common vein wall incision, the lower edge of the continuous suture 2-pin, left a pin for traction, continuous suture margin. PTFE patch repair with atrial septal defect, the right edge of the appropriate patch forward, and then the left vertical vein ligation. Cited the inflow of the coronary sinus total anomalous pulmonary venous drainage, with a small bougie from the coronary sinus do I insert a guide, atrial septal defect removal coronary sinus and the mouth of the divide, with 4-0 prolene margin suture line rough surface, atrial septal defect will be expanded to more than 3.0 cm, with a larger patch of autologous pericardium patch, will be separated into the pulmonary vein side of the left atrium. Placed according to the situation during temporary epicardial pacing wire.
Results No postoperative death, were followed up for 2-16 years, are back to normal cardiac function.
Conclusions The preoperative diagnosis of a clear design of the program operation is particularly important. Echocardiography can not specify

the time of diagnosis, should be carried out cardiac catheterization and cardiovascular imaging examination. Diagnosed the disease as soon as possible after the surgery. Surgical anastomosis of the key is large enough, smooth flow. Good perioperative management is to ensure successful operation.

20

The ED50 of Propofol for Successful Intubation without Neuromuscular Blockade in Children under 3 Years

Zhang XL, Wang WP, Xu JH

Cardiovascular Institute and Fu Wai Hospital, Chinese Academy of Medical Sciences and Peking Union Medical College, Beijing 100037 China

Objective To investigate the ED50 of propofol alone as an induction agent for endotracheal intubation for the children less than 3 years.

Methods We conducted a prospective, controlled trial of children under 3 years who required non-emergency endotracheal intubation in Fu Wai hospital (including ASD, VSD and PDA) Thirty-one unpremedicated ASA physical status Ⅰ or Ⅱ patients were anesthetized with propofol alone for induction. The ED50 of propofol for airway device placement was determined using Dixon's up-and-down method. The concentration of propofol for consecutive patients was determined by the response of the previous patient, using increments or decrements of 0.2 mg/kg. Intubating conditions were evaluated according to a scoring system described by Viby-Mogensen. The effective dose (ED50) of propofol enabling successful tracheal intubation was determined by calculating the midpoint concentration of all independent pairs of patients after at least seven crossover points (i. e. success to failure of tracheal intubation) were obtained. The ED50 was defined as the average of crossover midpoints in each pair. Blood pressure, heart rate, Bis and SpO2 were recorded during induction. Hemodynamic data changes were compared by repeated measures ANAOVA., and P-value <0.05 was significant.

Results The bolus ED50 of propofol required for successful tracheal intubation was 4.84 (0.28) mg/kg. From probit analysis, ED95 of propofol 5.84 mg/kg (95% confidence limits 5.40-9.72 mg/kg). With ED50 induction, MAP decreased 6.8% (70.1 ± 8.8 mmHg vs. 65.3 ± 8.2 mmHg, $P<0.05$), returned to baseline after intubation. No patients suffered from significant bradycardia or hypotension.

Conclusions The ED50 of propofol for successful intubation without neuromuscular blockade in children under 3 years e is 4.84 mg/kg. A higher induction dose of propofol alone in children than in adults, and no patients suffered clinically significant bradycardia or hypotension. It was safe to use higher dose of propofol alone to induct in children under 3 years.

21

Retrospective Analysis of Cardiac Arrest and Cardiopulmonary Cerebral Resuscitation in 100 Children after the Cardiac Operation

Zhang YB, Wang X, Liu YL, Li SJ, Yan J

Cardiovascular Institute and Fu Wai Hospital, Chinese Academy of Medical Science and Peking Union Medical College, Beijing 100037, China

Objective To evaluate the effect of Cardiopulmonary Cerebral Resuscitation (CPCR), survival resuscitation rate from Cardiac Arrest (CA).

Methods A retrospective analysis was carried out for 100 patients received CPCR after the cardiac operation in recent four years. 63 boys and 37 girls were included in this study, the average age was 19 months (0.5-84), and the average weight was 9 kg (2.8-23), 52 patients were mechanical ventilated when the CA happened. According to the AHA guideline of Pediatric Basic Life Support (PBLS) and Pediatric Advanced Life Support (PALS) 2005, C (circulation), D (drugs) and A (airway), B (breathing) were given at the same time by the members of resuscitation team. Bolus given of low-dose epinephrine, early cerebral and gastrointestinal protection and the usage of temporary pacemaker were the emphasis in our experience. Chest open and Extracorporeal Membrane Oxygenator (ECMO) were given to the appropriate patients failure of Restoration of Spontaneous Circulation (ROSC). Patients who only received positive pressure ventilation or resuscitation drugs but without chest compression were not included.

Results The successful ratio of initial resuscitation was 52%, 21 cases were given bedside chest open, and 11 of them were followed by ECMO (3 survived to hospital discharge). The main reasons caused CA in this group were hypoxemia (44%), ventricular fibrillation (23%),

Pulseless Electronic Activity (PEA, 20%), disorder of electrolytes (10%). Neither weight nor age affected ROSC. Severe hypoxemia and poor heart dysfunction were the main reasons responsible for the failure of the initial resuscitation.

Conclusions The higher ratio of initial resuscitation in this group was benefit from the timely aware of CA, the correct judgement of the cause of CA, the well-trained resuscitation group and the comprehensive treatment after the establishment of ROSC. ECMO were useful for the initial resuscitation and the long term result of CPCR.

22

Hybrid Technique: Single-stage Repair of Coarctation of the Aorta with Ventricular Septal Defect in Infants

Li SJ, Zhang Y, Zheng ZH
Center for Pediatric Cardiac Surgery the Department of Surgery, Fu Wai Hospital, Beijing, China

Objective The optimal surgical strategy for the repair of coarctation of the aorta (CoA) associated with a ventricular septal defect (VSD) is controversial. This study introduced a hybrid technique to repair CoA and VSD simultaneously through a sternotomy in infants.

Methods There were 4 severely ill infants presented with CoA-VSD from October 2008 to December 2008, who underwent complete repair by hybrid technique. All patients had large VSD. The VSD type was perimembranous, and the diameter was nearly 1 cm. All patients had a median sternotomy incision. Through an ascending aorta approach, aortic angiogram was performed. A balloon catheter was forwardly advanced through a guidewire previously positioned in the ascending aorta. Selection of balloon diameter was based on the immediate angiographic measurements of the mean value between isthmic and distal aortic segments. Then balloon angioplasty was performed to dilate coarctation of the aorta. VSD was closed with standard perfusion techniques and cardioplegic arrest.

Results Balloon angioplasty was performed successfully in all patients. No patients died. There were no complications during a mean follow-up 6 months (range 5 to 7 months). The blood pressure difference between the arms and legs was not significant.

Conclusions Balloon angioplasty through the ascending aorta approach and VSD closure simultaneous provided advantages to patients with CoA-VSD. It is a simple, safe and alternative method for infants with CoA-VSD, especially for those severely ill infants.

23

A Comparison of Long-term Outcome of Radial Artery with Saphenous Vein Graft in CABG

Zhu YP, Zhao Q, Chen AQ
Department of Cardiac Surgery, Ruijin Hospital, Shanghai Jiao Tong University, Shanghai 200025

Objective The left internal mammary artery (LIMA) has been shown to improve the outcome of coronary artery bypass grafting (CABG) and become the gold standard graft. However the benefit of the radial artery (RA) has not been determined. The aim of this retrospective study was to compare the long-term outcome of the radial artery with the saphenous vein graft in CABG.

Methods Between January 2004 and December 2005, 324 patients who were underwent isolated OPCAB composed this study. There were 79 patients received the radial artery graft (the RA group), of which 59 patients had total arterial grafts (LIMA and RA), 20 patients had standard procedure (LIMA to LAD, SVG to other target vessels) with RA (LIMA, SVG and RA). The other 245 patients who underwent CABG without RA (LIMA and SVG) composed the SVG group. A complete follow-up was obtained for 254 patients from 36 to 60 months after the operation (mean 41.6 months). Coronary artery CT or angiography were performed in 63 cases after the operation, including 18 cases with angina symptoms. Thus 63 LIMA, 29 RA and 142 SVG were followed up from 3 to 52 months (mean 32.1 months). Outcomes were evaluated by univariate analysis and survival analysis.

Results Clinic outcomes: The mean age of the RA group was younger. The clinic characters showed a significant higher prevalence of female, severe angina (CCS) and smoke in the RA group. The mean number of conduits in the RA group was fewer (RA 3.28 ± 0.88, SVG 3.62 ± 0.70; $p = 0.004$). The prevalence of taking exercise post-operatively was higher in the RA group (RA 58/67, 86.6%; SVG 118/170, 69.0%; $p = 0.006$). The actuarial survival, freedom from MACE (major adverse cardiac event) and angina at 12 months or 36 months were similar. The total survival curve showed significant benefit in the RA group ($p = 0.01$). The MACE-free survival curve also showed significant benefit in the RA group ($p = 0.044$). The angina-free survival curve showed no significant difference. As a subgroup analysis (age 60-70), there was no significant difference of the total survival curve, the MACE-free survival curve and the angina-free survival curve between two groups. Image study outcomes: Results of the LIMA grafts were all excellent. The overall patency of the RA graft was higher than the SVG (RA 27/29, 93.1%; SVG 103/142, 72.5%; p = 0.018). The rate of TVR (target vessel revascularization) of the RA graft was less (RA 0/29, 0%; SVG 24/142, 16.9%; p = 0.036). There was no difference in the patency rate at 12 months. The patency rate of the RA graft at 24 and 36 months were superior (RA 21/21, 100%; SVG 102/128, 79.7% at 24 months; p = 0.049; RA 17/18, 94.4%; SVG 79/115, 68.7% at 36 months; p = 0.023). The Long-term patency curve showed significant benefit in the RA group (p = 0.032).

Conclusions The RA graft improved survival and reduced MACE after CABG. The RA graft had superior patency. The long-term outcome of the RA was better than SVG.

24

Strategy for Surgical Management of Patients with Non-committed Ventricular Septal Defect Double-outlet Right Ventricle

Li SJ, Hu SS, Zheng ZH, Liu ZG, Zhang HL, Wang D, Liu YL, Shen XD, Ya J

Department of Cardiac Surgery, Cardiovascular Institute and Fu Wai Hospital, CAMS and PUMC, Beijing 100037, China

Objective Depending on the relationship of ventricular septal defect (VSD) with arterial valves, double-outlet right ventricle (DORV) can be divided into four subtypes: subaortic VSD, subpulmonary VSD, doubly committed VSD and non-committed VSD (DORVncVSD), of which the last is defined when the superior edge of the VSD is distant for both arterial valves from a distance greater than an aortic valve diameter. So far, DORVncVSD remains challenge for cardiac surgeons. This study reports our experiences with this subset, and focus on its anatomic characters, surgical options and outcomes, especially the newly developed double root translocation (DRT) for DORVncVSD with pulmonary stenosis.

Methods From Jan 1996 to Feb 2009, 123 DORVncVSD patients (90 males, 33 females) under 7 years old were underwent surgical repair. The mean age at surgery was 3.1 ± 2.1 years (range, 3 months to 7 years) and the mean body weight was 12.2 ± 4.5 kg (range, 4 to 20 kg). There were 65 single ventricular repair (51 Fontan type procedures and 14 others) and 58 biventricular repair (33 intraventricular tunnel repair, 9 Rastelli, 9 artery switch operation, 2 REV and 5 DRT). For most patients with biventricular repair, VSDs were superiorly enlarged. According to the period at surgery, the patients were divided into early group (from Jun 1996 to Dec 2004) and late group (from Jan 2005 to Feb 2009).

Results There were 19 operative deaths, with overall mortality of 15.4% (19/123). The operative mortality rate in early and late group were 26.2% (16/61) and 4.8% (3/62) (p < 0.01). In early group, biventricular repair mainly consist of intraventricular tunnel repair (IVR) and Rastelli procedures, with biventricular repair rate of 42.6% (26/61) and its mortality rate of 26.9% (7/26). In late group, more options were used for biventricular repair. In this group, the biventricular repair rate was 50% (31/61) and mortality rate of biventricular repair was 6.5% (2/31). There was no significant different biventricular repair rate between early and late group, however, less mortality rate was found in late group (p < 0.05). Modified Fontan procedure contributed to most single ventricular repair. The mortality rate of single ventricular repair were 25.7% (9/35) and 3.2% (1/31) in early and late group, respectively, (P < 0.01).

Conclusions With improvement of surgical technique and knowledge for DORVncVSD, several procedures were developed for its biventricular repair. DORVncVSD patients should undergo biventricular repair as far as possible, according to its better surgical outcomes than single ventricular repair. By resecting part infundibulum, superiorly enlarging VSD, complete left ventricular outflow tract relief and double root translocation, DRT provide an option of true meaning anatomic repair for DORVncVSD patients with pulmonary stenosis.

25

Arterial Switch Operation for the Surgical Management of Ventriculoarterial Discordance with Left Ventricular Outflow Tract Obstruction: Results and Fellow Up

Li SJ[1], Hu SS, Liu ZG[1], Zheng Z[1], Wang D[1], Li YQ[2], Zhang YJ[1]
1Department of Pediatric Cardiovascular Surgery, the National Cardiovascular Center and Fu Wai Hospital, Beijing, Chinese Academe of Medical Science and Peking Union Medical College
2Department of Echocardiography, the National Cardiovascular Center and Fu Wai Hospital, Beijing, Chinese Academe of Medical Science and Peking Union Medical College

Objective Surgical management of ventriculoarterial discordance with left ventricular outflow tract obstruction (LVOTO) remains challenge. This study aims to evaluate the results of arterial switch operation (ASO) for this subgroup of patients.
Methods Between Jun 2004 and June 2009, 11 of 110 consecutive patients with ventriculoarterial discordance (transposition of great artery and Taussig-Bing syndrome) and LVOTO undertook ASO and LVOT relief (the other surgical options including Rastelli procedures in 22, REV in 23, double root translocation in 54). Median age and weight were 20 months (range, 4 to 64 months) and 14 kg (range, 4.6 to 24.0 kg). The causes of anatomic LVOTO, preoperative pressure gradient and their surgical treatments are summarized in table 1, with the median preoperative peak systolic pressure gradient of 36.0 mmHg (range, 10.2 to 46.2 mmHg). The ASO was performed according to our standard technique with LVOT resection and/or pulmonary valvotomy as required.
Results There was no perioperative death. The median gradient across LVOT at predischarge was 10.2 mmHg (range, 3.2 to 27 mmHg) with no neoaortic insufficiency detected. Follow-up ranged from 3 months to 4 years. During 172 patient-months of follow-up time, no late deaths occurred and no reoperation was required. One patient currently developed mild neoaortic insufficiency which, however, was hemodynamically insignificant. Median LVOT gradient at last follow-up was 5.8 mmHg (range, 3.2 to mm 16 Hg). All patients were in NYHA class I.
Conclusions In selected patients with ventriculoarterial discordance/LVOT abnormalities, the ASO can be performed with satisfactory survival and functional status if LVOTO is resectable in absence of hypoplastic pulmonary annulus. Relief of LVOTO appears to be sustained at medium-term follow-up.

26

Aortico-left Ventricular Tunnel: A Different Finding and New Experience

Wang W, Sun HN, Song YH, Xu JP, Sun HS, Hu SS
Department of cardiac surgery, Cardiovascular Institute and Fu Wai Hospital, Chinese Academy of Medical Science and Peking Union Medical College, Beijing 100037, China

Objective To describe some new findings of aortic-left ventricular tunnel (ALVT) about clinical features, anatomy, treatment and follow-up.
Methods We reviewed Clinical, diagnostic methods and surgical details of patients well-documented case from June 1995 to May 2009 in Fu Wai hospital and excluded the data reported previously, analysis the data of follow-up. And compared with previous descriptions found in literature published in English.
Results 5 patients were diagnosed as aortic-left ventricular tunnel and tunnels lay above or from the non-coronary sinus Valsalv. Associated lesions occurred in 3 patients, all patients underwent surgery under standard cardiopulmonary bypass. ALVT can be diagnosed accurately by Magnetic resonance imaging (MRI), Surgical methods include direct suture, patch closure and aortic valve replacement (AVR). At follow-up, 4 patients were in NYHA class I, 1 in Class II-III. No aortic regurgitation in1, mild to moderate in 1. The aortic mechanical valve is normal in 1 paravalvular leakage in 1 and recanalization of tunnel in 1.
Conclusions We first describe the aortic orifice of the tunnel arose above or from the non-coronary sinus on the world since 1963, most patients presented in adulthood, besides echocardiography, MRI is a helpful and noninvasive tool to diagnose the lesion, Three-dimensional echocardiography was used in follow-up of ALVT for the first time and gave an accurate diagnosis. Long-term follow-up is essential, a special attention should be paid to those who underwent AVR, the character of anatomy, natural history, diagnosis and treatment should be reconsidered.

27

An Outcome Analysis of Bidirection Glenn Procedure on Children within 12 Months with Complex Congenital Heart Disease

Yan J, Shi Y, ZHang J, Wang Q
Chinese Academy of Medical Sciences Fu Wai Hospital Surgical Department, Beijing 100037, China

Objective To analyse the results of bidirectional Glenn procedure on children within 12 months with complex congenital heart disease.
Methods 34 patients with complex cyanotic congenital heart defects underwent a bidirectional Glenn shunt between January 1998 and December 2008. There were 21 male and 13 female patients, the mean age was 0.66 ± 0.21 years. The mean transcutaneous oxygen saturation was 73% ± 9% and the mean pulmonary pressure was 12.19 ± 3.68 mmHg before the operation. 16cases were performed on pump and 18cases were performed off pump.
Results There were 2 patients died and 5 patients suffered severe complications. After operation mean operation time was 173.55 ± 42.16 minutes, and mean vena cava pressure was 17.74 ± 3.62 mmHg, mean transcutaneous oxygen saturation was 84 ± 16% after operation. Follow-up echocardiography showed functioning Glenn shunts without any obstruction at the anastomosis.
Conclusions Bidirectional glenn procedure showed satisfied effect on surgical treatment for children within 12-month with complex congenital heart disease on children within 12 months. This procedure can improve the oxygen supply and pulmonary vessel growth for whom can't get total correction procedure.

28

Outcome of Aggressive Pulmonary Annulus Preservation Strategy in Complete Tetralogy Repair

Hua ZD
Cardiovascular Institute and Fu Wai Hospital, Beijing 100037

Objective To assess the operative and mid-term outcome of a very aggressive pulmonary annulus preservation strategy which achieved 95% freedom of transannular patch in complete tetralogy repair.
Methods From Aug 2006 through May 2009, 139 consecutive patients underwent repair of tetralogy of Fallot at a median age of 6.5 months, with median weight 7.2 kg. None of the patients had a prior shunt. One hundred thirty-two patients (95%) had pulmonary valve annulus-sparing procedures, predominantly through a transatrial and transpulmonary approach (n = 120, 86.3%). Special techniques including generous pulmonary Supra-valve patch, bicuspid pulmonary leaflets plasty or augmentation to maximally preserve pulmonary annulus. Intraoperative measurements included the pulmonary valve annulus, pressure of postbypass pulmonary artery, right ventricular outlet and left ventricle. All survived patients were closely followed up.
Results Only seven patients had a transannular patch (5.0%). Among them, 5 (71.4%) had subpulmonary ventricular defect. None of tricusp pulmonary valve needs TAP. Preoperative size of pulmonary annulus less than-6 is associated with TAP ($p < 0.001$). Twelve (13.7%) patients needed repump to either do a ventriculotomy and patch the incision or TAP to relieve residual stenosis. One patients needed a third pump run to do a TAP. The operative mortality was 0.7%, and there was one late death due to hemoptysis. The pulmonary regurgitation of non-TAP patients were less than mild in 105 (79.5%), mild to moderate in 27 (20.5%). 3 patients had peak gradient greater than 50 mmHg across right ventricle and pulmonary artery at 1 month follow-up, but the gradient dropped to less than 50 mmHg in 2 patients at 6 month follow-up. One patient had a persistent 50-55 mmHg gradient across pulmonary valve and he is under close follow-up.
Conclusions Excellent outcome can be achieved even with 95% freedom of TAP in complete repair of tetralogy. Functions of most patients' pulmonary valve were well preserved.

29

Operative and Mid-Term Outcome of Congenitally Corrected Transposion of Great Artery

Hua ZD, Hu SS, Pan XB, Shen XD, Li SJ, Yan J, Liu YL, Wu QY, Wang X
Center of Pediatric Cardiac Surgery, Cardiovascular Institute and Fu Wai Hospital, CAMS and PUMC, Beijing 100037, China

Objective To retrospectively analyze the surgical and mid-term outcomes of 107 patients with corrected congenital transposition of great arteries (CCTGA) who underwent surgical treatment in one Hospital.

Methods A total of 107 CCTGA patients with surgical treatment from 1996 to 2005 were studied. There were 72 male and 35 female, with the mean age of 11.5 years and mean body weight of 31 kg. Among the cohort, 81 were levocardia, 23 dextrocardia, 3 mesocardia. Initial surgical procedure included single ventricle repair in 14 patients, conventional biventricular repair in 75, double switch in 17 patients, and senning and nikadoh in 1 patient. 93% patients were followed-up with the mean time of 47.8 months.

Results Operative mortality was 4.76%, with single ventricle repair 0%, conventional biventricular repair 4%, atrial-arterial double switch 0%, atrial-ventricular double switch 40%. The risk factors for operative mortality were lesions with double outlet left ventricle combined with pulmonary stenosis ($P < 0.05$), and Rastelli procedure ($P < 0.05$). 12 patients (12.6%) died during follow-up period, among them 10 (83.3%) were in conventional repair group, 2 (16.7%) in single ventricle repair group, no death in double switch group. The risk factors for follow-up mortality were conventional biventricular repair, Rastelli procedure and tricuspid regurgitation.

Conclusions Conventional biventricular repair had a disappointing outcome in both peri-operative and mid-term follow-up period. Patients suitable for single ventricular repair had fair short-and mid-term outcomes. Atrial-arterial double switch procedure had good operative and mid-term results.

30

Early Rescue Therapy of High Frequency Oscillation in Pediatric Patients with Severe Hypoxaemic Respiratory Failure after Congenital Heart Surgery

Wang X, Duan LL, Zeng M, Zhang YB, He Y
Center of Pediatric Cardiac Surgery, Cardiovascular Institute and Fu Wai Hospital, CAMS and PUMC, Beijing 100037, China

Objective In order to determine the optimum timing and strategy for the application of HFOV in pediatric patients with severe hypoxaemic respiratory failure after congenital heart surgery.

Methods and **Results** HFOV was instituted in 30 patients ranging in age from 7 days to 5 years with congenital heart disease meeting pulmonary criteria for severe hypoxaemic respiratory failure ($PaO2/FiO2 < 100$). The whole patients were divided into two groups according to the time of HFOV. Early initiation group ($n = 19$) was defined as using HFOV within 6 h after the $PaO2/FiO2 < 100$. Arterial blood gases, oxygenation index (OI) and PaO2/FiO2 ratio were prospectively recorded prior to HFOV (oh) and at 1 h, 4 h, 8 h, 12 h, 24 h, 48 h respectively. After 1 hour of treatment, PaCO2 significantly decreased ($P < 0.01$) and remained within the target range thereafter in the early initiation group. There were significant increase in PaO2/FiO2 ratio from 4 hours of HFOV ($P < 0.05$) and until 48 hours. But in late initiation group ($n = 11$), The PaO2/FiO2 ratio was not showed a significant increase except the 12 h point. There were significant changes between the two groups in PaO2/FiO2 ratio ($P < 0.01$) at predetermined intervals throughout the course of the HFOV protocol. 15 patients (78.95%) were weaned from the HFO ventilator in the early initiation group and 13 patients (68.42%) survived. But in the late initiation group only 2 patients (18.18%) survived. 5 patients were transferred to ECMO after failing HFOV support in the whole group, but only 1 survival.

Conclusions In pediatric patients with severe hypoxaemic respiratory failure after congenital heart surgery, Early initiation of HFOV (less than 6 h after the $PaO2/FiO2 < 100$) improves ventilation and gas exchange in a rapid and sustained fashion and provided a good outcome. For those patients who failing HFOV support more than 48 h, it may be no use to be transferred to ECMO support again.

31

Pediatric Extracorporeal Membrane Oxygenation Support: Managements and Considerations in ICU

Wang X, Zhang YB, He Y
Department of Cardiac Surgery, Cardiovascular Institute and Fu Wai Hospital, CAMS and PUMC, Beijing 100037, China

Objective To evaluate the clinical outcomes of postoperative ECMO support following congenital cardiac surgery in our hospital. In order to establish the important predictors of outcomes.

Methods Retrospective review of 28 children requiring ECMO support after cardiac surgery at out hospital from Dec. 2004 to Jun. 2009.

Results 28 patients all had biventricular repair. The specific indications for ECMO included inability to separate from cardiopulmonary bypass in OR ($n = 14$), serious low cardiac output syndrome on maximal inotropic support or cardiac arrest in PICU ($n = 11$) and postoperative LV support for primary ASO whose LV/RV ratio between 0.5 to 0.6 ($n = 3$). Median age of the patients was 17.83 months (1 month to 6 years) and median weight was 8.79 kg (4-17 kg). The average duration of ECMO was 142 hours (range: 8-302 hours). 16 children (57.14%) survived >3 days after decannulation and 13 (46.43%) survived to discharge. In this series, 10 patients died of irreversible ventricular failure, 2 were serious bleeding and 3 were sepsis and acute renal failure. Length of time on ECMO, inotrope score at ECMO initiation and serum lactate within 24 hours of ECMO were not significantly different between the survivor and nonsurvivor. The only difference between the two groups was the inotrope score after ECMO 24 hours later. The survivor group have a much lower score ($P < 0.05$).

Conclusions ECMO support is an effective mechanical support for cardiopulmonary failure in the postcardiotomy pediatric patient. Inability to separate from ECMO support and the development of acute renal failure may have an increased risk of death. ECMO for TGA/IVS patients may be good indication.

32

One Stage Repair of Pulmonary Atresia with Ventricular Septal Defect

Li SJ, Deng XC, Liu YL, Sheng XD, Jun Y, Hu SS
Center for Pediatric Cardiac Surgery, Cardiovascular Institute & Fu Wai Hospital, Chinese Academy of Medical Sciences, Beijing, China
Department of Cardiac Surgery, Cardiovascular Institute & Fu Wai Hospital, Peking Union Medical College, Chinese Academy of Medical Sciences, 167 Beilishilu, Beijing 100037

Objective To introduce the application of Rastelli procedure (conduit connection), patch and modified Rev procedure in the surgical management of pulmonary atresia with ventricular septal defect and comparison among them so as to get a better understanding of one stage repair of pulmonary atresia with ventricular septal defect.

Methods From November 1992 to October 2008, 74 patients with pulmonary atresia with ventricular septal defect underwent one stage repair in Fu Wai Hospital. There were 40 males and 34 females, aged from 8 months to 27 years (Median: 2.6 years), 54 cases of type I, 6 cases of type II, 14 cases of type III by Castaneda classification. All patients underwent preoperative echocardiography and angiocardiography and evaluated by the same team. There were 3 types operations: the patch group, in patients with membraneous atresia and relatively good developed main pulmonary arteries, transannular valved patches were utilized (35 cases); conduit group, in type II or with vestigial main pulmonary arteries, a conduit connecting between right ventricle and main pulmonary artery was utilized (28 cases); modified Rev group, in patients with poor developed main pulmonary artery, but only lower segmental atresia not longer than 1.5 cm, the left and right pulmonary arteries were dissected, the atresic segment were excised and the main pulmonary arteries were anastomosed to the right ventricular incision with a valved path (11 cases); the major aortopulmonary collaterals with communication to native pulmonary arteries were surgical ligated (6 cases) or interventional occluded (5 cases). ANOVA was used in comparison among the groups.

Results The mean values of all patients: McGoon: 1.67 ± 0.50, Nakata index (mm2/m2): 155.38 ± 84.955. Early postoperative echo showed no statistical difference among the three groups; complications: 7 cases in the patch group, 7 cases in the conduit group, 2 cases in the modified Rev group, no significant statistical difference. There were 53 cases of long-term followed up with duration from 7 months to 8 years (mean 5.2 years). There were 25 cases in NYHA I, 18 cases in NYHA II and 7 cases in NYHA III of heart function, 3 late deaths, 2 in the conduit group and 1 in the patch group. 3 cases were reoperated on due to conduit degeneration or relatively small size. Echocardiography showed the pulmonary flow velocity was significantly slower in both of the patch and modified Revgroups than in the conduit group ($p < 0.05$), albeit no statistical difference among them.

Conclusions Clear and definitive diagnosis of patients with pulmonary atresia with ventricular septal defect should be got before operation. One stage repair should strictly comply with surgical indications. Different procedures should be applied according to the development of main and branch pulmonary arteries. Modified Revprocedure avoids utilization of conduits so as to decrease or avoid degeneration and deficit of growth in xenografts which warrants better near and intermediate outcomes whereas further study should be taken to find out its long term effect.

33

Consecutive 154 Patients Heart Transplantation: Experience in Fu Wai Hospital

Huang J, Hu SG, Song YH, Wang W, Feng L
Cardiovascular Institute and Fu Wai Hospital, PUMC & CAMS, Beijing 100037, China

Objective To summarize single center experience in consecutive 154 heart transplants.

Methods From June 2004 to June 2009 154 patients (147 orthotopic and 7 heterotopic 44.3 ± 14.2 years (range13-72 years, ≤18 years 13 cases, ≥60 years 22 cases),) underwent heart transplantations. Inclusion criteria were cardiomyopathy (67.5%) Ischemic cardiomyopathy (22.9%), and others 9.6%. Twenty-three patients (14.9%) mean left ventricular diastolic diameter were 71.8 ± 13.0 mm mean left ventricular ejection fraction were 27.8 ± 9.4%. The preoperative level of Pro-BNP averaged 2842.7 ± 1535.2 fmol/ml (normal range < 400 fmol/ml). Basiliximab was administered to all recipients as induction agent as an induction agent. Maintenance immunosuppressive regimen consisted of cyclosporine A (CsA)/tacrolimus, mycophenolate mofetil/azathioprine and predisone. Sirolimus was given to renal dysfunction patient and CsA/tacrolimus dose was reduced simutatently to 1/2 - 2/3 original target concentration. EMBs were routinely performed 3w, 3 months, 6 months and 12 months after transplantation. Acute rejection ≥grade II were treated with optimization of immunosuppressant doses. Acute rejection ≥grade III need intravenous methylprednisolone and additional EMBs 2-3 weeks later.

Results Mean follow-up time were 27.8 ± 16.1 (range 0-60) months. 12 patients died, 6 patients died within 3 months, and 6 died late (> 3 months). 2 patients died of acute rejection. The 1-, 2-, 3-, 4-and 5 year survival rates (K-M curves) were 98.6%, 94.5%, 93.4%, 84.8% and 77.7%, respectively. 142 recipients (%) survived with good cardiac condition. The grades of the acute rejection in 482 biopsy specimens were as follow: Grade (G) IIIb in 1 (0.2%) patient, G IIIa in 19 (3.9%) patients, G II in 54 (11.2%) patients, G I + 0 in 409 patients.

Conclusions Endometrial biopsy immunosuppressive regimen and follow-up mode ensures excellent median-term survival rate of heart transplantation

34

Light Preconditioning: a Novel Modality for Enhancing Early Survival of Implanted Bone Marrow Mesenchymal Stem Cells

Hou JF, Zhang H, Yuan X, Wei YJ, Hu SS
Department of Surgery, Research Center for Cardiac Regenerative Medicine, Ministry of Health, Cardiovascular Institute and Fu Wai Hospital, Chinese Academy of Medical Sciences and Peking Union Medical College

Objective Recent years have witnessed a growing interest and enthusiasm in the application of bone-marrow derived stem cell-based therapies to repair or regenerate damaged myocardium. However, progress in stem cell therapy is hampered by the poor survival of implanted cells. We hypothesized that low-level laser irradiation (LLLI) preconditioning prior to bone-marrow mesenchymal stem cells (BMSCs) transplantation might remodel the hostile milieu of infarcted myocardium and subsequently enhance early survival and therapeutic potential of implanted cells.

Methods BMSCs were isolated from male donor rat. Myocardial infarction was induced by left anterior descending artery ligation in female rats. Three weeks later, female rats were randomly divided for LLLI preconditioning study and the following LLLI preconditioning and cell survival study. After chest-opened, a 635 nm, 5 mW diode laser was performed with energy density of 0.96 J/cm^2 for 150 seconds for the purpose of myocardial preconditioning. In LLLI preconditioning study, vascular endothelial growth factor (VEGF), glucose-regulated protein 78 (GRP78), superoxide dismutase (SOD) and malondialdehyde (MDA) in the infarcted myocardium were evaluated at 1 hour, 1 day and 1 week after laser irradiation. In cell survival study, 2 millions male BMSCs or no-serum culture media was injected into infarcted myocardium with or without LLLI preconditioning. Cell survival was assayed with quantitative real-time polymerase chain reaction to identify Y chromosome gene and apoptosis was assayed with TUNEL staining. Capillary density, myogenic differentiation and left ventricular function were tested at 1 week.

Results After LLLI preconditioning, increased VEGF and GRP78 expression, as well as the enhanced SOD activity and inhibited MDA production, was observed.

35

Pulmonary atresia with ventricular septal defect in elder children and adults

Xu JP, Shi Y, Yan J, Wang Q, Luo GH

Chinese Academy of Medical Sciences Fu Wai Hospital Surgical Department, Beijing 100037, China

Abjective One-stage and multistage surgery culminating in completed hemodynamic repair is now performed for pulmonary atresia with ventricular septal defect (PA-VSD). This paper is to evaluate the effects of two surgical approaches.

Methods 39 elder children and adults with PA-VSD in the Fu Wai Hospital Adult Congenital Heart Disease Center Registry from Octomber 1996 through October 2008 formed the basis for this study. Of 39 patients, 23 were corrected by one-stage repair and 16 by staged repair. 3 patients with MAPCAs underwent unifocalization operation and one-stage repair. 3 patients with MAPCAs underwent unifocalization operation and staged repair.

Results For one-stage repair, 4 patients died with a mortality of 17.4%. For staged repair, 2 patients died with a mortality of 12.5%. The results of the follow-up were satisfactory from 17 months to 9.2 years.

Conclusions The precise evaluation of pulmonary and MAPCAs is the pivotal factor to choose the reconstructive procedures. Staged hemodynamic repair can be performed with a low surgical risk in properly selected adults with PA/VSD.

Basic Research

1

Inhibition of Atorvastatin on C-reactive Protein-induced Inflammatory Response in Pulmonary Artery Smooth Muscle Cells by Nuclear Factor-B Pathway

Li J, Li JJ, He JG, Nan JL, Guo YL, Xiong CM
Department of Cardiology, Fu Wai Hospital, Chinese Academy of Medical Sciences, Peking Union Medical College, Beijing 100037, China.

Objective C-reactive protein (CRP) is a well-known marker of inflammation, and has been recognized as a risk predictor of pulmonary arterial disease. Although statins have a beneficial effect in animal models and patients with pulmonary arterial hypertension (PAH), the underlying mechanisms of their action have less been investigated. We, therefore, examined the effects of CRP on the expression of interleukin-6 (IL-6) and monocyte chemoattractant protein-1 (MCP-1), and the possible mechanisms of atorvastatin on CRP-induced IL-6 and MCP-1 production in cultured human pulmonary artery smooth muscle cells (PASMCs).
Methods In a preliminary study, the human PASMCs were stimulated by a varity of concentration of CRP (5-200 μg/ml) at different time points (0, 3, 6, 9, 12, 18 and 24 hours) to determine the dose-and time-dependent effects of CRP on inflammatory response of the cells. Then, the cells were pre-incubated for 2 hours with atorvastatin (0. 1-10 μmol/l) in the presence of CRP. The supernatant levels of IL-6 and MCP-1 secretion were examined by ELISA. The cellular IL-6 and MCP-1 mRNA expression and nuclear factor-κB (NF-κB) activity were determined by real-time reverse transcription and polymerase chain reaction (RT-PCR) and electrophoretic mobility shift assay (EMSA), respectively.
Results CRP induced a dose-and time-dependent IL-6 and MCP-1 secretion and mRNA expression. In addition, CRP also significantly activated the NF-κB pathway. Pre-incubation of 0. 1-10 μmol/l atorvastatin significantly decreased the secretion of IL-6 and MCP-1 induced by CRP, and increased IL-6 and MCP-1 were completely abrogated by 10 μmol/l of atorvastatin by attenuating the activation of NF-κB.
Conclusions The present study demonstrated that inhibited effect of atorvastatin on CRP-induced inflammatory response presented as IL-6 and MCP-1 enhancement in cultured PASMCs was associated with NF-κB pathway. This pathway might represent a promising target for controlling CRP-induced inflammatory response in pulmonary arterial disease.

2

A Proteomic Approach to Investigate Atherosclerotic Plaques from Human Coronary Arteries

Li L, Zhao H, Wang HY
Department of pathology, Cardiovascular Institute and Fu Wai Hospital, Chinese Academy of Medical Sciences, Peking Union Medical College, Beijing 100037, China

Objective To analyze the proteins relating to atherogenesis applying the proteomic approach and clarify the mechanism atherosclerosis.
Methods Coronary arteries were obtained from patients who were undergone the allogenic heart transplantation for coronary artery disease and

primary cardiomyopathy without atherosclerosis (as control group). Proteins were extracted from finely minced specimens (1 atherosclerotic artery and 1 normal artery) and separated by two-dimensional gel electrophoresis. Coomassie Blue-stained gels were analyzed using PD-Quest software.

Results A total of 18 distinct spots corresponding to 10 proteins were identified by matrix assisted laser desorption/ionization mass spectrometry using NCBI database. The expression level for some proteins were down-regulated in atherosclerotic arteries, such as small heat shock protein HSP27, transgelin and profilin, the others were up-regulated, that were nexilin, cyclophilin A and serum albumin precursor compared to normal. The decreased level of transgelin in atherosclerotic artery was further confirmed by immunohistology.

Conclusions Trangelin, profilin and HSP27 were known to play important roles in the dynamics of actin cytoskeleton and maintaining the phenotype differentiation of vascular smooth muscle cells (VSMC). The decreased expressions of them suggested the phenotype modulation of VSMC that may be one of major factors on atherogenesis. Cyclophilin A was a protein secreted by VSMC response to inflammatory stimuli and a chemoattractant for T cells, monocytes and eosinophils, monocytes and neutrophils. This suggested an important role, as a proinflammatory molecule, in the pathogenesis of atherosclerosis. Nexilin was F-actin binding protein, located at cell-matrix adherens junction and might be involved in the linkage between the actin cytoskeleton and cell-matrix adherens junction. Therefore, Nexilin might also be a biomarker for vascular injury. In conclusions, many proteins differentially expressed in atherosclerotic coronary artery are playing important roles in inflammation and phenotypic modulation of smooth muscle. They would be involved in ACS events relating to atherogenesis.

3

Construction and Assessment of Short-hairpin RNA Eukaryotic Expression Vector Targeting TGF-β1 Labeled by GFP

Li N, Han YL, Kang J, Qi YM, Guo L, Yan CH
Department of Cardiology, Shenyang Northern Hospital, Shenyang 110016

Objective To construct short hairpin RNA (shRNA) eukaryotic expression vectors targeting TGF-β1 for further research on the effects of TGF-β1 on vasculogenesis and angiogenesis.

Methods Three pairs of siRNA target sequences coding from the mRNA of TGF-β1 gene provided by GenBank were designed and three pairs of nucleotides were synthesized. After annealing, the double-strand DNA products were ligated into the pEN_mH1c entry vector, and in turn into the shRNA eukaryotic expression vector pDS_hpEy labled by GFP through the LR recombination reaction. The three resulting TGF-β1 shRNA expression vectors were named pDS_Ta, pDS_Tb and pDS_Tc respectively. After sequencing successfully, the vectors were transfected into the mouse fibroblast cell line (NIH/3T3), and then cell clones stably expressing TGF-β1 shRNA were screened. Reverse Transcript-Polymerase Chain Reaction (RT-PCR) and Western Blot were used to detect the mRNA and protein expression.

Results RT-PCR and Western Blot showed that pDS_Tc down regulated TGF-β1 mRNA and protein expression markedly in NIH/3T3 cells.

Conclusions ShRNA eukaryotic expression vectors targeting TGF-β1 were successfully constructed which can be used for further investigation on the mechanism through which TGF-β1 regulates vasculogenesis and angiogenesis.

4

Cyclooxygenase-2 (COX-2) G-765C is a Protective Factor for Coronary Artery Disease but not for Ischemic Stroke: a Meta-Analysis

Li WL
Cardiovascular Institute and Fu Wai Hospital, Chinese Academy of Medical Science and Peking Union Medical College, Beijing 100037, China

Objective Cyclooxygenase (COX) catalyzes the first two steps in prostanoid production. COX-2 is highly expressed in chromic inflammatory diseases including atherosclerosis. Previous case-control studies suggested the variant of COX-2 gene (G-765C) is associated with coronary artery disease (CAD) and ischemic stroke. However, other studies did not confirm this relationship. We assessed the relationship between COX-2 G-765C and diseases such as CAD and ischemic stroke, using a meta-analysis.

Methods Databases, including PubMed, EMbase, CBM and CNKI, were searched to get the genetic association studies. Data were extracted by two authors and pooled odds ratio (OR) with 95% confidence interval (CI) was calculated.
Results The meta-analysis included 4930 CAD patients and 17997 controls, as well as 1628 ischemic stroke patients and 17653 controls. For CAD, the pooled OR of-765C was 0.80 (95% CI: 0.65-0.98) compared with wild type allele in recessive model, and was 0.99 (95% CI: 0.92-1.06) in dominant model. For ischemic stroke, the pooled OR of-765C was 1.11 (95% CI: 0.88-1.42) in recessive model compared with wild type allele, and was 1.05 (95% CI: 0.93-1.18) in dominant model. No publication bias was found in this meta-analysis.
Conclusions The synthesis of available evidence supports that the COX-2-765C is protective for CAD. However, it is not associated with ischemic stroke.

5

Lysophosphatidic Acid Inhibits Hypoxia and Serum Deprivation-induced Apoptosis in Mesenchymal Stem Cells Involving Endoplasmic Reticulum Stress Pathway

Li ZW, Wei H, Cong XF, Chen X
Research Center for Cardiac Regenerative Medicine, the Ministry of Health, Cardiovascular Institute and Fu Wai Hospital, Chinese Academy of Medical Sciences and Peking Union Medical College, Beijing 100037, China.

Objective Previously we demonstrated that hypoxia and serum deprivation (hypoxia/SD) induced MSCs apoptosis through the mitochondrial apoptotic pathway and lysophosphatidic acid (LPA) protected MSCs from mitochondrial dysfunction through activation of ERK and PI3K/Akt pathways. Here, we investigated whether the endoplasmic reticulum (ER) apoptotic pathways were involved in hypoxia/SD-induced apoptosis of MSCs and the inhibitory roles of LPA on these pathways.
Methods MSCs were exposed to hypoxia/SD for 6 hours to reproduce MSCs apoptotic model. The normal control group, the hypoxia/SD apoptotic group and the preincubation with SB202190 (p38 inhibitor), SP600125 (JNK inhibitor) or LPA followed by hypoxia/SD groups were included in the following experiments. Apoptosis of MSCs was detected by Hoechst 33342 staining and Annexin V-FITC flow cytometric analysis. The mitochondrial membrane potential ($\Delta\Psi m$) in MSCs was assessed with flow cytometry after incubating cells with fluorescent probe JC-1. Activation of p38 and JNK, cleavage activation of procaspase-3, translocation of cytochrome c and Bax between mitochondria and cytosol, and ER stress-related procaspase-12 cleavage and CHOP expression were all detected by Western Blot.
Results Cleavage activation of procaspase-12 and CHOP expression, both mediators of ER stress-induced apoptosis, were induced in MSCs during hypoxia/SD treatment. Meanwhile, phosphorylation of p38 also occurred in MSCs, and the inhibition of p38 activation by SB202190 resulted in a dramatic decrease in apoptosis accompanied by partly reversed-decrease of $\Delta\Psi m$ and reduced mitochondrial release of cytochrome c. In addition, inhibition of p38 by SB202190 also suppressed the cleavage of procaspase-12. These results suggest that p38 involves in the activation of both mitochondrial and ER caspase-12 apoptotic pathways. Activation of p38 and its downstream cleavage of procaspase-12 could be also inhibited by LPA. However, unlike p38 inhibitor SB202190 which enhanced hypoxia/SD-induced phosphorylation of JNK and CHOP expression, LPA inhibited both JNK activation and CHOP expression.
Conclusions Our findings suggest that LPA antagonizes hypoxia/SD-induced apoptosis of MSCs at least in part through inhibition of p38-dependent mitochondrial and ER apoptotic pathways as well as inhibition of JNK and CHOP activation, indicating the novel molecular targets by LPA to inhibit hypoxia/SD-induced apoptosis in MSCs.

6

Interactions among Genetic Variants from SREBP2 Activating-Related Pathway on Risk of Coronary Heart Disease in Chinese Han Population

Liu XL, Lu XF, Gu DF
Department of Evidence Based Medicine and Division of Population Genetics, Cardiovascular Institute and Fu Wai Hospital, Peking Union Medical College and Chinese Academy of Medical Sciences, Beijing, China

Objective Sterol regulatory element binding proteins (SREBPs), as a family of membrane-bound transcription factors, control the metabolism of cholesterol and fatty acids. We conducted a case-control study to investigate whether the common variants of genes from the SREBP2 activating-related pathway, involving SREBP2, SCAP, INSIG1 and INSIG2 genes, were associated with coronary heart disease (CHD) of Chinese Han population individually or interactively.

Methods We recruited 853 cases with CHD from patients hospitalized at the Fu Wai Hospital and Cardiovascular Institute (Beijing, China). The 948 controls were judged to be free of ischemic changes by ECG, without symptoms of chest pain and to be free of CHD by medical history, the Rose questionnaire and clinical examination. Three, four and two single nucleotide polymorphisms (SNPs) from the INSIG1, INSIG2 and SCAP genes were chosen as heliotype-tagging SNPs (htSNPs), respectively, and one nonsynonymous coding SNP was selected from SREBP2. The selected SNPs were genotyped using standard polymerase chain reaction and restriction-fragment-length polymorphism methods. The logistic regression model was performed to examine the independent effect of the each polymorphism on CHD. The gene-gene interaction was examined using both the Multifactor Dimensionality Reduction (MDR) program and logistic regression model.

Results The results from MDR indicated that there existed the SNP-SNP interactive effect of INSIG1 gene on CHD (best prediction accuracy = 56.09%, $p = 0.002$ on 1000 permutations). The results from LRM also identified the 2-locus interaction model (adjusted $p \leqslant 0.001$ for interaction) as well as the 3-locus gene-gene interaction (adjusted $p = 0.026$ for interaction). Single polymorphism analysis showed that the rs4822063 of SREBP2 was associated with LDL-C in the controls. The genotype CC carriers had higher LDL-C than the major allele G carriers (3.44 ± 0.90 mmol/L versus 3.17 ± 0.84 mmol/L, adjusted $p = 0.038$).

Conclusions The results suggested that the INSIG1 gene was associated with CHD; there might be potential interactive effect on CHD among genes from SREBP2 activating-related pathway. Further studies are warranted to replicate our results in other people and to elucidate the biological mechanism.

7

The Effects of Combined Amlodipine and Atorvastatin on the Balance of Myocardial MMPs/TIMPs System in SHR

Lu JC, Cui W, Liu DM, Liu F, Yang XH, Xie RQ, Gu GQ
Second Hospital of Hebei Medical University, Shijiazhuang City, Hebei Province Road 215 peace

Objective To explore the effect of amlodipine, atorvastatin, and their combination on the balance of myocardial MMPs/TIMPs system, we investigate the changes of MMP-2, MMP-9 as well as TIMP-1, TIMP-2 expression in SHR.

Methods 36-week-old SHR were randomly allocated into four groups: a vehicle-treated control group; an amlodipine (10 mg/kg/day)-treated group; an atorvastatin (10 mg/kg/day)-treated group; and a group treated with a combination of amlodipine and atorvastatin (both at 10 mg/kg/day). In addition, WKY rat was chose as control group of normal blood pressure. Drugs were administered by oral gavages every morning for a period of 12 weeks before hearts were harvested for analysis. Geltin zemography was used to evaluate the activity of MMP-2 and MMP-9. RT-PCR was used to observe the gene expression of MMP-2, MMP-9 as well as TIMP-1, TIMP-2.

Results Gelatin demography showed the activity of MMP-2, MMP-9 was higher in SHR than that in WKY (each $P < 0.05$). Either amlodipine or atorvastatin lowered the activity of MMP-2 and MMP-9 of SHR (each $P < 0.05$) ; furthermore, combination therapy had the best lowering effect ($P < 0.05$). RT-PCR showed the mRNA expression levels of MMP-2 and MMP-9 in SHR were all obviously increased in contrast to that in WKY (each $P < 0.05$). The mRNA expression levels of MMP-2 and MMP-9 in the amlodipine or atorvastatin administration groups were obviously reduced compared with that in SHR group (each $P < 0.05$). The mRNA expression levels of MMP-2 and MMP-9 in the combined amlodipine and atorvastatin group were even lower than that in the single amlodipine or atorvastatin groups (each $P < 0.05$). The mRNA expression levels of TIMP-1 in SHR were obviously increased in contrast to that of WKY (each $P < 0.05$). Nevertheless, either amlodipine or atorvastatin as well as combination therapy did not alter myocardial TIMP-1 levels in SHR (each $P > 0.05$). The mRNA expression levels of TIMP-2 in SHR were not different from that in WKY (each $P > 0.05$). Either amlodipine or atorvastatin as well as combination therapy did not alter myocardial TIMP-2 levels in SHR (each $P > 0.05$).

Conclusions Both amlodipine and atorvastatin decreased the activity, mRNA?

8

The Effects of Combined Amlodipine and Atorvastatin on Myocardial Proinflammatory Cytokine in SHR

Lu JC, Cui W, Liu F, Liu DM, Xie RQ, Yang XH, Du J
The department of cardiology, the second hospital of Hebei medical university

Objective To explore whether activated proinflammatory cytokine network may play some role in the additive beneficial effects of amlodipine, atorvastatin, and their combination on cardiac hypertrophy, through examining the effects of each drug and co-administration therapy on circulatory levels of hs-CRP, TNF-α, IL-1β, and the protein expressions of myocardial TNF-α, IL-1β in SHR.

Methods 36-week-old SHR were randomly allocated into four groups: a vehicle-treated control group; an amlodipine (10 mg/kg/day)-treated group; an atorvastatin (10 mg/kg/day)-treated group; and a group treated with a combination of amlodipine and atorvastatin (both at 10 mg/kg/day). In addition, WKY rat was chose as control group of normal blood pressure. Drugs were administered by oral gavages every morning for a period of 12 weeks before hearts were harvested for analysis. Left ventricular mass index (LVMI) was assessed by morphology measurement. The levels of serum hs-CRP were detected with ELISA. The serums TNF-α, IL-1β were detected by radioimmunity assay (RIA). Cardiac inflammatory cell infiltration was observed by HE staining. The protein expressions of TNF-α, IL-1β were detected with Western blot technique.

Results LVMI and cardiac inflammatory cell infiltration in SHR was higher than that in WKY rat. Treatment with amlodipine or atorvastatin alone significantly decreased LVMI and inhibited local inflammatory cell infiltration in cardiac tissue, and combination therapy inhibits further compared with each monotherapy. The serum levels of hs-CRP, TNF-α, IL-1β were significantly higher in SHR control group than that of WKY control group (each $P<0.05$). The serum levels of hs-CRP and TNF-α in the amlodipine or atorvastatin administration group were significantly dropped compared with SHR control group (each $P<0.05$), and those in the combined drug group were even dropped down further than that of the single drug group ($P<0.05$). Both amlodipine and atorvastatin slightly but not significantly decreased serum IL-1β concentration (each $P>0.05$), and combination therapy significantly decreased serum IL-1β concentration compared with SHR control group ($P<0.05$). Compared with that of same aged WKY, the protein expressions of TNF-α, IL-1β were proved to be enhanced in SHR control group by western blot (each $P<0.05$). Furthermore, all the proteins were reduced markedly after amlodipine or atorvastatin intervention (each $P<0.05$), and that of the combined drug group was even lower than that of the single drug groups (each $P<0.05$).

Conclusions By way of down regulation for systemic inflammation and myocardial TNF-α, IL-1β, amlodipine and atorvastatin may obviously reverse cardiac hypertrophy. Amlodipine combined with atorvastatin may have additive effects on inhibition of myocardial inflammatory response.

9

In Vivo Detection of Bone Marrow Mesenchymal Stem Cells (MSCs) after Intracoronary Infusion Using Magnetic Resonance Imaging: An Experimental Study of a Novel Method to Trace the Transplanted Cells

Lu MJ, Zhao SH, Song P, Jiang SL, Liu YQ
Cardiovascular Institute and Fu Wai Hospital, PUMC & CAMS, Beijing 100037, China

Objective This study was designed to use MRI to observe the cell distribution after intracoronary infusion (ICI) in variations of heart status in a swine myocardial infarction model.

Methods Twenty-four Chinese mini-pigs were divided into 4 groups ($n=6$). After inducing a myocardial infarction, iron oxide labeled male cells (1×108) were infused through the coronary artery of the beating swine heart in Group 1. In Group 2, cardiopulmonary bypass (CPB) was set up and then the same volume of cells was infused after cardiologic arrest. In Groups 3 and 4, the animals underwent either beating or arrested ICI with the same volume of saline. Three days later, cell distribution was assessed by T2 * change with magnetic resonance imaging and

Results T2 * change of the heart in the cell infusion groups was significantly higher than that of saline infusion groups. However, in the MRI visualization of myocardium with a short axis slice of mid-left ventricular, signal void corresponding to the ventricular septum between Groups 1 and 2 were not visible. Group 1 had less T2 * change than Group 2 in the spleen (16.72 ± 2.83 versus 22.18 ± 3.98, $P<0.05$) and liver (2.4 ± 0.44 versus 5.32 ± 3.40, $P<0.05$). However, there was no statistical significance of T2 * change between two groups in the kidney.

Conclusions The majority of BMSCs transplanted by ICI would be entrapped by the extracardial organs. The arrested heart with CPB during ICI does not favor more cell retention in the injured myocardium. The optimal approach of delivery of BMSCs still needs further investigation. Qualitative and quantitative in vivo cell-tracking and monitoring of organ distribution of intracoronary infusion of MSC (SPIO labeled) in AMI is feasible in MRI.

10

The 11-15 Domain of M6P/IGF2R Mediate the Bio-function of Recombinant Human CREG Protein to VSMC

Luan B, Han YL, Guo P, Yan CH, Guo L, Kang J
Department of Cardiology, Shenyang Northern Hospital, Shenyang 110016

Objective Our earlystudyhad suggested the transmembrane insulin-like growth factor II receptor (M6P/IGF2R) might take part in the CREG protein regulating VSMC in This study, we will analyse the bio-function of CREG glycoprotein and the role of every domain of M6P/IGF2R.
Methods 1. The eukaryotic expression vectors, pcDNA3. 1 myc-His/wt/mCREG, were constructed. The recombinant wt/mCREG protein was purified with Ni-NTA column according to 6 × His affinity chromatographic theory. The protein were analyzed by PNGaseF digestion and Western blot. 2. The effect of recombinant wt/mCREG protein on VSMC proliferation, migration and differentiation were studied. To analyze if wt/myCREG protein bind directly to M6P/IGF2R, M6P/IGF2R anti-body blocking test, double immunofluorescence staining and co-immunoprecipitation method were used. 3. The domains protein was gained by Ni-NTA affinity chromatography and purified. The affinity of wt/mCREG to M6P/IGF2R domains was analyzed. The competitive binding test was used to identify the direct binding of CREG to IGF2R domains.
Results 1. The recombinant wtCREG protein was identified as a glycoprotein because the molecular weight of fusion protein decreased from 30KD to 25KD after PNGaseF digestion. The recombinant mCREG protein was unglycosited because the molecular weight of fusion protein unchanged after PNGaseF digestion. 2. The wt/mCREG protein depressed the proliferation, migration, excreting the extro-cell material and promote differentiation of VSMC. The biologic power of wtCREG is stronger than that of mCREG. The wt/mCREG protein binded directly to M6P/IGF2R. 3. The wtCREG protein had high affinity to 7-10 domain and 11-15 domain M6P/IGF2R. Whereas, the mCREG protein had high affinity to 11-15 domain. M6P blocked the binding of wtCREG to 7-10 domain. The 11-15 domain protein blocked the bio-function of wt/mCREG to VSMC. THE 7-10 domain protein blocked only the bio-function of wtCREG.
Conclusions The bio-function of wt/mCREG protein to VSMC was mediated by M6P/IGF2R which is independent on glycosides. The glycosides may strengthen the function of CREG protein. The 11-15 domain of M6P/IGF2R is the functional domain of CREG protein.

11

A Functional Variant of Nedd4l Is Associated With Hypertension, Antihypertensive Response and Orthostatic Hypotension

Luo F, Wang YB, Wang XJ, Sun K, Zhou XL, Hui RT
Cardiovascular Institute and Fu Wai Hospital, Beijing 100037, China

NEDD4L is involved in the regulation of plasma volume and blood pressure by controlling cell surface expression of the kidney epithelial Na^+ channel. Previously, the cryptic splice variant rs4149601 (G/A) an allele of NEDD4L, generating isoform I, was estimated to decrease blood pressure by down regulating Na^+ reabsorption. However, a recent functional study showed that isoform I should lead to abnormal Na^+ reabsorption increases by antagonistically down regulating ENaC activities. To determine whether the variant rs4149601 A allele is a risk factor for hypertension, has an impact on the antihypertensive response to hydrochlorothiazide and is associated with orthostatic hypotension, we performed a case-control study of hypertension (n = 1686), a 4-week clinical trial (n = 542) and a case-control study of orthostatic hypotension (n = 793) in Chinese, respectively. We found that the allele was significantly associated with hypertension after appropriate adjustment (OR, 1. 39; 95% CI, 1. 13 - 1. 72; P = 0. 002). The blood pressure reduction in A carriers after hydrochlorothiazide treatment was greater than that in GG carriers, with differences of 6. 1 mmHg (P = 0. 009) in SBP and 2. 7 mmHg (P = 0. 027) in DBP. The allele was significantly associated with orthostatic hypotension after adjustment for cardiovascular risk factors (OR, 0. 68; 95% CI, 0. 48 - 0. 98; P = 0. 039). In conclusions, rs4149601 is a genetic risk factor for hypertension, a protective factor against orthostatic hypotension in hypertensive subjects, and the antihypertensive response to hydrochlorothiazide is more sensitive in an allele carrier than in GG carriers. Consequently, the A allele may be a useful marker for predicting hypertension,

12

The Impact of Chronic Intermittent Hypoxia on Cardiac Function in Rats

Luo Q, Liu ZH, Zhao ZH
Cardiovascular Institute and Fu Wai Hospital, PUMC & CAMS, Beijing 100037, China

Objective Sleep apnea is associated with congestive heart failure. The aim of this study is to investigate the impact of chronic intermittent hypoxia (CIH) on left ventricular function in rats.
Methods Twenty adult male Sprague-Dawley rats (body weight about 200 g) were randomly divided into experimental (CIH) and normal controls (NC). During daylight hours, the O2 concentration was decreased to 6 ~ 7% every 60 seconds (CIH) or was left unchanged (NC). Exposure was performed 8 hours/day for 5 weeks. Animals were weighed weekly. At the end of the exposure, systolic arterial blood pressure and heart rate were measured by tail cuff plethysmograph. At last, animals were anesthetized for echocardiography and cardiac catheterization.
Results At the end of the 5-weeks exposure, there were no differences in weight between the groups. Blood pressure was greater in CIH than in NC (122.3 ± 4.1 mmHg vs. 136.3 ± 6.8 mmHg, $P < 0.001$). LV weight/body weight was greater in CIH than in NC (3.04 ± 0.24% vs. 2.82 ± 0.21%, $P < 0.001$). Left ventricular ejection fraction measured by echocardiogram was lower in CIH than in NC (73.0 ± 5.6% vs. 86.0 ± 4.3%, $P < 0.001$), and left ventricular fractional shortening decreased in CIH group (37.5 ± 4.5% vs. 50.6 ± 5.2, $P < 0.001$). Mean arterial pressure by cardiac catheterization was greater in CIH than in NC (86.7 ± 4.7 mmHg vs. 80.7 ± 3.2 mmHg, $P = 0.013$). Compared with the NC group, left ventricular end-diastolic pressure was higher (6.2 ± 3.0 mmHg vs. 13.6 ± 1.0 mmHg, $P < 0.001$), and the maximal rates of left ventricular pressure in systole and diastole were lower in CIH. There were no significant differences in heart rate between the groups (380.2 ± 39.8 beat per minute vs. 382.3 ± 45.4 beat per minute, $P = 0.524$).
Conclusions Chronic intermittent hypoxia may lead to left ventricular myocardial dysfunction.

13

Association of Interleukin-18 Gene Promoter Polymorphisms with Risk of Acute Myocardial Infarction in the Northern Chinese Han Population

Pei F, Han YL, Zhang XL, Yan CH, Kang J
Department of Cardiology, Shenyang Northern Hospital, Shenyang 110016

Objective IL-18 plays an important role in the pathogenesis of acute myocardial infarction (AMI). Variations in the DNA sequence in the IL-18 gene promoter may influence IL-18 production and/or activity, and so this can modulate an individual's susceptibility to AMI. To test this hypothesis, we investigated the relationship of IL-18 gene promoter-607C/and-137 G/C polymorphisms and their heliotypes with the risk of AMI in northern Chinese Han population.
Methods We performed a case-control study including 244 patients who survived an AMI and 220 age-and sex-matched controls. Using sequence specific primer-polymerase chain reaction (PCR-SSP), the-607C/and-137 G/C polymorphisms were identified.
Results Two polymorphisms, -607C/A and-137G/C, were in linkage disequilibrium (LD). Significant differences were observed in the genotype and allele distribution of-607C/a polymorphism of the IL-18 gene among cases and controls. The-607CC genotype and the C allele at position-607 in the promoter region of the IL-18 in AMI were significantly higher than those in the controls (OR = 2.100, 95% CI 1.376-3.206, $P < 0.001$ and OR = 1.659, 95% CI 1.280-2.151, $P < 0.001$, respectively), while the-607AA genotype in AMI was markedly lower than that in controls (OR = 0.557, 95% CI 0.362-0.855, $P = 0.009$). After adjustment for conventional risk factors, multivariate logistic regression analysis showed that the C allele carrier (CC + CA) of-607C/A was an independent risk factor for AMI (OR = 1.666, 95% CI 1.064-2.609, $P = 0.026$). Consistent with the genotyping analyze results, the-607C/-137G heliotype conferred an increased risk of AMI (53.2% vs. 42.7%, OR = 1.522, 95% CI 1.174-1.973, $P = 0.001$).

Conclusions This study shows for the first time that the IL-18 gene promoter-607C/a polymorphism may be considered as a genetic risk factor for AMI in the northern Chinese Han population.

14

Association of IL-17F His161Arg Polymorphism with Risk of Acute Myocardial Infarction in the Northern Chinese Han Population

Pei F, Han YL, Zhang XL, Yan CH, Kang J
Department of Cardiology, Shenyang Northern Hospital, Shenyang 110016

Objective There is growing evidence that coronary atherosclerosis and its most severe phenotype, myocardial infarction (MI), are chronic inflammatory diseases. Interleukins (ILs) are important mediators and modulators of inflammation. The His161Arg polymorphism in the gene encoding of IL-17F has recently been consistently found to be associated with chronic inflammatory disorders. In this study, we explore the hypothesis that the variant also affects the risk of MI.
Methods We conducted a case – control association study on a cohort of 513 unrelated MI patients and 477 age-and sex-matched control subjects in a Chinese Han population.
Results Differences in the genotype distributions and allele frequencies of this polymorphism between cases and controls were insignificant ($P = 0.38$ and 0.57, respectively). Further stratification for age, gender, the number of diseased coronary arteries and other cardiovascular risk factors did not affect the negative findings.
Conclusions This study indicates for the first time that unlike other chronic inflammatory diseases, the IL-17F His161Arg polymorphism is unlikely to be a major contributor to the pathogenesis of MI.

15

Salvianolic Acid B blocks the Transient Outward Potassium Current in Isolated Ventricular Myocytes of Rat

Ran YQ, Li N, Wang RR, Wang HT, Wu YL, Pu JL
Center for Cardiac Arrhythmia, Fu Wai Hospital, Chinese Academy of Medical Science and Peking Union Medical College, Beijing 100037, China.
Hebei Yiling Pharmaceutical Research Institute, Shijiazhuang 050035, China.

Objective To investigate the effects of Salvianolic acid B, an aqueous component of Danshen (Salvia miltiorrhiza), on transient outward potassium current (Ito) in rat ventricular myocytes.
Methods Ventricular myocytes were isolated from male Sprague-Dawley rats using enzymatic dissociation method. Whole cell patch-clamp technique was used to detect the Ito in ventricular myocytes. Solution of Salvianolic acid B with a concentration of 100 μM was added into the suspension of myocytes.
Results Using the standard protocol for recording Ito, we recorded the Ito presented as an outward peak current, which was the fast competent of Ito (Itof); and a maintained current, which was the slow component of Ito (Itos). At the concentration of 100 μM, Salvianolic acid B blocked the peak current of Ito and shifted down the current-voltage curve from membrane voltage-20 mV to 60 mV. At membrane voltage 30 mV, the drug decreased the peak Ito from 12.38 ± 3.06 (pA/pF) to 9.11 ± 2.22 (pA/pF), with a decrease rate of $25.91\% \pm 10.52\%$ ($n = 8$, $P < 0.05$). Moreover, Salvianolic acid B reduced Itof but had little effect on Itos. When subtracted the Itos, Salvianolic acid B blocked Itof more significantly. The peak current of Itof was decreased from 9.55 ± 3.29 (pA/pF) to 6.36 ± 2.36 (pA/pF) at the membrane voltage 30mV, with a decrease rate of $33.17\% \pm 11.7\%$ ($n = 8$, $P < 0.05$).
Conclusions Salvianolic acid B blocks Ito channels, mainly blocking the fast component of Ito.

16

Phenotype Alterations of Rat Peripheral Blood Mononuclear Cells during the Differentiation into Endothelial Cells

Sun L, Chi YF, Hou WM, Sun ZD, Niu ZZ, Sun Y, Sheng W
Qingdao Municipal Hospital, Qingdao cardiac surgery on the 5th Middle East China Sea

Objective To study the changes of stem cell markers and endothelial cell phenotype during the differentiation of rat peripheral blood mononuclear cells into endothelial cells.

Methods Mononuclear cells were in vitro cultured in fibronectin culture medium and induced by vascular endothelial growth factors (VEGF) and basic fibroblast growth factors (bFGF) in order to stimulate a differentiation into endothelial cells.

Results The expressions of CD31, CD34, Flk-1, vWF on adherent cells were different in different time durations. The expressions of CD31 and CD34 started on the 2nd day of culture, reached the peak on the 4th day, gradually decreased and even disappeared on the 6th day. While, Flk-1 expressed on the 3rd day of culture, gradually increased, and reached at the peak on the 7th day. vWF expressed gradually until 100% on the 7th day.

Conclusions The differentiation of peripheral blood stem cells into endothelial progenitor cells is characterized by the appearance of endothelial cell phenotypes and the disappearance of stem cell markers, both in the manner of gradual progression.

17

Protective Effects Of Relation of Heat Shock Protein 70 to Immature Cardio protection Induced by Norepinephrine

Sun ZD, Gao SZ, Mao ZF, Wang ZW, Wu ZY
Department of Cardiovascular Surgery, Qingdao municipal Hospital, Medical College of Qingdao University, Qingdao 266011

Objective To investigate the protective effects of heat shock protein 70 (HSP70) for immature myocardium.

Methods Thirty rabbits (aged 14-21 days) were randomly divided into 5 groups. Control group (C) was underwent isolated working rabbit heart model at 24 h after distilled water was injected intreaperitoneally. E4h group, E12h group, E24h group and E48h group were also underwent isolated working rabbit heart model at 4 h, 12 h, 24 h, 48 h after norepinephrine was injected intreaperitoneally respectively. The HSP70 level, lactate dehydrogenase (LDH) and creatine kinase (CK) leakage, adenosine triphosp hate (ATP) and malondialdehyde (MDA) level, superoxide dismutase (SOD) activity, hydroxyproline (HP) and endothelin (ET) level myocardial cell Ca^{2+} content, Ca^{2+}-ATPase activity of mitochondria ([Ca^{2+}-ATPase]m) and itsCa^{2+} levelt ([Ca^{2+}]m), synthesizing ATP activity of mitochondria ([ATP]m) and myocardial ultratructure were tested.

Results The cardiac function recovery was better in E24h group than that of other groups ($P < 0.05$). The HSP70 content, ATP content (11.64 ± 1.87), SOD activity (235.83 ± 12.30), HP (6.45 ± 1.53), [Ca^{2+}-ATPase] m activity (18.46 ± 1.95) and [ATP] m activity (106.26 ± 9.42) in E24h group were higher than that of other groups ($P < 0.01$). The MWC (72.48 ± 1.36), LDH (37.28 ± 3.26) and CK leakage (57.38 ± 4.75), MDA content (1.17 ± 0.12), ET (76.84 ± 10.37), myocardial cell Ca^{2+} content (2.54 ± 0.34) and [Ca^{2+}]m content (38.37 ± 3.61) in E24h group were lower than that of other groups ($P < 0.01$). The myocardial ultra structure injuries in E24h group were less than that of other groups.

This study demonstrates that HSP70 is related to immature cardioprotection by norepinephrine.

18

The Expression of Connexin43 in Rats with Pulmonary Arterial Hypertension Induced by Monocrotaline and the Effect of Treatment with Bosentan

Tan XY, He JG
Department of Internal Medicine, Cardiovascular Institute and Fu Wai Hospital, Chinese Academy of Medical Sciences and Peking Union Medical College, 167 Beilishi Rd, Beijing 100037, China.

Objective It is critical for the development of effective treatments to understand the mechanism of pathogenesis of pulmonary arterial hypertension (PAH). We explored the role of connexin43 (Cx43) in the pathogenesis of PAH in a rat model.
Methods Two weeks after rats were injected with saline or 60 mg/kg monocrotaline (MCT), they received vehicle or 300 mg/kg/day of a dual endothelin (ET) receptor antagonist (bosentan) which was gavaged once daily for 3 weeks. The rats were divided into three groups, control (n = 10), MCT (n = 35), and MCT + bosentan (n = 22). Then we used immunofluorescence to investigate the changes of Cx43 and Cx37 expression in the smooth muscle and endothelial cells of the small pulmonary artery.
Results Comparing with the control group, mean pulmonary arterial pressure and the percent medial wall thickness (% WT) of small pulmonary arteries were markedly increased in the MCT group, and they were significantly decreased by the subsequent treatment with bosentan. The Cx43 expression was not detected in the endothelial cells of small pulmonary artery of the control rats, but was significantly high in the MCT and MCT + bosentan treated rats. The expression of Cx43 was significantly lower in the MCT + bosentan treated rats than those in the MCT treated rats. The Cx37 expression was detected in the endothelial cells of all three groups of rats, and there was no significant difference among them.
Conclusions The highly expression of Cx43 in endothelial cells of small pulmonary artery might be associated with the occurrence of PAH. One of the probable mechanisms of the protection of bosentan could be the inhibition of Cx43 expression in the endothelial cells of small pulmonary artery.

19

The Effects of Cellular Repressor Of E1A-Stimulated Genes on Human Vascular Endothelial Proliferation and Migration

Tao J, Han Y, Yan CH, Guo P, Luan B, Wu GZ, Wang ZS
Department of Cardiology, Northern Hospital, Shenyang 110016, China

Objective We has identified that cellular repressor of E1A-stimulated genes (CREG) can promote differentiation of human vascular smooth muscle cells (VSMCs) and inhibit their proliferation and apoptosis in vitro. These findings suggested that CREG is an important endogenous factor in regulating VSMCs homeostasis. Although CREG has been extensively investigated in VSMCs, roles of CREG in regulating function of arterial endothelial cells (ECs) remain unclear. The aim of this study was to investigate the effects of CREG on ECs migration and proliferation.
Methods (1) Phoenix 293 cells were transected with sense-CREG retroviral vector (pLNCX-CREG), RNA interference CREG retroviral vector (pLNCX-shRNA-CREG) or green fluorescent protein (GFP) expressing control retroviral vector (pLNCX-GFP) by liposome method respectively. Then ECs were infected with packaged viruses collected from transfected phoenix 293 cells. Single ECs clones stably infected with different viruses were selected with corresponding antibiotics (G418 or puromycin). (2) Antibiotic genes expression was detected through RT-PCR and CREG expression of ECs before or after its being infected by retrovirus was detected Western blot. (3) Effects of CREG on ECs migration were investigated by scrape injury analysis and Transwell migration model. Zymography was performed to investigate the change of gelatinases. (4) Cell counting and flow cytometry were performed to detect the ECs proliferation in different groups.
Results (1) three kinds of retroviruses, packaged by phoenix 293 cells transfected with pLNCX-GFP, pLNCX-CREG and PLXSN-shRNA-CREG vectors, were used to infect ECs and after selection with G418 or puromycin, single cell clones were picked up and replanted for amplification. The ECs with GFP expression, CREG over expression or suppression were obtained. (2) The transected ECs clone transcript G418 or puromycin resistance genes respectively, which were identified by RT-PCR assay. Western blot analysis showed that CREG expression in-

creased in ECs infected by pLNCX-CREG retrovirus, decreased obviously in ECs infected by pLNCX-shRNA-CREG retrovirus compared to normal group. (3) Overexpression of CREG promoted ECs migration. a. The scrape injury assay and Tran swell migration model suggested that CREG over expression enhanced but its suppression attenuated migration of ECs compared to the normal and GFP expression control groups. b. Gelatin zymography indicated that expression of gelatin rose in CREG over expression ECs compared to CREG suppression ECs, but it made no statistics difference in comparison with normal and GFP expression groups. (4) The cell count and Flow cytometry assay results showed that proliferation of ECs was enhanced in CREG over expression group and attenuated in the CREG suppression group.

Conclusions Over expression of CREG can promote the migration and proliferation of ECs in vitro. Our study showed that CREG facilitates migration and proliferation of ECs and contributes to the maintenance of vascular homeostasis. This may provide a promising approach for the prevention and treatment of ISR and late stent thrombosis after PCI.

20

Identification and Function Assessment of Smooth Muscle Cells Derived from Mouse Embryonic Stem Cells

Tian XX, Han YL, Kang J, Yan CH, Qi YM, Li N, Tao J, Wu GZ
Department of Cardiology, Shenyang Northern Hospital, Shenyang 110016

Objective To investigate the phenotype and function of ESCs derived SMCs.

Methods ①Induced differentiation and selection: Embryoid bodies were made from SPIE-ESCs and cultured suspended for 5 days. On day 6 embryonic bodies were attached to plates. On day 7 all-trans retinoic acid (10-8 mol/L) was used to induce differentiation for 4 days. On day 11 we observed the differentiation character under fluorescence scope and performed puromycin (10 μg/mL) selection for 2 days; ②Phenotype identification: Selected SMCs' morphology was observed. Immunofluorescence Staining and Western Blotting of SM α-actin, SM22α, SM-MHC were made; ③Contractility: Carbachol (10-5 mol/L) treatment of selected SMCs for 30 min; ④In vitro vasculogenesis: Selected SMCs was mixed with equal amount of endothelial cells and then cultured on Matrigel to observe the recruitment of SMCs to endothelial lumen like structure.

Results ①Differentiated SMCs lay in periphery of embryoid body; ②Selected SMCs were positive for SM α-actin, SM22α, SM-MHC staining. The expression level of SM α-actin, SM22α was comparable to rat primary aortic SMCs, except that SM-MHC expression level was low; ③Selected SMCs showed contractility stimulated by Carbachol; ④Selected SMCs were recruited to endothelial lumen like structure.

Conclusions SMCs derived from ESCs are similar to mature SMCs in phenotype and function. With conquer of ethical and immunorejective issues in their clinical application, these cells may serve as promising seeding cells for tissue-engineered blood vessels.

21

Construction and Expression in Mouse Embryonic Stem cells of Vector SM22α-PAC-IRES2-EGFP used for Purification of Smooth Muscle Cells

Tian XX, Han YL, Kang J, Yan CH, Qi YM, Li N, Tao J, Wu GZ
Department of Cardiology, General Hospital of Shenyang Military Region, Shenyang 110016

Objective To construct a double expression vector of puromycin resistance (Pac) gene and enhanced green fluorescence protein (EGFP) gene driven by smooth muscle specific SM22α promoter (pSM22α-PAC-IRES2-EGFP), paving the way for further purification of ESCs derived SMCs.

Methods SM22α promoter was cloned from pSM22α-EGFP by PCR. CMV promoter of pIRES2-EGFP vector was replaced by SM22 promoter to establish pSM22α-IRES2-EGFP. Pac gene, excised from pSM2C by HindIII/ClaI digestion, was subcloned into pSuper. basic to establish pSuper-PAC. After BglII/AccI enzyme digestion of pSuper-PAC, pac gene fragment was obtained, which was further subcloned into pSM22α-IRES2-EGFP to produce pSM22α-PAC-IRES2-EGFP. ESCs were transfected with pSM22α-PAC-IRES2-EGFP using lipofectamine. Positive clones were selected by G418 and induced to differentiate and further indentified by amplification of pac gene by RT-PCR. Differentiated cells were immunostained by SM α-actin, and expression of SM α-actin and EGFP was observed at the same time under fluorescence microscope.

Results Sequencing results showed that pSM22α-PAC-IRES2-EGFP vector was successfully constructed. Amplification of pac gene identified 4

ESCs clones successfully transfected. After induction of differentiation, partial portion of differentiated cells expressed EGFP, accompanied by positively stained by SM α-acting antibody.

Conclusions PSM22α-PAC-IRES2-EGFP vector was successfully constructed. ESCs clones transected with this vector expressed Pac gene and EGFP gene, and the expression of EGFP is smooth muscle specific.

22

Functional Analysis of the C-reactive protein (CRP)-Gene 717A > G Polymorphism Associated with Coronary Heart Disease

Wang LY, Lu XF, Li HF, Chen SF, Gu DF

Department of Evidence Based Medicine and Division of Population Genetics, Cardiovascular Institute and Fu Wai Hospital, Chinese Academy of Medical Sciences and Peking Union Medical College, Beijing, China

National Human Genome Center at Beijing, Beijing, China

Objective Atherosclerosis underlies the major pathophysiological mechanisms of coronary heart disease (CHD), and inflammation contributes to all phases of atherosclerosis. C-reactive protein (CRP), a sensitive, but nonspecific marker of inflammation has been shown to play proatherogenic roles in the process of atherosclerosis. Our previous report showed that rs2794521 (-717A > G), located in the promoter of the CRP gene, was independently associated with CHD in Chinese subjects. In the present study, we tried to investigate the biological significance of this genetic variation in vitro.

Methods The influence of G to A substitution at the site of rs2794521 on the transcriptional activity of the promoter of the CRP gene was assessed by luciferase reporter assay. The protein binding to the site of rs2794521 was detected by EMSA assay.

Results The G to A exchange at the site of rs2794521 resulted in an increased transcriptional activity of the promoter of CRP gene, and glucocorticoid receptor (GR) protein factor bound drastically differently to the A and G alleles at the site of rs2794521.

Conclusions These results provided functional evidence supporting the association of the SNP rs2794521 of the CRP gene with CHD probably through regulating the expression level of CRP by different variations of rs2794521.

23

Promotion of Bone Marrow Stem Cells Angiogenesis by Ginsenoside Rg1 after Myocardial Infarction in Rabbits

Ning Y, Wang NY

Beijing Hospital of Integrated Traditional and Western Medicine, Beijing, China

Objective To investigate the effects of ginsenoside Rg1 X on the heart function and the size of myocardial infarct in Japan white rabbits with myocardial infarction (MI).

Methods In rabbits (control group n = 10; Rg1 group n = 8), the bone marrow mononuclear cells (BM-MNC) were extracted from the hip bone marrow with ficoll, labeled with 1. 1'-dioctadecyl-1 to3, 3, 3', 3'-tetramethylindocyanine perchlorate (DiI) and reinjected into the hip bone cavities. One day later, MI was induced by 30-min ischemia followed by 14 day reperfusion of the coronary artery. Saline or 10 mg/kg/d of ginsenoside Rg1 was injected from 1 to 5 days after MI. The left ventricular function and infarct size in 1 week and 2 weeks after infarction were measured. The DiI (a bone marrow mononuclear cell marker) positive cells and CD31 (a endothelial cell marker) positive cells were detected by confocal microscopy. Peripheral EPCs number and measure blood NOx were measured. In other group myocardial interstitial G-CSF levels during ischemia and reperfusion were measured.

Results Rg1 significantly reduced the infarct size (control group: Rg1 group = 18. 5 ± 2. 2 : 11. 8 ± 1. 9, %, $p < 0.05$) and improved cardiac function (EF control group: Rg1 group = 50. 0 ± 5. 8 : 69. 2 ± 9. 0, %, $p < 0.01$). Rg1 raised the peripheral EPCs number (control group : Rg1 group = 0. 34 ± 0. 08 : 0. 75 ± 0. 10, %, $p < 0.05$) and the NOx concentrations (control group: Rg1 group = 21. 8 ± 1. 34 : 28. 2 ± 2. 1, μmol/l, $p < 0.05$) of serum. Rg1 significantly increased the level of myocardial interstitial G-CSF during ischemia (control group: Rg1 group = 22. 3 ± 1. 9 : 28. 6 ± 2. 3, ng/ml, $p < 0.01$) and reperfusion (control group : Rg1 group = 22. 1 ± 1. 6 ng/ml : 29. 5 ± 2. 8, ng/ml, $p < 0.01$). Confocal microscopy revealed that significant increases of endothelial cells with positive DiI (control group : Rg1 group = 4. 4 ± 0. 6 :

6.7 ± 0.8, %, $p < 0.05$) and capillary density (control group : Rg1 group = 1050 ± 71.7 : 1359.8 ± 86.6, /mm2, $p < 0.05$) in Rg1, suggesting enhanced angiogenesis by Rg1.

Conclusions Ginsenoside Rg1 reduced the area of myocardial infarction and improved cardiac function of rabbit model with myocardial infarction. it is supposed that, Rg1 multiplies EPCs of peripheral blood, promotes its release of NO and stimulates the secretion of G-CSF of cardiac muscle tissue.

24

Effect of Local Injection Of Ginsenoside Rg1 On Angiogenesis of Japanese White Rabbits with Ischemic Lower Limbs

Ning Y, Wang NY
Beijing Hospital of Integrated Traditional and Western Medicine, Beijing, China

Objective To observe the effect of local injection of Rg1 on angiogenesis of ischemic lower limbs in rabbits,

Methods Ischemic lower limbs were induced byligating right femoral artery of rabbits. Rabbits were randomly divided into control group ($n = 8$) and Rg1 treatment group ($n = 8$). The CD31 (an endothelial cell marker) positive cells were investigated by confocal microscopy, serum NOx and interleukin-1-β levels were measured by ELISA.

Results Rg1 alleviated ischemic symptoms of lower limbs, and increased capillary density significantly (control group vs. Rg1 group = 257.5 ± 46.2 mm2 vs. 603.8 ± 81.7 mm2, $P < 0.01$), serum concentration of Nox (control group vs. Rg1 group = 20.4 ± 2.3 μmol/l vs. 27.3 ± 2.2 μmol/l, $P < 0.05$) and interleukin-1-β (control group vs. Rg1 group = 0.135 ± 0.043 pg/ml vs. 0.331 ± 0.033 pg/ml, $P < 0.05$).

Conclusions Rg1 increased local capillary angiogenesis and alleviated ischemic symptoms of ischemic lower limbs of Japanese white rabbits, and its mechanism might be related to up-regulation of serum NO and interleukin-1 concentration.

25

Association of Rs3753921 Polymorphism of the CREG Gene And Coronary Artery Disease in the Han Population of North China

Wang T, Han YL, Zhang XL, Yan CH, Kang J
Department of Cardiology, Shenyang Northern Hospital, Shenyang 110016

Objective The purpose of the present study was to assess the possible association between cellular repressor of E1A-stimulated genes (CREG) and coronary artery disease (CAD) in the Han population of North China.

Methods A case-control study was conducted in 338 patients with angiographically documented CAD and 287 control subjects free from CAD who had normal coronary angiograms. The rs3753921 single nucleotide polymorphism was selected and genotyped.

Results The genotype frequencies of TT, CT and CCof rs3753921 polymorphism were 65.7%, 30.2% and 4.1% in CAD patients, 59.2%, 35.5% and 5.2% in the controls respectively ($P = 0.248$). The frequencies of C allele in cases and controls were 19.2%, 23.0%, respectively ($P = 0.103$). Subsequent stratified analysis by gender and age also showed no statistical significance in the genotype frequencies and allele frequencies between the two groups.

Conclusions The result suggests that rs3753921 polymorphism of the CREG gene might not be associated with CAD in the Han population of North China.

26

H2O2 Induced Apoptosis of Rat Mesenchymal Stem Cells Through Both ER Stress and A Mitochondrial Death Pathway

Wei H, Li ZU, Chen X, Cong XF
Cardiovascular Institute and Fu Wai Hospital, 167 Beilishilu, Beijing 100037

Objective Low viability of mesenchymal stem cells (MSCs) transplanted into infarcted heart is a limit for the improvement of heart function and neovascularization after myocardial infarction. Sustained oxidative stress in infarcted heart resulted from the increase of reactive oxygen species (ROS) might be an important factor to induce apoptosis of MSCs. In order to establish the base for screening bioactive molecule or drug to prevent apoptosis, a in vitro model of oxidative stress was established to mimic the environment And the effect, and the mechanism of H2O2 on MSC apoptosis were studied.
Methods Rat MSCs treated with various concentration of H2O2 were stained with Hoechst33342 or evaluated by flow cytometric analysis of cell apoptosis. The optimal concentration and treatment time of H2O2 were determined to establish apoptosis model of oxidative stress in vitro. After MSCs were treated with 1.2 mM H2O2 for 24 h, the related protein expressions were determined by western blot, the mitochondrial membrane potential ($\Delta\Psi m$) of cells was analyzed with JC-1, and the specific inhibitors of signaling pathways were used to reveal the roles of different signalling pathways in H2O2 induced MSC apoptosis.
Results Apoptosis of MSCs was observed obviously after the cells were treated with more than 0.9 mM H2O2 for 12-24 hours. H2O2 treatment resulted into decrease of mitochondrial $\Delta\Psi m$, release of cytochrome C from mitochondria to cytosol and bax translocation from the cytosol to the mitochondria in MSCs. Caspase-3 was cleaved at 3 hour of the treatment, and its inhibitor Z-DEVD-FMK prevented the early and late apoptosis of MSCs. In addition to dysfunction of mitochondria, H2O2 treatment also led to activation of caspase-12 which was a specific regulator to endoplasmic reticulum stress-induced apoptosis. Z-ATAD-FMK, a specific inhibitor of caspase-12, prevented the early and late apoptosis of MSCs. H2O2 increased phosphorylation of JNK from 30 min to 1 hour of treatment, and phosphorylation of p38 reached the maximum at 3 hour of treatment. Moreover, p38 inhibitor SB202190 prevented the early apoptosis of MSCs, while JNK inhibitor SP600125 inhibited the late apoptosis of the cells. In addition, the loss of mitochondrial $\Delta\Psi m$, release of cytochrome C and bax translocation were prevented by SB202190 but not by SP600125.
Conclusions H2O2 induces apoptosis of rat MSCs in a dose and time dependent manner. Both ER stress and a mitochondrial death pathway involve apoptosis of the cells in which caspase-3 and caspase-12 play important roles. H2O2 treatment also activate the JNK/p38 pathway, among which p38 contributes to the early apoptosis of MSCs by regulating mitochondrial pathway, and JNK involves the late apoptosis through other pathway.

27

Cellular Repressor of E1A-Stimulated Genes Inhibits Human Vascular Smooth Muscle Cell Apoptosis via Blocking P38/JNK MAP Kinase Activation

Wu GZ, Han YL, Deng J, Tao J, Guo L, Tian XX, Kang J, Zhang XL, Yan CH
The Cardiovascular Research Institute and Department of Cardiology (Y. H., J. D., J. T., L. G., X. T, J. X. C. Y.), Shenyang Northern Hospital, Shenyang, China;
Department of Cardiology (G. W.), Xijing Hospital, Fourth Military Medical University, Xi'an, China.

Objective Vascular smooth muscle cell (VSMC) apoptosis accelerates atherosclerosis and promotes restenosis following vascular injury. Cellular repressor of E1A-stimulated genes (CREG) has recently been shown to play a critical role in maintaining tissue homeostasis. However, its role in VSMS apoptosis remains unknown. The present study examined whether CREG may regulate VSMC apoptosis and further investigated the mechanism involved..
Methods VSMCs were isolated from human internal thoracic artery and apoptosis was induced by serum starvation or apoptotic inducers (STS and VP-16). Treatment with STS significantly reduced CREG expression and caused caspase-3 activation. The time course of CREG downregulation and caspase-3 cleavage was inversely related, suggesting that reduced CREG expression may contribute to VSMC apoptosis. To obtain di-

rect evidence in supporting this notion, expression of CREG was down regulated (CREG-DW) by retrovirus expressing CREG shRNAs or up-regulated (CREG-UP) by retroviral infection with vector pLNCX-CREG. CREG-DW significantly increased VSMC apoptosis, whereas CREG-UP significantly reduced apoptosis induced by serum starvation and apoptotic inducers. To further explore the mechanisms involved, the effect of CREG-DW and CREG-UP on activation of several apoptotic regulating molecules was determined. Among these proteins, p38 and JNK mitogen-activated protein kinase were found to be significantly upregulated in CREG-DW and significantly reduced in CREG-UP VSMCs, whereas no significant change was observed in ERK and PI3K activation. Moreover, CREG-DW induced VSMC apoptosis was blocked by a p38-specific inhibitor (SB203580) or by overexpression of a dominant negative P38α (p38α AGF). In addition, CREG-UP increased expression of the VSMC differentiation markers SM α-actin and SM-MHC, and reduced cell-associated fibronectin and laminin-1 in cultured VSMCs. Finally, balloon injury-induced vascular caspase 3 activation was significantly inhibited whereas SM α-actin and SM-MHC expression was significantly increased by treatment with recombinant CREG protein.

Conclusions These results demonstrate for the first time that CREG plays a key role in modulating VSMC apoptosis through the p38 and JNK signaling transduction pathways in vitro and in situ.

28

Role of TWEAK on the Expression of LOX-1 in THP-1 Cell

Wu YB, Xu CS, Zeng HS

Department of Cardiology, Tongji Hospital, Huazhong University of Science and Technology, Wuhan 430030, China

Objective The expression of TWEAK was detected in regions rich in macrophage/foam cells in atherosclerotic plaques and TWEAK can induce various molecular mediators of atherogenesis, such as IL-6, IL-8, MCP-1 and MMP-9. The aim of this study was to investigate the expressions of LOX-1 in THP-1 cells by TWEAK.

Methods and Results Stimulation of LOX-1 expression by TWEAK. The effects of different concentration of TWEAK on the mRNA expression of LOX-1 were determined by semi-quantitative RT-PCR in THP-1 cells. Changes in the expression of LOX-1 protein at different concentration of TWEAK were determined by Western Blot. We found upregulation of LOX-1 expression in THP-1 in a dose-and-time-dependent manner after incubation with TWEAK.

Conclusions The results suggest that TWEAK is involved in atherosclerosis by inducing LOX-1 expression in monocytes.

29

Folic Acid Influences Plasma Homocysteine Levels And Arterial Endothelial Function in Patients with Unstable Angina

Xing YB, Guo HY, Chi JF, Wang P

Shaoxing City, Zhejiang Province, Shaoxing City, Zhejiang Province People's Hospital, City Center North Vietnam No. 568

Objective To assess whether folic acid supplementation could produce improvements in Hcy levels and arterial endothelial function in the patients with unstable angina and hyperhomocysteinemia.

Methods The plasma Hcy levels of 52 cases with UA and 30 age and sex-matched control subjects were measured by using high-performance liquid chromatography with fluorescence detection, plasma folic acid and VitB12 levels were measured with immunoassay. The patients with hyperhomocysteinemia were treated with 5 mg of folic acid for 8 weeks, rechecked the plasma levels of Hcy, folic acid and VitB12 at the end of 4th and 8th week. Arterial endothelial function was measured as flow-mediated dilation of the brachial artery using high-resolution B-mode ultrasound in 22 cases with UA and hyperhomocysteinemia.

Conclusions Hcy level is elevated in patients with UA. Folic acid can reduce the plasma Hcy levels and improve arterial endothelial function in the UA patients with hyperhomocysteinemia.

30

Expression of CREG Protein in Mice Embryogenesis

Yang GT, Han YL, Yan CH, Kang J
Department of Cardiology, Shenyang Northern Hospital, Shenyang 110016

Objective The cellular repressor of E1A stimulated genes (CREG), as a novel transcriptional regulator, was cloned originally from a HeLa cDNA library. It can antagonize the E2F-dependent transcriptional activation and the oncogenic transformation of primary cells induced by the Adenovirus E1A oncoprotein cooperating with the oncogene ras. It Has been shown that CREG is widely expressed in adult tissues such as brain, heart, lung, liver, intestine, and kidney of mice. To further clarify the relationship between the expression of CREG and cellular differentiation, in this study, we used immunohistochemistry, Western blot and RT-PCR methods to detect the expression of CREG in mice embryogenesis and the distribution of the expression in 18. 5-dpc (days post coitus) embryos. We also observed the relationship between CREG and vasculogenesis in order to provide necessary evidence for studying function of CREG in the future.

Methods The pregnant mice were killed at different time after the day of post coitus and embryo mice were obtained. The samples were imbedded in paraffin and then were cut into sections, stained with HE, finally observed by microscopy. ②Using immunohistochemistry, we detected the expression and distribution of CREG in embryo mice of different stage. ③Western blot was used to detect the expression of CREG in mice embryogenesis and in 18. 5-dpc embryos. ④Total RNA was extracted by Trizol from embryo mice. Reverse transcriptase-PCR was used to measure the expression change of CREG mRNA at different stage in embryo mice. ⑤Sections were stained to observe the morphology change of vasculogenesis in embryo. ⑥The relationship between SM α-actin and CREG was detected in vasculogenesis at different stage. ⑦The expression of CREG was also observed in vessels of different adult organs.

Results Expression of CREG protein in different stage mouse embryo: Immunohistochemistry analysis at different stage of mouse embryos showed that the earliest time point of CREG expression was the day of 5. 5 pc, which was located in primitive ectoderm. Neither inner cell mass nor trophectoderm was found CREG protein at day 4. 5 embryos. At day of 6. 5 and 9. 5 development, CREG protein was found most widely expressed in endoderm, mesoderm and ectoderm. When mouse development entered into the phase of organogenesis and histogenesis, CREG protein was distributed in different organs with different initated time point. At day of 13. 5 and 15. 5 pc, CREG protein was detected in heart, brain, and liver, but not in lung, intestine and kidney. Up to the day of 18. 5 pc, the expression of CREG was observed in all above organs. Western blot and RT-PCR analysis identified that the expression of CREG was gradually increased and reached to the highest in the 18. 5-dpc embryos. ②The distribution of CREG protein in organs of 18. 5-dpc embryos: The result showed that the CREG protein was expressed at the higher level in brain, heart, intestine and kidney in 18. 5-dpc embryos than that in lung and liver. By immunohistochemistry, we observed that CREG protein was located in colloid cells, myocardial cells, alveolar epithelial cells, hepatic cells, intestinal mucosa cells and renal tubule epithelia cells which were dark brown homogeneous in cytoplasm, but not in nuclus. ③Morphology characteristic of vessels in embryogenesis mice and the location of CREG protein: In 9. 5-dpc embryos, vessel wall was composed of one-layer endothelial cells. The gap of cells was large and blood cells were located in vascular lumens. Immunohistochemistry showed that CREG was expressed (+ +) only in the endothelial cells associated with the initial formation of vascular lumens, SM α-actin was not detected. In 10. 5-dpc embryos, vessels are surrounded with two-layer or multi-layer cells which were arranged loosely. Both the expressions of SM α-actin and CREG protein were found (+) with co-localization in adventitial cells in 10. 5-dpc embryos vessels. Besides in the endothelial cells and VSMCs, CREG protein was also detected in the adventitial cells (+ +). The expressions of SM α-actin and CREG proteins were much stronger in 12. 5-dpc than that in 10. 5-dpc. From 15. 5-dpc to 18. 5-dpc, endomembrane, tunica media and adventitia are much clearer and lumens are much larger than ever with vessel development. Meanwhile, SM α-actin protein was expressed (+ + +) either in 15. 5-dpc or in 18. 5-dpc. However, compared to the SM α-actin protein, CREG expression which reached to maximum in 15. 5-dpc embryos vessel (+ + +), was found to reduce slightly (+ +) and keep on from 18. 5-dpc embryos vessel to adults ones. ④Expression of CREG in vessels of different organs: The CREG protein expression with different quantity was identified to lie not only in large vessel but also in micro vessel of different organs such as heart, lungs, spleen and kidneys in the adult mice. The expression of CREG proteins were much stronger in coronary (+ + +) than that in lung, spleen and kidney (+).

Conclusions The earliest time point of CREG expression was in the 5. 5-dpc embryos. The level of CREG was gradually increased and the highest in the 18. 5-dpc. The distribution of CREG in organs in 18. 5-dpc embryos was similar to that in adult mice. These results suggest that CREG was expressed in mice embryogenesis and probably participate in differentiation of these organs. In 9. 5-dpc embryos, CREG was expressed only in the endothelial cells associated with the initial formation of vascular lumens. With the differentiation and recruitment of the

VSMCs into the embryonic vascular structures, the expressions of both SM α-actin and CREG were found to increase gradually from 10. 5-dpc embryos to adult vessels. These results provide the evidence for the suggestion that CREG might play an important role in regulation of murine vasculogenesis by inducing and holding the differentiation of vascular cells, especially in VSMCs.

31

Relationship between the Interleukin 8 Gene-251A/T Polymorphism and Coronary Heart Disease in Northern Han Chinese

Zhang BH, Han YL, Zhang XL
Department of Cardiology, Shenyang Northern Hospital, Shenyang 110016, China

Objective IL-8 plays an important role in the pathogenesis of coronary heart disease (CHD). This study was to investigate the relationship between interleukin 8 (IL-8) gene-251A/T polymorphism and coronary heart disease (CHD) in northern Chinese Han population.
Methods A total of 268 CHD patients and 205 control subjects were enrolled in this study for determination of IL-8 gene-251A/T polymorphism by polymerase chain reaction-restriction fragment long polymorphism (PCR-RFLP) approach.
Results The genotype frequencies of IL-8-251A/T polymorphism AA, AT and TT genotype have no significant difference between CHD and control subjects (X2 = 2. 152, $P > 0.05$). The frequencies of IL-8-251A/T polymorphism A, T allele also have no significant difference between two groups (X2 = 2. 019, $P > 0.05$). For analysis on the subgroups, the genotype frequencies of IL-8-251A/T polymorphism AA, AT, and TT have no significant difference between patients with unstable angina pectoris (USAP) and control subjects (X 2 = 0. 496, $P > 0.05$). The frequencies of A, T allele also have no significant difference between the USAP and control subjects (X 2 = 0. 472, $P > 0.05$). After adjustment for conventional risk factors, including, age, smoking status, hypertension, diabetes mellitus, hypercholesterolemia, a binary logistic-regression analysis suggested that no difference was demonstrated between the IL-8 gene-251A/T polymorphism and CHD in northern Chinese han population. ($P > 0.05$).
Conclusions IL-8 gene-251A/T polymorphism is not correlated with an increased risk of CHD in northern Chinese han population.

32

Is Ezetimibe Causes an Increase in the Risk of Cancer—From Meta-analyses of Ezetimibe Trials

Dan Z
Fu Wai-Oxford Collaborative Centre for Cardiovascular Health, Cardiovascular Institute and Fu Wai Hospital, CAMS and PUMC, Beijing 100037, China

The combination of ezetimibe and statin is the only product to treat both sources of cholesterol; absorption in the intestine and production in the liver. In some clinical studies, it was shown that the combination of ezetimibe and statin was superior to Lipitor in lowering LDL-C. But, the cancer signal first arose in the SEAS, a trial presented at ESC last year made people worry about the safety of ezetimibe's long-term using.
SEAS (Simvastatin and Ezetimibe in Aortic Stenosis) triall, during a median follow-up of 4 years, simvastatin and ezetimibe did not reduce the composite outcome of combined aorticvalve events and ischemic events in patients with aortic stenosis, but associated with an increase in any new onset of cancer (101 vs. 65, 95% CI, 1. 13 to 2. 12, $P = 0.006$). But, a meta-analyse based on two large and long-scale clinical trial has a different result. In SHARP and IMPROVE-IT combined2, there was no overall excess of cancer (313 vs. 326, 95% CI, 0. 82 to 1. 12, $P = 0.61$, a non-significant difference). Even so, when newly diagnosed (i. e. incident) cancers in all three trials were considered together, there was still no significant excess (414 vs. 391 95% CI, 0. 92 to 1. 22; $P = 0.46$).
In aggregate, the hypothesis-testing SHARP and IMPROVE-IT trials involve about four times as much information about the incidence of cancer as does the hypothesis-generating SEAS trial. In the analysis of SHARP and IMPROVE-IT (or of all three trials together), there was no significant excess incidence of cancer, either overall or at any particular site, and there was no suggestion of an emerging trend with longer treatment and follow-up periods. When the results of all the trials are analyzed properly, no particular type of cancer is significantly increased and there is no significant excess of death from any particular type of cancer. The SEAS result appears to have been a chance finding.
Above all, the available results from these three trials do not provide credible evidence of any adverse effect of ezetimibe on rates of cancer. In

future, follow-up of longer duration (such as SHARP and IMPROVE-IT) will permit the balance of risks and benefits to be determined more reliably.

33

The Relationship between Levels of Biomarkers and Anxiety in Patients with Heart Failure

Zhang DL, Zhang J
Department of Heart Failure, Cardiovascular Institute and Fu Wai Hospital, PUMC and CAMS, Beijing 100037, China

Objective To study the levels and roles of biomarkers in heart failure patients with anxiety.
Methods Heart failure patients who were admitted to Heart Failure Care Unit and Intensive Care Unit were consecutively enrolled into this study. Anxiety was evaluated by Self-Rating Anxiety Scale (SAS) and depression was evaluated by Self-Rating Depression Scale (SDS). Biomarkers, including C-reactive protein (CRP), High-sensitivity C-reactive protein (hs-CRP), Big endothelin (Big-ET), NT-proBNP, ESR, total bilirubin, creatinine and uric acid, were measured within 3 days after the patients finished the SAS and SDS evaluation. Demographic and clinical data were recorded.
Results Six hundred and eighty-four patients with heart failure were included in this study, in which 137 cases (20.03%) had anxiety. The levels of Hs-CRP and Big-ET were higher in heart failure patients with anxiety than those in patients without anxiety and depression (321.72 vs. 287.87, P = 0.044; 279.63 vs. 243.90, P = 0021). The level of CRP or NT-proBNP was not significantly different between these two groups.
Conclusions Anxiety is a particularly common finding in inpatients with heart failure, while heart failure patients with anxiety have higher inflammation and Big-ET levels.

34

The role of HDL-C Prospect From the Evidence-based Medicine

Zhang HB
Fu Wai-Oxford Collaborative Centre for Cardiovascular Health, Cardiovascular Institute and Fu Wai Hospital, CAMS and PUMC, Beijing 100037, China

We know that HDL cholesterol has an inverse association with the incidence of coronary heart disease from many clinic epidemiological studies1. In the Prospective Studies Collaborative meta-analysis of 60 observational studies, each 0.2 mmol/L higher HDL cholesterol was associated with about one-third lower risk of CHD death2. If raising HDL cholesterol can reduce the risks of cardiovascular events has become a new focus in this field.

Coronary Drug Project study showed that the Niacin group made a significant 19% reduction in non-fatal myocardial infarction or coronary death, as compared with the placebo3. But the widespread use of niacin has been limited by flushing resulting from the cutaneous vasodilation. A new randomized trail HPS2-THRIVE is to assess the effect of raising HDL-cholesterol with ER niacin/laropiprant 2 g versus matching placebo on the time to first major vascular event. ER niacin/laropiprant is a new drug which can reduce flushing. The results will be published in about 3 years. ILLUMINATE study was stopped prematurely because of an excess of deaths in patient receiving torcetrapib plus atorvastatin, but further analysis showed that torcetrapib was associated with an increase of mean systolic blood pressure. This may not be related to the drug's mechanism4. A new generation of CETP inhibitor is being studied now.

Above all, more clinic trails should be done to detect if HDL cholesterol can really produce cardiovascular benefits. The results of HPS2-THRIVE study and other trails related to the new generation of CETP inhibitor that would be done in the future will provide significant evidence in this field.

35

Inhibition of Rac1 Activity Hinders Vasculogenesis during Early Embryonic Development

Zhang J1), Han YL1), Kang J1), Zhang XL1), Li SH2), Yan CH1)
(1) Department of Cardiology, Shenyang Northern Hospital, Shenyang 110016, China;
(2) Department of Pathology and Laboratory Medicine, Robert Wood Johnson Medical School, Piscataway, NJ 08854, USA

Background Whether Small G Protein Rac1 plays a role in regulating blood vessel formation, especially endothelial cells (ECs) differentiation during early embryonic vascular development remains unclear.

Methods To observe the effects of Rac1 on the differentiation and migration of ECs murine embryonic stem cells (ESCs) lines stably expressing the constitutively active Rac1 mutant (Rac1G12V) or dominant negative Rac1 mutant (Rac1T17N) and the resulting embryoid bodies (EBs) were established as models.. We used contrast phase microscope to observe the development and differentiation features of EBs; pull-down assay to analyze the expression of Rac1 activity; immunofluorescence staining and western blot to inspect the differentiation markers of ECs; matrigel model to observe the assembly of endothelial network.

Results It showed that neither increase nor suppression of Rac1 activity significantly affect the differentiation of EBs to form the typical primitive germ layers. Expression of dominant negative Rac1 did not affect ECs differentiation, but it significantly inhibited cell migration, furthermore completely blocked the assembly of vessel network. Actin stress fibers were largely absent in Rac1T17N-expressing cells. Expression of Rac1T17N inhibited FAK activity while Rac1G12V did not affect it compared with control group.

Conclusions These results indicated that the effect factor of Rac1 on the vasculogenesis of EBs was to inhibit cell migration, which was probably mediated by F-actin mechanism.

36

A monocyte Chemoattractant Protein-1 Gene Polymorphism was not Associated with Coronary Artery Disease in Han Chinese population

Zhang XL, Han YL, Kang J, Yan CH
Department of Cardiology, Shenyang Northern Hospital, Shenyang 110016

Background Coronary artery disease (CAD) is one of the most common forms of heart diseases. Monocyte chemoattractant protein-1 gene (MCP-1, CCL2) has been considered one of the candidate genes that play a role in atherogenesis of CAD. Recently, the association of a single nucleotide polymorphism (SNP) in the MCP-1 gene promoter (-2518A > G) and CAD has been investigated with controversial results.

Methods In the present study, -2518A > G polymorphism of MCP-1 was determined in 502 CAD patients and 410 control subjects to investigate the possible involvement of MCP-1 in CAD.

Results No significant differences in the genotype or allele frequencies were revealed between subjects with and without CAD ($P = 0.581$ and 0.310, respectively). Further stratification analysis by gender or age and analysis of clinical features in relation to myocardial infarction also yielded negative results.

Conclusions 2518A > G polymorphism of MCP-1 does not seem to contribute substantially to CAD in Han Chinese.

37

The Association of Serum Total Bilirubin, Plasma NT-proBNP, C reactive Protein and Invasive Hemodynamic Parameters in Patients with Heart Failure

Zhang YH, Zhang J, Wang D
Department of Cardiology, Cardiovascular Institute and Fu Wai Hospital, Chinese Academy of Medical Sciences and Peking Union Medical College, Peking 100037, China

Objective To explore the correlation of serum total bilirubin (T-Bil), invasive hemodynamic parameters, plasma N-terminal proBNP (NT-proBNP) and C reactive protein (CRP) in patients with heart failure.

Methods Invasive hemodynamic parameters derived from Swan-Ganz catheter, T-Bil, plasma NT-proBNP and CRP within 12 hours after hospital admission were analyzed in 130 patients with chronic heart failure[New York Heart Association (NYHA) class Ⅱ-Ⅳ].

Results Incidence of hyperbilirubinemia was 67.69% in this patient cohort. Compared with those in non-hyperbilirubinemia group, right atrial pressure, right ventricular pressure, pulmonary artery pressure, pulmonary capillary wedge pressure (PCWP) pulmonary vascular resistance, NT-proBNP and left ventricular ejection fraction were different significantly in total hyperbilirubinemia and hyperbilirubinemia Ⅰ and Ⅱ group ($P < 0.01$ or $P < 0.05$, respectively). The left ventricular diastolic diameter and the level of serum CRP were higher in total hyperbilirubinemia group than those in non-hyperbilirubinemia group ($P = 0.03$, $P < 0.01$). The serum T-Biles increased significantly in higher PCWP, right atrial pressure and NT-proBNP groups than those in lower level groups ($P = 0.02$, $P < 0.01$, $P < 0.01$, respectively). Partial correlation analysis showed serum T-Bil was associated with PCWP, right atrial pressure, pulmonary vascular resistance and NT-proBNP, respectively ($r = 0.21$, $P = 0.02$; $r = 0.33$, $P < 0.01$; $r = 0.20$, $P = 0.04$; $r = 0.37$, $P < 0.01$, respectively). Multiple linear regression analysis showed both right atrial pressure and NT-proBNP correlated independently with serum T-Bil ($\beta = 0.39$, $P < 0.01$; $\beta = 0.29$, $P = 0.01$, respectively).

Conclusions For patients with heart failure, serum T-Bil correlate well with right atrial pressure, PCWP and NT-proBNP and is a valuable indicator of exact clinical evaluation for heart failure.

38

The Protective Effects of Hydrogen Sulfide to Neonatal Rat Cardiomyocytes Subjected to Hypoxia Injury

Zhang Y, Cheng WP
PUMC & CAMS, Department of Anesthesiology, Cardiovascular Institute and Fu Wai Hospital, Beijing 100037, China
Capital University of Medical Sciences, Department of Anesthesiology, An Zhen Hospital, Beijing 100029, China

Objective To observe the direct effect of hydrogen sulfide (H2S) with different concentrations on the neonatal rat myocardial cells subjected to hypoxia injury, and further to evaluate the protective concentration of hydrogen sulfide.

Methods Primary-cultured myocardial cells from neonatal rats were randomly divided into 6 groups: control groups and hypoxia groups. The hypoxia groups were divided into S0 group, S100 group, S200 group, S400 group and S800 group according to the concentration of NaHS that is 0 μmol/L, 100 μmol/L, 200 μmol/L, 400 μmol/L and 800 μmol/L in the solution of hypoxia, which subjected to hypoxia for 48 h. Then the number of survival cells and the activity of lactate dehydrogenase (LDH) were measured.

Results The number of survival cells was increased and the activity of LDH was decreased in S100 group、S200 group and S400 group comparing with S0 group ($P < 0.01$). While there were no significant differences ($P > 0.05$) between S0 group and S800group in the number of survival cells and the activity of LDH.

Conclusions NaHS solution of 100 μmol/L to 400 μmol/L may protect myocardial cells from hypoxia injury.

39

The Correlation of Red Blood Cell Distribution Width with Natriuretic Peptides, Hs-CPR and GDF-15

Zhao XY, Yang YJ, Zhang J
Cardiovascular Institute and Fu Wai Hospital, PUMC & CAMS, Beijing 100037, China

Objective Red blood cell distribution width (RDW), a numerial measurement of the variability in size of circulating erythrocytes, has recently been shown to be a strong predictor of adverse outcomes in patients with heart failure independent of anemia and in patients with coronary artery disease, but the underlying mechanism is unknown. The aim of the study was to evaluate the correlation of RDW-Standard deviation (RDW-SD) and RDW-Coefficient of variation (RDW-CV) with New York Heart Association (NYHA) functional class and echocardiographic functional parameters in heart failure patients, (NT-proANP), high-sensitivity C-reative protein (hs-CRP), and to analyze the correlation between the increased RDW and natriuretic peptides, and growth-differentiation factor. 15 (GDF15)

Methods We measured the RDW-SD、RDW-CV and plasma levels of NT-proANP, NT-proBNP, NT-proCNP, hs-CRP. And GDF-15 in 102 consecutive left ventricular heart failure patients and 38 normal control subjects. The correlation analysis was made between RDW-SD, RDW-

CV with NYHA functional class, left atrium diameter (LAD), left ventricular end-diastolic diameter (LVEDD) and left ventricular ejection fraction (LVEF), respectively. And we further analyzed the correlation between the RDW-SD, RDW-CV with GDF-15, hs-CRP, NT-proANP, NT-proBNP and NT-proCNP.

Results In heart failure group, the level of RDW-SD and RDW-CV were significantly higher than those in control group ($P < 0.05$). There was a correlation between RDW-SD, RDW-CV and NHYA functional class in heart failure patients. In the analysis of RDW with echocardiographic functional parameters, the RDW-SD and RDW-CV were positively related to LVEDD (both $p < 0.05$) and negatively related to LVEF. However there was no significant correlation between the RDW and LAD. In heart failure group, RDW-SD and RDW-CV has a positive correlation with NT-proANP, NT-proBNP, GDF-15 and hs-CRP, respectively.

Conclusions In heart failure patients, the level of RDW was significantly increased. RDW has a good correlation with NYHA functional class and the echocardiographic functional parameters. We found that increased RDW could reflect meurohumoral activation and the inflammatory state, and Growth-differentiation factor-15 (GDF-15) might affect the variability in size of circulating erythrocytes in heart failure patients.

40

The Prognostic Value of GDF-15 in Heart Failure Patients

Zhao XY, Yang YJ, Zhang J
Cardiovascular Institute and Fu Wai Hospital, Beijing 100037, China

Objective The aim of the study was to evaluate the prognostic value of GDF-15 in heart failure patients and compare it with NT-proBNP.

Methods We measured the plasma level of GDF-15 and NT-proBNP by enzyme immunoassay method in 102 left ventricular heart failure patients. All the patients were followed up for about 16.6 months. The primary clinical end points were cardiac death, heart transplantation or first re-admission for CHF. We used the area under the ROC curve (AUC) to evaluate the discriminative power of GDF-15 and NT-proBNP's for cardiac events in heart failure group. Univariant and multivariate Cox regression analysis were used to find the predictors of the cardiac events.

Results The plasma level of GDF-15[1588.86 (1146.12, 2719.01) pg/ml] in cardiac event group was significantly higher than that in the none cardiac event group [1125.81 (780.40, 1841.13) fmol/ml] ($P < 0.01$). The AUC of NT-proBNP [0.778 (95% confidence interval: 0.676 to 0.879; $P < 0.01$] is bigger than that of GDF-15[0.642 (95% Confidence interval: 0.518 to 0.765; $P < 0.05$]. According to univariant COX analysis including the following factors: GDF-15, NT-proBNP, age, gender, NYHA classification, LVEF, Atrial fibrillation/atrial flutter, Ventricular tachycardia and diabetes, GDF-15, LogNT-proBNP, NYHA classification, LVEF and Ventricular tachycardia were correlated to the adverse outcomes. But in multivariate COX analysis, only LogNT-proBNP [B (SE): 1.804 (0.452), $P = 0.000$] was the significant independent predictor of the cardiac events.

Conclusions GDF-15 can predict the cardic death, readmission and heart transplant in heart failure group and decompensated heart failure group, but it's prognostic value seems not to be better than NT-proBNP.

41

The Correlation of GDF-15 with Cardiac Function, Echocardiographic Functional Parameters and N-terminal Natriuretic Peptide in Heart Failure Patients

Zhao XY, Yang YJ, Zhang J
Cardiovascular Institute and Fu Wai Hospital, Beijing 100037

Objective Growth-differentiation factor-15 (GDF-15), a member of the transforming growth factor-β cytokine superfamily, was initially cloned from an activated macrophage cell line. The aim of the study was to evaluate the correlation of plasma GDF-15 with New York Heart Association (NYHA) functional class and echocardiographic functional parameters. As the natriuretic peptide is thought to be the classic biomarker of heart failure, we compare the correlation between the GDF-15 with NT-proANP、NT-proBNP and NT-proCNP in heart failure patients.

Methods We measured the plasma levels of GDF-15, NT-proANP, NT-proBNP and NT-proCNP with enzyme immunoassay method in 102 left ventricular heart failure patients and 38 normal control subjects. The correlation analysis was made between GDF-15 and NYHA functional class, NT-proANP, NT-proBNP, NT-proCNP, left atrium diameter (LAD), left ventricular end-diastolic diameter (LVEDD) and left ventricular ejection fraction (LVEF), respectively.

Results In heart failure group, the plasma concentration of GDF-15 [1231.9 (798.8, 2038.6) vs. 615.8 (413.0, 765.26) pg/ml, $P < 0.01$] was significantly higher than in control group. The plasma GDF-15 of heart failure patients were gradually and significantly increased with the NYHA functional class except to the patients between NYHA I and NYHA II. Correlation analysis showed that there were correlation between GDF-15 with NT-proANP ($r = 0.389$, $p = 0.000$), NT-proBNP ($r = 0.413$, $p = 0.000$) and NT-proCNP ($r = 0.245$, $p = 0.013$). In univariant analysis, GDF-15 was positively related to NYHA and LVEDD (both $P < 0.15$), and negatively related to LVEF. According to multivariate stepwise regression analysis including the following six factors: age, gender, NYHA classification, LAD, LVEDD and LVEF, only NYHA classification [B(SE): 0.155 (0.029); $P = 0.000$] was the independent correlative maker for GDF-15.

Conclusions In heart failure patients, the plasma concentration of GDF-15 is significantly increased and it correlated with NT-proANP, NT-proBNP and NT-proCNP. GDF-15 shows a good correlation with the cardiac function and echocardiographic functional parameters.

42

The Correlation of NT-proANP、NT-proBNP and NT-proCNP with Renal Function in Heart Failure Patients

Zhao XY, Yang YJ, Zhang J
Cardiovascular Institute and Fu Wai Hospital, Beijing 100037

Objective Now we know the natriuretic peptides are activated in both heart failure patients and severe renal insufficiency patients. But it is not clear whether there is a correlation between the natriuretic peptides and the renal function in heart failure patients with mild renal insufficiency. The aim of the study was to observe whether there was a correlation between the NT-proANP、NT-proBNP、NT-proCNP and the renal function in heart failure patients who had serum creatinine (Cr) lower than 2 mg/dl.

Methods We measured the serum creatinine, blood urea nitrogen (BUN), and plasma NT-proANP, NT-proBNPand NT-proCNP in 112 heart failure patients and 44 normal control subjects. We analyzed the correlations between NT-proANP, NT-proBNP, NT-proCNP and Cr, BUN, eGFR respectively.

Results The serum levels of Cr [85.50 (73.00, 101.00) μmol/L] and BUN [5.10 (4.20, 6.70) mmol/L] in heart failure group were significantly higher than those in the control group {Cr [75.50 (65.00, 88.00) umol/L], BUN [4.65 (3.86, 5.99) mmol/L}, respectively (both $P < 0.05$). Meanwhile thee GFR [87.59 (71.33, 102.69) ml/min] in heart failure group was significantly lower than that in the control group [94.42 (79.96, 112.60) ml/min] ($P < 0.05$). In heart failure patients, NT-proANP, NT-proBNP and NT-proCNP were positively correlated with Cr and BUN, respectively (all $P < 0.05$); and negatively correlated with eGFR (all $P < 0.05$). – According to multiple step wise regression analysis, when including the following five factors: age, gender, Cr, BUN and eGFR, only BUN was the independent correlative maker for NT-proANP and NT-proBNP; while Cr was the independent correlative maker for NT-proCNP. When plus NYHA and diuretic as the addition factors, the results revealed that NYHA, BUN and diuretic were the independent correlative maker for NT-proANP and NT-proBNP; while only Cr was the independent correlative maker for NT-proCNP.

Conclusions The serum levels of Cr and BUN in heart failure patients ($Cr < 2$ mg/dl) were significantly increased, while the eGFR significantly decreased. Even in the heart failure patients without obviously increased renal function, the level of NT-proANP, NT-proBNP and NT-proCNP were effected with renal function.

43

The Correlation of NT-proANP、NT-proBNP and NT-proCNP with Bilirubin in Heart Failure Patients

Zhao XY, Yang YJ, Zhang J
Cardiovascular Institute and Fu Wai Hospital, Beijing 100037

Objective To observe whether NT-proANP, NT-proBNP and NT-proCNP correlate with the bilirubin and other liver function indicators in heart failure patients. And to analysis the correlation between bilirubin and the cardiac function as well as echocardiographic parameters.

Methods The plasma NT-proANP, NT-proBNP, NT-proCNP and bilirubin were measured in 112 left ventricular heart failure patients and 44 normal control subjects. Elisa kits from BIOMEDICA company was applied to test the plasma levels of NT-proANP, NT-proBNP and NT-proC-

NP. The Pearson correlation analysis was done and multiple stepwise regression was used to analysis the association between bilirubin with clinical cardiac function and echocardiographic parameters.

Results The serum levels of total bilirubin (TBIL), direct bilirubin (DBIL), indirect bilirubin (IBIL), γ-glutamyltransferase (GGT), alkaline phosphatase (ALP) were significantly higher in heart failure group than those in control group (P all <0.05). Glutamic oxalacetic transaminase (GOT) and glutamic pyruvic transaminase (GPT) showed no significant difference between the two groups ($P>0.05$). In heart failure patients, LogNT-proANPand LogNT-proBNP were positively correlated with LogTBIL, LogDBIL, LogIBIL, LogGGT and LogALP, respectively. However, the LogNT-proCNP showed no correlation with bilirubin and other liver function indicators. In univariate analysis, LVEF and age were negatively related with bilirubin, while NYHA classification, LAD, LVEDD were positively related with bilirubin in heart failure patients. However, in multiple regression analyses, only age and NYHA were independently associated with LogTBIL, LogDBIL and LogIBIL, respectively. NYHA was the strongest impact factor.

Conclusions The bilirubin level was significantly increased in heart failure patients, and positively correlated with NT-proANP and NT-proBNP. However, the NT-proCNP showed no correlation with bilirubin. The bilirubin level in heart failure patients had good correlation with the cardiac function and echocardiography parameters. In multiple regression analysis, only NYHA and age were independently correlated with bilirubin.

44

Prognostic Value Comparison of NT-proANP, NT-proBNP and NT-proCNP in Heart Failure Patients

Zhao XY, Yang YJ, Zhang J
Cardiovascular Institute and Fu Wai Hospital, Beijing 100037

Objective C-type natriuretic peptide (CNP) belongs to the natriuretic peptide family and is structurally related with a 17 amino-acid ring linked by a disulfide bond. But the prognostic value of CNP is not clear yet. So we compare the prognostic values of NT-proANP, NT-proBNP and NT-proCNP for cardiac events in heart failure patients.

Methods The NT-proANP, NT-proBNP and NT-proCNP in the blood plasma were measured using enzyme immunoassay method in 112 left ventricular heart failure patients. All the patients were followed up for about 16.8 months. The primary clinical end points were cardiac death, heart transplantation or first re-admission for CHF.

Results The plasma levels of NT-proANP [6.56 (4.54, 8.61) vs. 3.62 (2.64, 5.49) nmol/l] and NT-proBNP [165.55 (78.62, 271.96) vs. 43.28 (12.94, 105.91) fmol/ml] in cardiac event group were significantly higher than those in the none cardiac event group (both $P<0.05$). Meanwhile, The level of NT-proCNP had a tendency of increase in cardiac event group [6.25 (4.03, 8.39) vs. 5.22 (4.09, 7.20) pmol/l], but had no statistics meaning ($P>0.05$). From the ROC curve, we could found that NT-proANP and NT-proBNP could distinguish the cardiac events in heart failure patients, and the value of NT-proBNP is better. NT-proCNP could not predict the cardiac events in heart failure patients. NT-proANP, NT-proBNP, NT-proCNP, age, gender, NYHA classification, LAD, LVEDD, LVEF, Atrial fibrillation/atrial flutter, ventricular tachycardia and diabetes were introduced as evaluation factors. LogNT-proANP、LogNT-proBNP、NYHA classification、LVEF、LVEDD and Ventricular tachycardia were revealed associated with the adverse outcome in univariant COX analysis But in multivariate COX analysis, only LogNT-proBNP [B (SE): 1.103 (0.539); $P=0.041$] and LVEF[B (SE): -0.042 (0.021); $P=0.046$] were significant independent predictors of the cardiac event.

Conclusions In the three natriuretic peptides, NT-proANP and NT-proBNP can predict the cardic death, readmission and heart transplantation in heart failure patients. Meanwhile NT-proCNP shows poor predict value in heart failure patients.

45

Cardioprotection of Cardiomyopeptidin in Mini-swines with Myocardial Ischemia-reperfusion Injury

Tang Y, Qian X, Tian Y, Yuan WM, Peng P, Zhang BJ, Wu AL
Chinese Acad Med Sci, Peking Union Med Coll, Fu Wai Hosp & Cardiovasc Inst, Animal Experimental Center, Beijing 100037, China

Objective To observe whether cardiomyopeptidin can protect myocardium in mini-swines with myocardial ischemia-reperfusion injury
Methods Twelve pigs were used and their myocardial ischemia-reperfusion injury resulted from the balloon inflation in the distal one third of the left artery descending for 90 minutes and then deflation through femoral artery. Sixty minutes after inflation, 2 ml of cardiomyopeptidin per minute was administered in test group (six pigs) while 0.9% sodium chloride was injected in control group (six pigs) at the same speed. Before ischemia, at the end of and 24 hours after cardiomyopeptidin or 0.9% sodium chloride injection, plasma myocardial enzyme level was measured and the heart function was evaluated by echocardiography. After 24 hrs of reperfusion, animals were sacrificed. Necrosis area was measured with triphenyhetrazolium chloride (TTC) staining and histopathology was described and scored.
Results Ten pigs of twelve survived. At the moment of the balloon inflation, S-T raised in the electrocardiogram which meant the myocardial ischemia. After the acute myocardial ischemia, the plasma levels of CK, CK-MB and LDH were increased and higher than before ($p < 0.05$). However, the test group does not differ to control group ($p > 0.05$) at one and twenty-four hours after medicine administration. It is a pity that we could not find difference between the two groups in left ventricular end systolic volume/left ventricular end diastolic volume (LVESV/LVEDV), interventricular septal thickness of end-systole, wall motion score index and left ventricular end systolic pressure/left ventricular end diastolic pressure (LVESP/LVEDP), although the wall motion score index decreased and LVEDV of test group were bigger than those of control group after ischemia. The score of infarction size with TTC staining was 0.30 ± 0.17 in test and 0.29 ± 0.07 in control ($p > 0.05$). The score of myocardial injury with light microscope had no statistic difference ($p > 0.05$) between the two groups by pathologist.
Conclusions In this study, we cannot certify the cardioprotection of cardiomyopeptidin in the myocardial ischemia-reperfusion injury model of mini-pigs. It might because the infarction was too serious to recover. The mini-pig model of myocardial ischemia-injury replicated by the balloon is little invasive and more stable than the thoracotomy. Therefore it is suitable for the study of the treatment and mechanism of myocardial ischemia-injury.

46

IGF-1, Epigenetic Regulation and Cardiovascular Disease

Yang X, Li YX
Texas Heart Institute, Houston, TX, USA

Cardiovascular diseases are the leading cause of morbidity and mortality in the Western world, and no effective therapy has been established. The malleability and dynamic nature of the epigenetic code, in contrast to the static genetic code, make therapeutic intervention in cardiovascular disease an enticing and high priority. Epigenetic includes 3 distinct, but highly interrelated, mechanisms: DNA methylation, histone modifications, and microRNAs (miRNAs) regulated RNA-based mechanisms. Insulin-like growth factor-1 (IGF-1) system exerts multiple physiological effects on the vasculature and heart through both endocrine and autocrine/paracrine mechanisms, and the effects of IGF-1 are mediated principally through the IGF-1 receptor (IGF-1R). However, the interactions of IGF-1 system and epigenetic regulation in cardiovascular disease are not known. Glucose toxicity is an important initiator of cardiovascular disease, contributing to the development of diabetic complications and cardiomyocyte death. We investigated whether high glucose (HG) state could induce apoptosis of H9C2 rat ventricular cells through microRNA regulated IGF-1 signaling pathway. We found that H9C2 cells exposed to HG had increased miR-1 expression level, decreased mitochondrial membrane potential, increased cytochrome-c release, and increased apoptosis. Glucose induced mitochondrial dysfunction, cytochrome-c release and apoptosis were blocked by IGF-1. Using prediction algorithms, we identified 3′-untranslated regionof IGF-1 gene is the target of miR-1. MiR-1 mimics, but not mutant miR-1, blocked the capacity of IGF-1 to prevent glucose-induced mitochondrial dysfunction, cytochrome-c release and apoptosis. In conclusions, we demonstrate that IGF-1 inhibits HG-induced mitochondrial dysfunction, cytochrome-c release and apoptosis and that IGF-1's effect is regulated by miR-1. Moreover, incubating H9C2 ventricular cells in HG resulted in decreased the levels of IGF-1R mRNA and IGF-1R protein when compared with H9C2 incubated in normal glucose. The effects of HG on reduced expression of IGF-1R and increased apoptosis were blocked by silencing p53 with small interference RNA but not by non-targeting scrambled siRNA. In addition, HG negatively regulated IGF-1R promoter activity as determined by ChIP analysis, which was dependent on p53 since siRNA-p53 attenuated the effects of HG on IGF-1R promoter activity. HG also increased the association of p53 with histone deacetylase 1 (HDAC1), and decreased the association of acetylated histone-4 with the IGF-1R promoter. Furthermore, trichostatin A, a specific HDAC inhibitor, relieved the repression of IGF-1R and prevented apoptosis of H9C2 following HG state. These results suggest that HG-induced repression of IGF-1R is mediated by the association of p53 with the IGF-1R promoter, and by the subsequent enhanced recruitment of chromatin-modifying proteins, such as HDAC1, to the IGF-1R promoter-p53 complex. In conclusions, our data demonstrate that HG exposure decreases expression of IGF-1R and decreases the association of acetylated histone-4 with the IGF-1R promoter, and suggest that enhancing acetylation of histone 4 and IGF-1R expression may be a useful strategy to prevent diabetic cardiomyopathy. In summary, our data yield new insight into the interactions of IGF-1 system and epigenetic regulation in cardiovascular disease, and may lead to the development of a novel therapeutic strategy for cardiovascular disease.

47

Novel Genetic Insights into the Mechanisms of Cardiomyopathies and Heart Failure

Ahmad F
Cardiovascular Institute, Departments of Medicine and Human Genetics, University of Pittsburgh, Pittsburgh, PA 15213, U. S. A.

5' AMP-activated protein kinase (AMPK) is a widely expressed heterotrimeric enzyme that serves as a cellular energy gauge, maintaining fuel supply by regulating energy-generating and energy-consuming pathways in response to metabolic needs. It comprises a catalytic α and regulatory β and γ subunits. In 2001, we discovered the first mutation in the gene PRKAG2, encoding the $\gamma 2$ subunit of AMPK, in families with cardiac hypertrophy and ventricular pre-excitation, and other mutations were quickly identified. We then showed that the cardiac hypertrophy was a manifestation of intracellular glycogen accumulation. Transgenic mouse models of the Thr400Asn (TGT400N) and the Asn488Ile (TGN488I) mutations in PRKAG2 recapitulate the human cardiomyopathy and exhibit an initial inappropriate activation of AMPK. In vivo cardiac glucose uptake is elevated early in TGT400N and TGN488I mice, and the increased glucose entry is directed toward glycogen synthesis. Despite active investigation by several laboratories, the mechanism of increased cardiac glucose uptake has remained unknown.

There are two families of cellular glucose transporters: the facilitated-diffusion glucose transporter (GLUT) family; and the sodium-dependent glucose transporter (SGLT) family. SGLTs transport glucose by a secondary active transport mechanism which uses the sodium concentration gradient established by Na +/K + ATPase pump. Classically, it has long been thought that only the GLUT isoforms GLUT1 and GLUT4 are responsible for glucose uptake in cardiac myocytes. However, we have determined that the SGLT isoform SGLT1 is present at the protein level in cardiac myocytes, and is largely localized to the sarcolemma. Furthermore, we have found that inappropriate AMPK activation leads to up-regulation of SGLT1 in TGT400N cardiac myocytes, which in turn is responsible for the increase in glucose uptake.

Our discovery of the functional significance of SGLT1 in a genetic cardiomyopathy also has potentially major implications in acquired heart failure. Cardiac SGLT1 expression is upregulated 2-to 3-fold in humans and mouse models with type 2 diabetic cardiomyopathy. In humans with severe heart failure, functional improvement following implantation of left ventricular assist devices leads to a 2-fold increase in cardiac SGLT1. SGLT1 expression is increased 2-to 3-fold in both human subjects and mouse models of cardiac ischemia, and inhibition of SGLT1 in mice exacerbates ischemic injury. Acute administration of leptin, a hormone with cardioprotective properties in ischemia, to mice increases cardiac SGLT1 expression -7-fold. Furthermore, SGLT1 mediates at least part of the increased cardiac glucose uptake in response to insulin and leptin. AMPK is known to be rapidly activated during ischemia, leading to stimulation of glucose uptake, glycolysis, and free fatty acid (FFA) oxidation. Whereas AMPK activation of glucose uptake and glycolysis is beneficial, its activation of FFA oxidation may be harmful. Therefore, a therapeutic strategy that mimics the effect of AMPK on glucose uptake through SGLT1, but not its effect on FFA oxidation during ischemia may be optimal.

48

Propranolol Blocks Cardiac Sodium Channels-A New Mechanism for Antiarrhythmic Effect

Wang DW, Alfred L, George JR
Department of Medicine and Pharmacology, Vanderbilt University Medical Center, Nashville, Tennessee

Antiarrhythmic drugs have been most commonly classified into four (class I-IV) categories. Those that block beta-adrenergic receptors are considered class II drugs and belong to nontraditional antiarrhythmic drugs. Propranolol is a widely used, nonselective beta-adrenergic receptor blocker with proven efficacy in reducing mortality after myocardial infraction and in the congenital long QT syndrome (LQTS), and more recently demonstrated efficacy in the primary prevention of sudden cardiac death in patients with congestive heart failure. At higher plasma concentrations, propranolol exhibits antiarrhythmic effects that are not fully explained by beta-blockade. We investigated the effects of propranolol on heterologously expressed recombinant human cardiac sodium channels (NaV1.5 encoded by SCN5A) to test the hypothesis that this drug directly interacts with this channel. Propranolol showed tonic and use-dependent block of NaV1.5 channels with IC50 values of 37.6 μM and 2.9 μM, respectively. Clinically used propranolol is a racemic mixture (R-and S-) but only the S-enantiomer has activity on the beta-adrenergic receptor. Our results indicated that both R-enantiomer and S-enantiomer have almost equal cardiac sodium channel blockade effects and the values of IC50 are very close to those of racemic mixture. In additional, we also studied the effects of propranolol on a novel malignant perinatal variant of long QT syndrome caused by a profoundly dysfunctional cardiac sodium channel (G1631D) that occurred de novo in unrelated and ethnically distinct newborns. Both cases survived after treatment with the combination of mexiletine and propranolol. The G1631D mutant exhibited 2.4-fold and 5-fold greater tonic and use-dependent propranolol block than wild-type channels. In summary, propranolol, R-propranolol and S-propranolol directly block human cardiac sodium channels in a dose-dependent manner and this new mechanism explains the beta-receptor independent antiarrhythmic effects of these drugs and may contribute to clinical efficacy in suppressing ventricular arrhythmia. We also show that certain mutation associated with LQTS exhibit enhanced sensitivity to propranolol, a potential mechanism whereby some patients may have greater benefit from beta-blockers that have membrane stabilizing properties.

49

A Mathematical Approach to Model Stroke Pathophysiology

Dronne MA
UK

Stroke is a major cause of morbidity and mortality in many countries. Moreover, no satisfactory treatment is currently available for all the ischemic stroke patients. Hundreds of neuroprotective drugs have been developed but, although they had showed very promising results in rodents in preclinical studies, they appeared to be ineffective in clinical trials. Many hypotheses have been advanced to explain this discrepancy but it remains difficult to understand. As rodent models don't seem well adapted in this case, we chose a complementary approach based on mathematical modelling and performing of in silico experiments.

We first built a model representing the precocious mechanisms of ischemic stroke: the decrease in ATP production due to the drop of cerebral blood flow, the increase of intracellular sodium and calcium concentrations, the increase of extracellular potassium concentration, the excessive release of glutamate in the extracellular space and the cell swelling. We validated this first model by comparing the simulation results with experimental results obtained in moderate or severe ischemia, with or without thrombolytic agent. We then used this model to study the role of several cell types during ischemia. The simulation results reinforced the hypothesis of a dual role of astrocytes: a protective role in moderate ischemia and an aggravating role in severe ischemia. We then used this model to simulate the effects of various neuroprotective agents such as channel blockers, receptor antagonists and transporter inhibitors. The simulation results suggested that the high proportion of white matter and of glial cells in human brain could contribute to explain the lack of efficacy of some of these neuroprotective agents (such as the blockers of sodium voltage-gated channels and the antagonists of NMDA receptors) during clinical trials.

We are currently adding to this model other models which represent some pathophysiological mechanisms appearing later in stroke such as the propagation of depolarisation waves, the inflammatory process, the synthesis of free radicals and the apoptotic cascade. This multi-scale global model of ischemic stroke is aimed at studying the effects of other neuroprotective agents such as anti-inflammatory drugs, free radical scavengers and anti-apoptotic drugs in order to better understand their lack of efficacy in stroke patients and to explore new therapeutic targets in stroke.

50

The Diabetic Rats Derived Bone Marrow Mesenchymal Stem Cells Have Impaired Abilities in Proliferation, Paracrine, Anti-apoptosis and Myogenic Differentiation

Jin PF, Zheng LC, Sun CC
The First Affiliated Hospital of Wenzhou Medical College, Wenzhou, PR China

Objective To study the diabetic condition inner environment effect on the biological properties of bone marrow-derived mesenchymal stem cells (BMSC).
Methods BMSCs were obtained from the streptozotocin (STZ) induced diabetic (N = 6) and normal rats (N = 6). Cell proliferation was evaluated by using cell counting kit-8 (CCK-8) assay. Production of vascular endothelial growth factor (VEGF) and insulin-like growth factor (IGF-1) were measured by enzyme-linked immunosorbent assay (ELISA). Apoptosis under the hypoxia and serum deprivation (hypoxia/SD) culture condition were detected by Hoechst33342 staining, TUNEL and flow cytometry. Myogenic differentiation, induced by 5-azacytidine (5-aza), was assessed by using immunocytochemical staining for the expression of sarcomeric α-actin and desmin.
Results The Proliferative abilities of diabetic rats derived BMSCs decreased significantly compared with the normal rats ($P < 0.01$). Similar results were also observed in the VEGF and IGF-1release ($p = 0.02$, $p < 0.01$ respectively). The myogenic differentiation were decreased significantly between diabetes group and the normal control group, the percents of sarcomeric α-actin and desmin positive cells in the two groups were 17.86 ± 1.58% vs. 13.72 ± 1.78%, $p < 0.01$; 19.61 ± 1.79% vs14.17 ± 1.36%, $p < 0.01$ respectively. The cell non-apoptotic rate was also decreased significantly between diabetes group and the normal control group ($p < 0.01$).
Conclusions BMSCs from the STZ induced diabetic rats could be successfully harvested and expanded in vitro culture condition. Although the morphology were uniform as normal individual, the proliferative and differentiation properties of diabetic rats derived BMSCs, as well as cytokine release and the anti-apoptosis ability were significantly impaired.

51

L-carnitine and Taurine Synergistically Inhibit the Proliferation and Osteoblastic Differentiation of Vascular Smooth Muscle cells

Xie H3, Yang B2, Zhou XM1, Song FL1, Li JM1, Zhou K1, Hu W1, Tang SY4, Yuan LQ3, Xiong SY3, Liao XB1
[1] **Department of Cardiothoracic Surgery, Second Xiang-Ya Hospital, Central South University, Changsha, Hunan 410011, People's Republic of China**
[2] **Department of Ultrasonic Diagnostics, Second Xiang-Ya Hospital, Central South University, Changsha, Hunan 410011, People's Republic of China**
[3] **Institute of Metabolism and Endocrinology, Second Xiang-Ya Hospital, Central South University, Changsha, Hunan 410011, People's Republic of China**
[4] **The School of Nursing of Central South University, Changsha, Hunan 410013, People's Republic of China**

Aim The regulation of vascular smooth muscle cells (VSMCs) function by l-carnitine (LC) and taurine (TAU) has been the subject of increasing interest and investigation. Previously we documented that taurine transporter (TAUT) is expressed in VSMCs and TAU inhibits osteoblastic differentiation of VSMCs via the ERK pathway. The aim of this study was to investigate the synergistic action of LC and TAU on proliferation and osteoblastic differentiation of VSMCs in vitro.
Methods and **Results** LC and TAU synergistically inhibited the proliferation and β-glycerophosphate (β-GP)-induced osteoblastic differentiation of VSMCs as evidenced by the decreasing [3H]thymidine incorporation, alkaline phosphate (ALP) activity and calcium deposition. Furthermore, LC stimulated TAU uptake and TAUT expression in VSMCs. Suppression of TAUT with small-interfering RNA (siRNA) abolished the synergistic action of LC and TAU in VSMCs.
Conclusions The synergistic inhibitory action of LC and TAU on proliferation and osteoblastic differentiation of VSMCs is attributable to the up-

regulation of TAUT expression and TAU uptake by LC.

52

Taurine Up-regulates Gas6 and Axl Expression in Vascular Smooth Muscle Cells via the ERK Pathway

Liao XB 1, Zhou XM 1, Yang B 3, Liu LM 1, Song FL1, Li JM 1, Zhou K 1, Meng JC 2, Yuan LQ 3, Xie H 2

1Department of Cardiothoracic Surgery, Second Xiang-Ya Hospital of Central South University, Changsha, Hunan 410011, People's Republic of China

2Institute of Metabolism and Endocrinology, Second Xiang-Ya Hospital of Central South University, Changsha, Hunan 410011, People's Republic of China

3Department of Ultrasonic Diagnostics, the Second Xiang-Ya Hospital, Central South University, Changsha, Hunan 410011, People's Republic of China

Aim Our previous studies demonstrated that taurine (TAU) inhibits osteoblastic differentiation of VSMCs via the extracellular signal-regulated kinase (ERK) pathway, but the mechanisms are not fully elucidated. The receptor tyrosine kinase Axl and its ligand Gas6 (growth arrest-specific protein 6) signaling has been reported to inhibit the calcification. The present study was undertaken to test the effect of the TAU on Axl and Gas6 production in VSMCs.

Methods Real-time quantitative RT-PCR and Western blot were performed. SPSS 13.0 was used for the statistical analyses. Comparisons were made using a one-way ANOVA.

Results Quantitative real-time RT-PCR analysis showed that treatment of cells with 5, 10, or 20 mM TAU for 6, 9 or 12 d partially reversed the decrease in Axl and Gas6 transcription induced by 10 mM β-GP in VSMCs. Treatment of VSMCs with PD98059, a specific ERK antagonist, reversed the stimulatory effect of TAU on Axl and Gas6 expression, suggesting that TAU appears to increase Axl and Gas6 production in VSMCs via ERK signaling pathway.

Conclusions These results suggest that an increase of Axl and Gas6 production caused by TAU may contribute to the inhibitory action of TAU on vascular calcification.

53

Endothelial Progenitor Cells and Salt-sensitive Hypertension

McGowan

Institute of Regenerative Medicine, University of Pittsburgh

USA

Endothelial progenitor cells (EPCs) are a circulating bone marrow – derived cell population that participate in both vasculogenesis and vascular homeostasis. Recent studies have shown that EPCs are reduced in hypertension that correlates inversely with its mortality rate. However, the molecular and cellular mechanisms underlying EPC reduction are poorly understood. Our current studies have focused on in vitro and in vivo studies of oxidative stress regulation of EPC function in hypertension. Our experimental observations suggest that endothelin-1 (ET-1)-induced oxidative stress contributes to EPC reduction in salt-sensitive hypertension. These findings may provide a mechanistic basis for developing new approaches to combat endothelial dysfunction in hypertension and other cardiovascular diseases (Original research work supported by extramural grants from NIH, AHA and ADA).

54

Dynamic Partnerships between KCNQ1 and Different KCNE Subunits-implication for the Regulation of Cardiac IKs channel Function

Tseng GN
Physiology & Biophysics, Virginia Commonwealth University, 1101 E. Marshall Street, Richmond, VA 23298, USA

The slow delayed rectifier (IKs) channel is an important determinant of action potential duration in human myocardium. The IKs channel consists of at least two components: KCNQ1 channel and KCNE1 auxiliary subunit. Mutations in kcnq1 & kcne1 genes have been linked to abnormalities in cardiac depolarization and increased risk for arrhythmias (long QT syndromes: LQT1 & LQT5, and short QT syndrome/familial atrial fibrillation or SQT2/fAF). Recent data from our lab and others have suggested that the subunit composition of cardiac IKs channels may be more complicated than previously believed. Transcripts of other members of the KCNE family (KCNE2-KCNE5) have been detected in human heart, and these KCNE subunits can all associate with the KCNQ1 channel to confer distinct channel phenotypes in heterologous expression systems. Can these additional KCNE subunits associate with the IKs (KCNQ1/KCNE1) channel complex to modify its function Can they sequester the KCNQ1 subunits into a low-conductance or non-functional state, so that fewer KCNQ1 subunits are available to form the IKs channels? We are particularly interested in KCNE2, because we have confirmed the presence of KCNE2 protein in human heart, and mutations in the kcne2 gene have been linked to LQT6 or fAF. We have shown that in heterologous expression systems, KCNE2 can associate with the IKs (KCNQ1/KCNE1) channel complex to reduce its current amplitude without changing its gating kinetics.

We have used a multidisciplinary approach of electrophysiology, molecular biology, protein biochemistry, and confocal microscopy to probe the relationship between KCNQ1, KCNE1 & KCNE2. Pulse-chase experiments in COS-7 cells showed that there was a KCNE1 turnover in the KCNQ1/KCNE1 complex, supporting the possibility that KCNE1 in the IKs channel complex can be substituted by KCNE2 when the latter is available. Biotinylation experiments in COS-7 cells show that, while KCNE1 relies on KCNQ1 coassembly for cell surface expression, KCNE2 can independently traffic to the cell surface, thus becoming available for substituting KCNE1 in the IKs channel complex. Injecting vesicles carrying KCNE1 or KCNE2 into KCNQ1-expressing oocytes leads to KCNQ1 modulation in the same manner as KCNQ1 + KCNEx ($x = 1$ or 2) cRNA co-injection. Thus, free KCNEx peptides delivered to the cell membrane probablyassociate with existing KCNQ1 channels to modulate their function. Finally, adenovirus-mediated KCNE2 expression in adult guinea-pig ventricular myocytes exhibits colocalization with native KCNQ1 protein and reduces the native IKs current density. We propose that in cardiac myocytes the IKs current amplitude is under dynamic control by the availability of KCNE2 subunits in the cell membrane. These observations suggest the intriguing possibility that the subunit composition of cardiac IKs channels is dynamic: KCNE1 functions as the major auxiliary subunit to set the IKs gating kinetics, while KCNE2 functions as a dynamic regulator to fine tune the IKs current amplitude.

Current experiments in the lab are designed to understand (1) the molecular details of KCNQ1 interactions with KCNE1 and KCNE2, (2) mechanisms of IKs remodeling during aging, and (3) impact on changes in the KCNE partners on IKs sensitivity to channel activators.

55

C-reactive Protein Decreases Interleukin-8 Production in Human Endothelial Progenitor Cells by Inhibition of p38 MAPK Pathway

Nan JL, Li JJ, Li J, Zhu CG
Department of Cardiology, Fu Wai Hospital, Chinese Academy of Medical Sciences, Peking Union Medical College, Beijing 100037, China.

Background C-reactive protein (CRP) has been reported to damage the vascular wall by inducing endothelial dysfunction and inflammation, and also been speculated to have a role in attenuating angiogenic functions of human endothelial progenitor cells (EPCs). Interleukin-8 (IL-8) is an important mediator of the paracrine mitogenic effect of EPCs, which has direct angiogenic effects on mature endothelial cells. We, herein, investigated the direct effect of CRP on IL-8 production and gene expression in cultured human EPCs.

Methods EPCs were isolated from the peripheral venous blood of healthy male volunteers. Cells were cultured in EndoCultTM liquid medium in the absence and presence of CRP at clinically relevant concentrations (5 to 25 μg/ml) for different durations (3 to 48 hours). IL-8 protein

and mRNA of cultured EPCs were evaluated using ELISA and real-time PCR.
Results The results showed that CRP at concentrations higher than 10 μg/ml significantly reduced IL-8 secretion of cultured EPCs with a peak at 25 μg/ml, and also decreased mRNA expression of EPCs with a peak at 12 hours. In addition, preincubation of EPCs with SB203580 (an inhibitor of p38 MAPK) concentration-dependently decreased CRP-inhibited IL-8 release as well as mRNA expression at 24 hours in EPCs.
Conclusions Our study, for the first time, demonstrated that CRP directly inhibited EPCs IL-8 secretion, key player of angiogenesis induced by EPCs, which occurred in part via an effect of CRP to active EPCs p38 MAPK signal transduction pathway. The ability of CRP to inhibit EPCs IL-8 secretion may represent an important mechanism that further links inflammation to cardiovascular disease.

56

Organism-Dependent Features in Protein Structures Revealed by Computational Geometry Information Analysis

Yong LL, Vaisman II
Laboratory for Structural Bioinformatics
Department of Bioinformatics and Computational Biology
George Mason University
Manassas, Virginia 20110, USA

Recent research on organism-specific features of proteins has been mostly focused on analysis of their primary sequences, while the structural differences are far less explored. The organism-specific structural features in proteins are obscured by the strong structural similarity between the homologous proteins across genomes. In this work we implemented protein structure descriptors based on local amino acid residue environment derived from Delaunay tessellation of protein structures. Delaunay tessellation provides quadruplets of nearest neighbor residues, in which we enumerated all possible residue compositions using full 20 letter alphabet as well as a number of reduced alphabets. Feature vectors based on these descriptors were generated for several sets of pairs of homologous proteins from different organisms. We used supervised machine learning techniques to train classifiers which were enabled to discriminate between the structures of homologous proteins from different organisms with high accuracy. We have also shown that such discrimination cannot be achieved by using sequence composition alone and that subtle structural and topological adjustments are likely to play an important role in the evolutionary divergence of proteins.

57

Novel Approaches for Stem Cell Mobilization and Differentiation in the Ischemic Myocardium

Ashraf M
Department of Pathology, University of Cincinnati Med Ctr, Ohio 45267, USA

Myocardium begins to lose myocytes within an hour following myocardial infarction. Since the heart has limited regeneration capability, the discovery of pluripotent stem cells with the ability to repair the damaged tissues offers exciting possibilities in the treatment of injured myocardium. However, the cell based therapy has been limited due to lack of ideal cell type and survival of donor cells after transplantation in the infarcted heart. This study discusses several approaches to enhance regenerative capacity of transplanted stem cells. These include upregulation of cytoprotective proteins, overexpression of Wnt11 or CXCR4, gene therapy with survival genes, combined gene delivery and cell therapy, neuropeptide-Y (NPY)/NPY Y5R ligand/receptor interaction, stem cell based hedgehog gene delivery, simultaneous activation of diverse signaling pathways and reprogramming with microRNAs. The results suggest that activation of signaling pathways of preconditioning promotes the survival of stem cells by release of paracrine factors and upregulation of cell survival genes. Increased upregulation of these cells with cardiac transcription factors promotes their cardiomyogenic potential. Mesenchymal stem cells co-overexpressing Akt and angiopoietin-1 show extensive survival and engraftment in the infarcted rodent heart. Simultaneous over expression Ang-1 and Akt lead to mature blood vessel formation over extended period of time. Ex-vivo hedgehog gene delivery improves angiogenesis and RBF in the infarcted heart to preserve global heart function through the upregulation of multiple angiogenic cytokines including iNOS and netrin. Current and future directions in stem cell based therapy include guided stem cell differentiation, enhanced proliferation, and identification of factors which can accelerate mobilization, homing and survival of stem cells. Stem cell-based therapy & reprogramming of stem cells and designing "Smart cells" to enhance their survival and homing into the injured myocardium hold a bright future for regeneration of infarcted myocardium.

58

Cellular Retinol-Binding Protein-1 Is Expressed by Fibroblasts in Rat Model with Myocardial Infarction

Yu MY, Wu HY, Wu YJ, Zhang HT, Guo TT
Department of Internal Medicine, Fu Wai Hospital, Cardiovascular Institute, Peking Union Medical College, Chinese Academy of Medical Sciences, 167 Beilishilu, Beijing 100037, China

Objective It has been reported that cellular retinol-binding protein-1 (CRBP-1) is transiently expressed in tissue repairing process. To understand the mechanism of ventricular remodeling of heart after myocardial infarction (MI), we have examined the expression of CRBP-1 in rat MI model.

Methods MI was produced in male Wistar rats by left coronary ligation. Rats were sacrificed to obtain the heart at 3, 6, and 15 days after operation. Heart were cut into four cross sections, fixed and embedded in paraffin. Sections were cut and stained with hematoxylin and eosin (HE), Masson's trichrome (MT), rabbit anti-CRBP-1 antibody and mouse anti-α-smooth muscle (SM) actin antibody. CRBP-1 and α-SM actin were also detected using Western blotting.

Results Forty-five Wistar rats developed MI with infarct size ranging from 45.6% to 56.2% (mean 48.6 ± 3.3%). Heart sections of MI with HE and MT staining showed a remarkable myocyte necrosis, collagen disposition and ventricular remodeling. CRBP-1 expression was detected at both of the endocardial and epicardial region of infarction, where fibroblasts infiltrated with myocyte necrosis 3 days and 6 days after operation. After 15 days, α-SM actin positive fibroblasts in the infarcted region expressed CRBP-1.

Conclusions We demonstrate that CRBP-1 is transiently and rapidly expressed by myofibroblast in rat model of MI. Our results suggest that CRBP-1 and possibly retinoic acid play an important role in ventricular remodeling after MI.

59

Toll-like Receptors and Cardiac Injury

Wei C
Department of Anesthesia and Critical Care, Massachusetts General Hospital, Harvard Medical School, USA

Toll-like receptors (TLRs) represent the first line of host defense against microbial infection and play a pivotal role in both innate and adaptive immunity. TLRs recognize invading pathogens through the "molecular pattern-recognition", transduce the signals via distinct intracellular pathways involving a unique set of adaptor proteins and kinases, and ultimately lead to activation of transcription factors and inflammatory responses. Among 10 TLRs identified in human, at least two exist in the heart, i. e., TLR2 and TLR4. Experimental data from our laboratory and other's has revealed that both TLR2 and TLR4 play an essential role in mediating cardiac dysfunction, modulates neutrophil functions and cytokine production, and contributes to high mortality during severe sepsis. Moreover, emerging evidence suggests that the TLRs can also recognize endogenous ligands and may play an important role in modulating cardiomyocyte survival and in ischemic myocardial injury. In animal models of ischemia-reperfusion (I/R) injury or in hypoxic cardiomyocytes in vitro, administration of a sub-lethal dose of lipopolysaccharide (LPS), which signals through TLR4, reduces subsequent myocardial infarction, improves cardiac functions, and attenuates cardiomyocyte apoptosis. By contrast, systemic deficiency of TLR2, TLR4, or MyD88, an adaptor critical for all TLR signaling, except TLR3, leads to attenuated myocardial inflammation, smaller infarction size, better preserved ventricular function, and reduced ventricular remodeling after ischemic injury. These loss-of-function studies suggest that both TLRs contribute to myocardial inflammation and ischemic injury in the heart although the exact contribution of cardiac (vs. circulatory cell) TLRs remains to be defined. These recent studies demonstrate an emerging role for TLRs as a critical modulator in both cell survival and tissue injury in the heart. This lecture will highlight our recent understanding of the complex role of TLRs in septic cardiomyopathy and ischemic myocardial injury. Defining the role of innate immune signaling in these critical cardiac conditions may have important therapeutic implication.

60

Sodium Channel Remodeling and Arrhythmias in the Post Infarction Heart

Wen DD, Boyden PA
Department of Pharmacology, Columbia University, New York, NY, USA

The epicardial border zone (EBZ) is a rim of surviving myocytes in the 5-day infarcted canine hearts. Reentry easily occurs in this substrate and its stabilization depends on the formation of functional lines of block. We first mapped reentrant circuits of sustained tachycardias in the EBZ to identify the central common pathway and outer pathway based on the block lines. Single cells were then dispersed from the central common pathway (IZc) and outer pathway (IZo) and used for voltage clamp studies. Although sodium current (INa) density was decreased in both IZc and IZo, the kinetic properties of INa in IZc were significantly altered comparing to those in IZo. Therefore, differences in INa remodeling in the EBZ help form the functional block lines that lead to reentry. To understand the molecular mechanisms of Na channel remodeling in these cells, we tested several intracellular modulators of Na channels to restore the reduced INa in IZs. We have shown that PKA stimulated increase in INa density in the remodeled IZs was due to augmentation of trafficking of channels to an active site on the membrane, but not due to directly phosphorylation of Na channels at the membrane. Recently, it has been shown that ankyrin-G (AnkG) helps target Na channels to excitable membranes. Therefore, we hypothesed that the infarction-induced remodeling of Nav1.5 may be associated with changes in AnkG in IZs. We found that AnkG protein showed a time-dependent (24 hr, 48 hr, 5 day) significant increase in the EBZ versus Remote regions of the infarcted heart, while Nav1.5 protein decreased. In addition, there was a change in AnkG subcellular location in IZs. Thus, in the acquired remodeling of INa in IZs, AnkG expression played an active role in myocyte electrical remodeling by influencing membrane protein cell surface targeting. Together these findings indicate that sodium channel remodeling plays a critical role in the post-MI arrhythmias, and that cellular AnkG and PKA may be related to the remodeling.

61

Character of Pacemaker Current in Mesenchymal Stem Cells Transfected with HCN4 Genes by LentiV

Zhou YF, Yang XJ, Li HX, Han LH, Song JP, Jiang Wp
Department of Cardiology, the First Affiliated Hospital of Soochow University, Jiangsu 215006

Objective To test if the pacemaker current can be elicited from mesenchymal stem cells (MSCs) transfected with HCN4 genes by LentiV.
Methods 1. MSCs of rabbit from the posterior iliac crest of rabbit were cultured at 37°C in a humidified atmosphere of 5% CO2. 2. The self-inactivating HIV-based lentiviral vector (LentiV) was used as transgenic delivery, which was constructed with plasmid hHCN4/pcDNA3. 3. Total RNA was extracted from control MSCs and those transfected with hHCN4, and RT-PCR was performed. 4. Whole-cell patch clamp was used to study membrane currents. If were elicited in the whole cell configuration by holding cells at-40 mV for 50 ms followed by 10-mV steps (2 s) to-130 mV and returned to-40 mV (50 ms) after each step. After the If was recorded, cells were superfused with extracellular solution containing 4 mM cesium chloride and the currents were measured accordingly.
Results 1. In addition to expressing characteristic hHCN4 protein, mHCN4-transfected hMSCs also express an anticipated high level of hHCN4 gene by RT-PCR and Western blot analysis. And immunofluorescence image is shown for GFP. Control MSCs were negative. 2. With the use of the whole cell configuration of the patch-clamp technique, If was elicited using hyperpolarizing steps in 10-mV increments from-40 mV to-140 mV from a holding potential of-40 mV and was voltage-dependent. The threshold of voltage for activation of If is around-80 mV. Remarkably, all hHCN4 positive cells exhibit a large cesium-sensitive If and it was significantly inhibited by 4 mM cesium chloride.
Conclusions The pacemaker current of If can be elicited from the mesenchymal stem cells transfected with HCN4 genes by LentiV. The genetically engineered MSC expressing hHCN4 is a demonstration of feasibility of preparing MSC-based biological pacemaker cells.

62

Mesenchymal stem Cells Transfected with HCN4 Genes by LentiV to Create Cardiac Pacemakers

Zhou YF, Yang XJ, Li HX, Han LH, Song JP, Jiang WP
Department of Cardiology, the First Affiliated Hospital of Soochow University, Suzhou 215006

Objective The study was to test if genetically engineered mesenchymal stem cells (MSCs) transfected with HCN4 genes can be modified to be cardiac pacemaker cells.

Methods 1. MSCs of rabbit were isolated from the posterior iliac crest of rabbit and were used from passages 2 to 4. 2. The self-inactivating HIV1-based lentiviral vector (LentiV) was used as transgenic delivery, which was constructed with plasmid hHCN4/pcDNA3. 3. Total RNA was extracted from control MSCs and those transfected with hHCN4, and RT-PCR was performed. 4. Membrane proteins were extracted from control MSCs and those transfected with hHCN4. Western blot analysis was performed. 5. Whole-cell patch clamp was used to study membrane currents. After the If was recorded, cells were superfused with extracellular solution containing 4 mM cesium chloride and the currents were measured accordingly. 6. MSCs transfected with either GFP alone or GFP-hHCN4 were cocultured with neonatal rabbit ventricular myocytes. The coculture beating rate of cardiac myocytes was measured after 3 days of coculture.

Results 1. In addition to expressing characteristic hHCN4 protein, mHCN4-transfected hMSCs also express an anticipated high level of hHCN4 gene by RT-PCR and Western blot analysis. 2. If was elicited using hyperpolarizing steps in 10-mV increments from-40 mV to-140 mV, and it was significantly inhibited by 4 mM cesium chloride. 3. The coculture beating rate of cardiac myocytes was 87 ± 11 bpm when MSCs were transfected with control plasmid (expressing only GFP) and 149 ± 14bpm when MSCs were expressing both GFP + hHCN4 ($P < 0.05$).

Conclusions The MSC expressing hHCN4 demonstrated that it is feasible to prepare MSC-based biological pacemaker cells. The study provides a platform for further investigating the possibility of modifying cardiac excitability with genetically engineered MSCs transfected with HCN4 gene by LentiV. MSCs transfected with hHCN4 genes by LentiV are capable of actively pacing ventricular cardiac myocytes and can be modified to be cardiac pacemaker cells.

63

Transplantation of Autologous Mesenchymal Stromal Cells Improves Left Ventricular Function in the Porcine Chronic Ischemic Model through Enhanced Angiogenesis and Neovascularization

Zhou YF, Wang SN, Yu ZX, Sachdev V, Arai AE, Horvath KA
Cellular Biology Section, Cardiothoracic Surgery Research Program, NHLBI, National Institutes of Health. Bethesda, MD, USA

Objective The use of cell based therapies to enhance angiogenesis in ischemic myocardium has demonstrated increased vascularity in treated tissue. A variety of cell types and methods have been employed with conflicting results. Whether direct injection of selected and expanded mesenchymal stromal cells (MSC) would not only enhance angiogenesis but improve the function of ischemic myocardium is unclear.

Methods In a porcine model at the time of ameroid constriction of the circumflex artery, adult bone marrow was harvested. The mononuclear cells were isolated via gradient centrifugation and cultured for 4 weeks. Sixteen animals underwent random treatment of the ischemic myocardium by direct intramyocardial injection (total 1.2 x 108 cells in 2.5 ml of saline) of autologous MSCs evenly divided into 25 injection sites for the cell treated group and equal volumes and injections sites of saline in the control group. Cine MRI and epicardial echocardiography were performed just prior to the injections and again 6 weeks later at the time of sacrifice at which point tissue was also analyzed.

Results Myocardial function as assessed by regional wall thickening (as measured by dobutamine stress echocardiograms) demonstrated a 40.9% improvement after cell treatment of the ischemic zone ($p = 0.016$) whereas the saline treated animals only had a 3.7% change ($p = 0.82$) compared to baseline. The left ventricular ejection fractions of MSC group showed 19.5% improvement from baseline $35.9 \pm 3.8\%$ to $42.9 \pm 5.8\%$ ($p = 0.049$). Increased vascularity was found in the MSC group compared to controls (0.86 ± 0.27 vs. 0.54 ± 0.16 capillary/myocyte ratio, $p = 0.018$). At 1 and 2 wks after MSC injection, clusters of injected cells close to the epicardium were seen. Higher magnification revealed many immature capillaries inside the cell cluster. Within the cluster area, cells were positive for vWF, smooth muscle actin and CD90, but negative for desmin, CD163 and CD68 suggesting that they were newly formed vessels derived from the injected MSCs, not inflammatory cells or regenerated myocytes. At 4 and 6 weeks, clusters of injected cells and mature vessels were also observed.

Conclusions Autologous injection of bone marrow-derived MSCs is safe. No observable side effects or abnormal cell proliferation were found in our study. Capillary density increased following cell treatment only. Echo and MRI analysis documented functional improvement following cell treatment as well. Direct injection of bone marrow-derived stem cells into ischemic myocardium led to the cells that differentiated into vascular endothelial and smooth muscle cells instead of cardiomyocytes, suggesting that the benefits of our cell-based therapy are mainly due to angiogenesis not the regeneration of cardiomyocytes.

64

Cardiovascular Tissue Repair and Regeneration in Coronary Heart Disease

Yong J, Geng YJ
Center for Cardiovascular Biology and Atherosclerosis Research, University of Texas Health Science Center at Houston and Texas Heart Institute, Houston, Texas, USA

During the development of coronary heart disease cardiovascular tissues are damaged and cells die by apoptosis or necrosis. In response to the injury, stem cells are mobilized and generate new cells to replace dead or malfunctional cells. However, stem cells from patient's own tissue may not be sufficient in number and quality to fulfill the need for tissue repair and regeneration because the disease may have advert impacts on stem cell function. A strong capacity of homing and traffic is critical for stem cells to enter and repair diseased organs and tissues. Recently we have characterized proteins that can help maintain stem cell survival and growth as well as traffic to the injured tissue. Apolipoprotein-J (ApoJ), a stress-responding, chaperone-like protein in high-density lipoprotein, may exert a protective effect on stem cells against oxidative injury. Recently, we have shown that expression of ApoJ by cDNA transfection markedly reduces apoptosis in fetal cardiac myoblast, and restores the mitochondrial membrane potential and prevents the release of cytochrome-C from mitochondria into cytoplasma. In this study, we further examined the role of ApoJ in cardiovascular progenitor gene expression. As determined by real-time PCR and by flow cytometry, ApoJ overexpression by cDNA transfection did not alter expression of c-kit, VEGFR2 and sca-1 but significantly increased expression of the chemokine receptor CXCR4 (receptor for stromal cell-derived factor-1, SDF-1). Moreover, Apo J markedly increased the migratory response of fetal cardiac myoblast to SDF-1 but not to VEGF. Incubation with anti-CXCR4 antibody inhibited the migration of stem cell enhanced by ApoJ. These data indicate that ApoJ increased stem cell migration is CXCR4 dependent. In addition, the ApoJ-induced increase in stem cell migration in response to SDF-1 was attenuated by PI3 kinase inhibitor LY294002 (0-5 uM) (ApoJ ± PI3 inhibitor compared to control = 1.02 ± 0.02 fold) but not by mitogen-activated protein/ERK kinase inhibitor PD98059 (0-30 uM) (ApoJ ± MAP kinase inhibitor compared to control = 2.18 ± 0.18 fold increase, $p = 0.02$). Our data indicate that Apo J increases stem cell migratory responses via CXCR4 chemokine receptor signaling which is PI3/Akt dependent. These findings provide a new paradigm for the biological role of ApoJ in regulation of stem cell functions and have implications for the development of a novel stem cell therapeutic strategy.

65

Simvastatin and Sildenafil Combine to Attenuate Pulmonary Hypertension

Zhao L
Experimental Medicine and Toxicology, Imperial College London, Hammersmith Hospital, UK

Statins have been proposed as a potential treatment for pulmonary arterial hypertension. If introduced into clinical practice, the statin would have to be used in conjunction with established therapy. We investigated the effects of combining simvastatin with a phosphodiesterase type 5 inhibitor, sildenafil, in the rat model of hypoxia-induced pulmonary hypertension. Our results demonstrated that the addition of simvastatin to sildenafil had a significant protective effect and significantly reverses hypoxia-induced pulmonary hypertension and remodelling. The effects, particularly the trophic effects on RVH and vascular remodelling, were more pronounced when the drugs were combined than when given alone. This response may be explained, at least in part, by an additive effect of simvastatin and sildenafil combination on eNOS expression and cGMP levels in lung and RV, and a more marked inhibition of RhoA activity. These data suggest that simvastatin can be usefully combined with sildenafil in the treatment of pulmonary arterial hypertension to achieve greater therapeutic benefit.

66

Role of Extracellular Matrix in Tissue Repair after Myocardial Infarction

Zhi QG, Zhao ZQ
Basic Biomedical Sciences, Mercer University Scholl of Medicine
Savannah, Georgia, USA

Left ventricular remodeling after myocardial infarction is characterized by progressive infarct expansion, wall thinning, and chamber dilation that contributes significantly to ventricular dysfunction and failure. Although much progress has been made to repair damaged myocardial tissue, and improve cardiac function through cellular transplantation, the techniques are plagued by limited cell retention, transplant survival and the clusters of the implanted cells between scar tissue and the cells distributed. The emerging field of tissue repair via reconstruction of extracellular matrix (ECM) has begun to provide promising alternative to the typical cellular transplantation technique. We tested the hypothesis that modulation of angiogenesis and cardiac function by a xenogegeic cellular matrix emulsion (EMU) is associated with recruitment of c-kit cells, myofibroblasts and macrophages after myocardial infarction. Study was performed in a rat model of 45 min ischemia followed by 3, 7, 21 and 42 days of reperfusion, respectively. EMU was harvested from the porcine small intestinal submucosa and injected into myocardium at reperfusion. Histological examination was performed by immunohistological staining, the tissue protein level was measured by Western blot and cardiac function was analyzed using echocardiography. Relative to saline injection, EMU injection significantly increased the population of c-kit positive cells in infarcted myocardium peaked at 7 days of reperfusion, consistent with significantly enhanced expression of 31 kDa stem cell factor. Along with this change, α-smooth muscle actin (α-SMA) expressing myofibroblasts and macrophages accumulated to a significant extent compared to the saline control. Increased VEGF protein level and strong immunoreactivity of VEGF expression were observed. Angiogenesis in the EMU area was significantly enhanced relative to the saline control, evidenced by increased density of α-SMA positive vessels. Furthermore, echocardiography showed significant improvements in fractional shortening, ejection fraction and stroke volume in the EMU group. The wall thickness of the infarcted middle anterior septum in the EMU group was significantly increased relative to the saline control. In conclusions, intramyocardial injection of an EMU into the ischemic/reperfused myocardium increases neovascularization and preserves cardiac function, potentially mediated by enhanced recruitments of c-kit positive cells, myofibroblasts and macrophages. These data provide experimental evidence to set a platform for translational research, and further support whether ECM modulation could be eventually used in a clinical application by targeting attenuation of remodeling-associated tissue injury after myocardial infarction.

67

The Effect of Lovastatin on the Expression of Serum Apoptosis-related Factor sFas and Caspase8

Chen GL
Peking Union Medical College and Chinese Academy of Medical Science, Beijing 100037, China

Objective Statins were shown to have cholesterol-independent properties such as increasing plaque stability, anti-inflammatory, improving endothelial cell function and anti-apoptosis activity. However, the specific mechanism has not been clarified. Soluble Fas (sFas), a marker of vascular injury, can increase the apoptosis of vascular smooth muscle cells. Caspase8 is a cysteine protease that participates in the signaling pathway for cell death induced by Fas. The purpose of this study is to observe the differences of plasma sFas, caspase8 between healthy controls and patients with hyperlipidemiaand the effect of fluvastatin on plasma sFas and caspase8.

Methods Thirty-six patients with hyperlipidemia took lovastatin 10 mg/d, orally for a total of eight weeks. Prior and after 8 weeks of treatment, venous blood was collected to measure the changes of blood lipids level. Westen blot was used to observe the difference between plasmasFas and caspase8.

Results Lovastatin could significantly reduce serum total cholesterol and LDL-C. The expression of sFas in patients with hyperlipidemia was higher than that in healthy controls ($p < 0.05$), but the caspase8 level had no significant difference ($p > 0.05$). After 8 weeks of medication, the expression of plasma sFas decreased significantly ($p < 0.05$), while caspase 8 had no significant change ($p > 0.05$).

Conclusions These results indicate that sFas is probably be involved in the atherosclerosis process and Lovastatin could decrease the level of blood lipid and sFas in patients with hyperlipidemia.

68

Effects of Lonic Contrast Media on Platelet Aggregation Function

Chen Q, Liu F, Cui W
Department of Cardiology, The Second Hospital of Hebei Medical University and Institute of Cardiocerebrovascular Disease of Hebei, Shijiazhuang 050000, China

Objective We study whether platelet aggregation function is associated with contrast media by measuring platelet aggregation in various inducers and the key ways of influence approaches.
Methods The study was performed in 22 patients (mean age 38.00 ± 15.01 years, 9 males and 13 females) undergoing radio frequency catheter ablation for paroxysmal supraventricular tachycardia. The criteria for exclusion include as the followings: hematological diseases, hemorrhagic disease and bleeding tendency; severe hepatorenal function insufficiency; receive the therapy of ticlopidine, clopidogrel, dipyridamole, warfarin, antifibrinolytic agents, standard heparin and low molecular weight heparin in four weeks; acute and subacute infection. After successful venipuncture ionic contrast media of compound meglumine diatrizoate were injected. Blood samples were obtained at pre-injection, post-injection 10 minutes and post-injection 20 minutes. Aggregation was assessed with a mobile four-channel impedance aggregometer (Chronolog-Log Corporation), which allowed measurement of aggregation beginning 1 hour after blood sampling. Platelet aggregation in the whole blood induced by ADP (10 μmol/L), arachidonic acid (10 μmol/L) and epinephrine (10 μmol/L). Continuous variables were expressed as the mean value plus or minus standard deviation (SD). The repeated measures engineered variance analysis was performed to compare differences for individual time points. Multiple comparisons were used LSD-t test. A P value of <0.05 was considered statistically significant.
Results In the arachidonic acid-induced platelet aggregation in the whole blood was lowest at pre-injection (10.68 ± 4.79 Ohms), highest at post-injection 10 minutes (13.09 ± 4.55Ohms). Multiple comparisons showed statistical difference between pre-injection and post-injection 10 minutes. In the epinephrine-induced platelet aggregation in the whole blood was also lowest at post-injection 10 minutes (8.83 ± 3.23 Ohms), highest at post-injection 20 minutes (10.75 ± 5.22 Ohms). But there were no statistical difference showed among three times. In the ADP-induced platelet aggregation at pre-injection (10.77 ± 5.58 Ohms) was higher than post-injection 10 minutes. But platelet aggregation at post-injection 20 minutes was the highest among three times. But there were also no statistical difference showed among three times.
Conclusions We used the impedance method for measuring aggregation in whole blood, showed that the arachidonic acid approach was the key way of contrast media influence platelet aggregation function.

69

Angiotensin II Type 1 Receptor Gene Polymorphisms and Hypertension in Han Chinese Population

Shu F, Chen SF, Gu FY, Gu DF
Cardiovascular Institute and Fu Wai Hospital, Beijing 100037

Objective The renin-angiotensin system (RAS) plays a critical role in blood pressure maintenance and is considered as an etiologic factor in the development of hypertension. Most of the known effects of angiotensin II, the major active component of RAS, are mediated by angiotensin II type 1 receptor (AGTR1). The AGTR1 is a member of the superfamily of G protein coupled receptors that have seven transmembrane domains. In 1994, Bonnardeaux et al. identified the 1166A > C (rs5186) polymorphism located in the 3' UTR of AGTR1 gene. Many subsequent studies investigated the relationship between rs5186, as well as SNPs, and essential hypertension with conflicting results. The present study aimed to assess the effects of variations in angiotensin II type I receptor (AGTR1) gene on the risk of essential hypertension in northern Han Chinese population.
Methods 502 (262/240, male/female) stage-2 hypertensive patients and 490 (257/233, male/female) age-, gender-and area-matched healthy normal controls were recruited. They came from three centers of northern China, namely Jilin, Beijing and Shandong province. Stage-2 hypertension was defined as an average systolic blood pressure (SBP) ≥ 160 mm Hg and/or diastolic blood pressure (DBP) ≥ 100 mmHg [11]. The control subjects had SBP < 140 mm Hg and DBP < 90 mm Hg and no history of hypertension. Three single nucleotide polymorphisms (rs275650, rs1492078 (C-521T) and rs5186 (A1166C)) were genotyped by polymerase chain reaction and restriction fragment length polymorphism method (PCR-RFLP). Associations between genotypes and blood pressure, glucose and lipid levels were conducted using gener-

al linear model adjusted for covariate variables of age, gender, BMI, smoking and drinking where appropriate. Haplo. stats software was used to estimate the effects of haplotypes on hypertension.

Results There were no significant deviations from Hardy-Weinberg equilibrium for three polymorphisms. Univariate analysis showed that the three polymorphisms were not associated with hypertension. These polymorphisms alone were not associated with hypertension after adjustment for effects from age, gender, BMI, smoking and drinking in logistic regression model. In the general linear model adjusted for the effects of covariates, there was no significant difference in the levels of blood pressure, glucose and lipids among three genotypic groups for each polymorphism in cases or controls. Haplotype analysis showed no association of common haplotype with hypertension.

Conclusions These results indicated that these three variations in the AGTR1 gene might not contribute to the risk of hypertension in the studied Chinese population.

70

MicorRNAs in Cardiovascular Diseases and the Application Prospect of MicroRNA in Clinical Examination

Chen X, Nie Y
Clinic Laboratory Center
Cardiovascular Institute and Fu Wai Hospital
Chinese Academy of Medical Sciences &. Peking Union Medical College
Beijing 100037, China

As a kind of endogenous non-coding RNA, microRNAs (miRNAs) play a pivotal role in many biological and pathological processes, including development, proliferation, differentiation, and apoptosis and so on. Almost thousands of unique miRNAs are encoded in the human genome, and they are predicted to regulate expressions of more than 30% of all human protein encoding genes. Interestingly, a subset of miRNAs is either specifically or highly expressed in heart; on the other, several miRNAs are aberrantly expressed in pathological condition. The connotation of several miRNAs in cardiovascular diseases has been well demonstrated. For example, miR-1, the cardiac specific miRNA in mammals, could slow conduction and depolarize the cytoplasmic membrane by post-transcriptionally reducing KCNJ2 (which encodes the K + channel subunit Kir2. 1) and GJA1 (which encodes connexin 43), and this likely accounts in part for its arrhythmogenic potential. MiR-21 regulates the ERK – MAP kinase signalling pathway in cardiac fibroblasts, playing a vital role in the pathogenesis of cardiac diseases. MiR-23a is involved in the pathogenesis of hypertrophy by down-regulating muscle specific ring finger protein 1 (MuRF1), an anti-hypertrophic protein. miR-29 family targets a series of mRNAs that encode proteins involved in fibrosis; enhancing miR-29 expression may have therapeutic value in the setting of post-MI cardiac remodeling. MiR-30c and miR-133 interact with 3' UTR of connective tissue growth factor (CTGF) directly; down-regulation of the both miRNAs is allied to myocardial fibrosis. MiR-320 aggravate ischemic heart disease by down-regulation of Hsp20 protein. Endothelial-specific miR-126 acts on the negative regulators of the VEGF and FGF pathway directly, including the Sprouty-related protein SPRED1 and phosphoinositol-3 kinase regulatory subunit 2 (PIK3R2/p85-beta), promoting the regeneration of blood vessels after myocardial infarction. Moreover, miR-126 inhibits vascular cell adhesion molecule 1 (VCAM-1) expression, then regulates the vascular inflammation indirectly. Thus, these miRNAs correlated with cardiovascular diseases may serve as some novel therapeutic target.

Besides searching the therapeutic target of cardiovascular disease, as novel biomarkers, miRNAs offer unique opportunities for prognosis, diagnosis and classification. Recently, miRNAs have been found in serum and other body fluids, called circulating miRNAs. Present studies have revealed that the level of miRNAs would change during the development and pathology. For instance, Serum levels of miR-141 can distinguish patients with prostate cancer from healthy controls. The ratio of miR-92a/miR-638 in plasma would decrease dramatically in leukemia patients, comparing with healthy body.

As the transcript, miRNAs could reflect the alteration of physiology more directly than proteins. Combining the important role of miRNAs in pathogenesis of cardiovascular diseases, screening miRNAs biomarkers is of significance in cardiovascular diseases prognosis, diagnosis and classification.

71

CREG Inhibits Migration of Human Vascular Smooth Muscle Cells by Mediating IGF-II Endocytosis

Cui JF, Han YL, Guo L, Kang J, Zhang XL, Yan CH
Cardiovascular Research Institute and Department of Cardiology, Shenyang Northen Hospital, Shenyang 110016, China

Background Cellular repressor of E1A stimulated genes (CREG), a secreted glycoprotein ubiquitously expressed in mammals, has originally been shown to act as a transcription repressor to antagonize transcription activation and cellular transformation induced by the adenoviral E1A oncoprotein. When overexpressed in human embryonic carcinoma cells, CREG enhances cellular differentiation and inhibits cell cycle progression. Our previous studies have shown that CREG is significantly down-regulated in the rabbit carotid artery after balloon injury. Furthermore, adenovirus-mediated CREG over-expression inhibits SMCs proliferation and attenuates neointimal hyperplasia in vitro and in vivo. It is therefore of interest to further defining if CREG also plays a role in SMCs migration and if IGF-II is involved in regulation of SMCs migration by interaction between CREG and its putative receptor protein M6P/IGF2R.

Methods We firstly performed gain-and loss-of-function analyses of CREG in cultured SMCs using Retrovirus CREG overexpression and knockdown CREG expression. Then, the scrape analysis, transwell assay and time-lapse analysis were used to investigate the relationship between CREG expression and vascular SMC migration. Meanwhile, Western blotting and Gelatin zymography analysis were used the MMP-2 and MMP-9 expression in cells. Furthermore, enzyme linked immunosorbent assay (ELISA) and endocytosis analysis were used to detect the IGF II secretion in cell medium.

Results CREG over-expression is identified to inhibit SMC migration associated with down-regulating activity of MMPs. Mechanistically, CREG knockdown attenuated the internalization of IGF-II and increased its secretion. Moreover, the effect of CREG knockdown on SMCs migration was blocked in a concentration-dependent manner by addition of anti-human IGF-II neutralize antibody. Despite the direct interactions between CREG and M6P/IGF2R have not yet been elucidated, our study indicated that M6P/IGF2R was involved in regulation of IGF-II endocytosis using both anti-human M6P/IGF2R neutralize antibody and recombinant M6P/IGF2R protein.

Conclusions These data demonstrate for the first time that CREG plays a critical role in SMCs migration by modulating IGF-II internalization, and that might provide a new therapeutic potential for vascular injury such as restenosis after angioplasty.

72

CREG Treatment Reduces Neointimal Hyperplasia in Human Arterial Organ Culture Model

Deng J, Han YL, Guo L, Yan CH, Liang M, Kang J, Liu HW
Department of Cardiology, Shenyang Northern Hospital, Shenyang 110016

Background We previously showed cellular repressor of E1A-stimulated genes (CREG) plays a critical role in the maintenance of SMCs in a mature, growth quiescent state in the normal artery and that CREG downregulation contributes to neointimal hyperplasia after vascular injury. We aimed to test the hypothesis that CREG protein treatment can reduce neointimal hyperplasia in cultured human arterial.

Methods The remnants of low limbs arteries from 6 patients undergoing amputation were collected. Sections were made at 3 mm intervals perpendicular to the vessel wall axis. The arterial segments were treated with 3 mm standard balloon-catheters for 60 s. After angioplasty, the organ segments were cultured in a mixture of DMEM, supplemented with 10% fetal calf serum. In the treatment group, CREG protein was added to the culture medium at different concentrations. After 28 days the organ cultures were fixed in 4% para-formaldehyde and embedded in paraffin. After staining with a modified HE technique the intimal wall thickening was analyzed with a computerized morphometric system. For the identification of smooth muscle cells (SMC) a monoclonal antibody against smooth muscle alpha-actin was used. Endothelial cells were identified using an anti-human CD31. PCNA-positive cells were detected in the neointima of the organ cultures, indicating mitotic activity in this area.

Results Treatment with CREG protein resulted in a lower intimal thickness growth above baseline levels, whereas untreated control arteries increased. The neointimal amount of the contractile protein smooth muscle actin (SMA) in CREG protein treated arteries was significantly higher than baseline values. The expression of proliferation marker PCNA decreased in CREG protein treated arteries. Elastic fibers were present in the media and intima before and after organ culture without significant differences between the groups. Collagen fibers were found abundantly in the inner longitudinal media, less commonly in the outer circumferential media, and they were absent in the intima without difference between the groups.

Conclusions Local CREG protein treatment reduces neointimal hyperplasia in cultured human arteries. CREG protein treatment leads to an increased amount of the contractile protein SMA and thus might have a therapeutic potential for the prevention of artery proliferation disease.

73

Association between ALOX5AP Gene Polymorphisms and Coronary Artery Disease in The Han Population of North China

Han YL, Li ZD, Zhang XL, Yan CH, Kang J
Department of Cardiology, Shenyang Northern Hospital, Shenyang 110016

Background Recent evidence has implicated specific gene polymorphisms of arachidonate 5-lipoxygenase – activating protein (ALOX5AP), and 2 at-risk haplotypes (HapA, HapB) in myocardial infarction and stroke, whereas other studies have been conflicting and to date, no data concerning coronary artery disease (CAD) are available in the Han population of North China. The aim of the present study was to investigate the possible associations between the variants of ALOX5AP gene and susceptibility to CAD in the Han population of North China.

Methods We sequenced the promoter, all of the exons, splite site region and 3′untranslated region of ALOX5AP gene, and 7 single nucleotide polymorphisms (SNPs) were found. Three (-1340T/G, + 8733T/C, + 20616G/C) of these polymorphisms were evaluated in 328 patients with angiographically proven CAD and 339 controls with normal coronary angiograms using polymerase chain reaction and restriction fragment length polymorphism (PCR-RFLP) assay. Allelic, genotypic and haplotypic association testing was performed using SHEsis and Phase version 2.1 software package. Multiple logistic regression was used to control for the presence of traditional risk factors including gender, age, body mass index, smoking, hypertension, diabetes mellitus and hyperlipidemia.

Results While none of the SNPs were found to be associated with CAD risk individually, there was an association between the 3 SNP haplotypes and CAD. We identified a protective haplotype-1340T, + 8733C and + 20616G ($P = 8.10e{-}005$, OR = 0.597, 95% CI = 0.462-0.773) and two different high-risk haplotypes-1340G, + 8733C and + 20616G ($P = 0.000546$, OR = 1.761, 95% CI = 1.274-2.434) and-1340T, + 8733C and + 20616C ($P = 0.034750$, OR = 2.206, 95% CI = 1.040-4.683). The frequencies of all alleles were in Hardy-Weinberg equilibrium.

74

Role of Irbesartan on the Expression of Cholesterol Transporters ABCA1/G1 in Macrophage

He T, Wu YB, Zeng HS
Department of Cardiology, Tongji Hospital, Huazhong University of Science and Technology, Wuhan 430030, China

Objective We investigated whether Irbesartan has the effect on the expression of ABCA1/G1 and underlined mechanisms.

Methods THP-1 cells were maintained in RPMI1640 containing 10% fetal bovine serum. The differentiation of THP-1 monocytes into macrophages was induced in the presence of 200 nM of phorbol 12-myristate 13-acetate (PMA) for 72 hours. First, cells were divided into five groups and stimulated individually by Irbesartan with concentrations of 0、5、10、50 and 100uM for 24 hours. The mRNA and protein level of ABCA1 and ABCG1 were detected by RT-PCR and Wester blot respectively. Then cells were divided into three groups and treated with the following reagents: Irbesartan 10uM, either Irbesartan 10uM or GW9662 30uM, and none of them. The mRNA level of ABCA1 and ABCG1 were detected by RT-PCR.

Results Irbesartan increased ABCA1 and ABCG1 mRNA levels in THP-1 macrophages in a dose-dependent fashion. It also increased ABCA1 and ABCG1 protein levels which was consistent with changes in mRNA levels. The minimum effective concentration of Irbesartan was 10uM. The PPARγ antagonist GW9662 could abolish the effects of Irbesartan on these genes.

Conclusions Our results showed that Irbesartan increased ABCA1 and ABCG1 expression via PPARγ dependent pathway.

75

Hypertension, Telomere Shortening and Stem Cell Aging

Zhen Y, Ju ZY
Max-Planck-Partner Group on Stem Cell Aging, Institute of Laboratory Animal Sciences, Chinese Academy of Medical Sciences, Beijing 100021, P. R. China

Telomere has been known as a mitotic clock that controls cellular ageing. Independent lines of evidence indicate that telomere dysfunction induces both cell intrinsic checkpoints and cell extrinsic checkpoint leading to an age-associated stem cell dysfunction. Telomere shortening induces a DNA damage response leading to cell cycle arrest or apoptosis. Deletion of p21, the downstream senescence checkpoint of p53, improved the life span of telomere dysfunctional mice without promoting cancer formation. In addition to the stem cell intrinsic defects, we have found that telomere dysfunction provokes defects of the hematopoietic environment that impair B-lymphopoiesis but increase myeloid proliferation in aging telomerase knockout (mTERC$^{-/-}$) mice. Capillary electrophoresis-time of flight-mass spectrometry (CE-TOF-MS) revealed four marker proteins (i. e., CRAMP, stathmin, EF-1α, and chitinase) upregulated in aging mTerc$^{-/-}$ mice. Orthologs of these proteins in human are also up-regulated in late-passage presenescent human fibroblasts and in early passage human cells in response to γ-irradiation. Analysis of blinded test samples validated the effectiveness of these biomarkers to discriminate between young and old, and between disease groups (MDS, cirrhosis) and healthy controls.

Accumulating evidence suggests that telomere length is a marker for biological aging of the cardiovascular system. Telomere length is determined by genetic and environmental factors. Studies in different racial populations are required to determine the prognostic value of telomere length in hypertension and cardiovascular diseases. To study the association between leukocyte telomere length and the risk and prognosis of hypertension in a Chinese population, we measured the relative telomere length of leukocytes by a quantitative PCR-based method in 767 subjects: 379 healthy controls and 388 hypertensive patients, ages 30 to 80 years. The median telomere length ratio, 0. 57 (interquartile range: 0. 48 to 0. 72), was shorter in hypertensive than in healthy normotensive subjects (0. 67; interquartile range: 0. 53 to 0. 93; $P = 0.001$). After 5 years of follow-up, subjects with shorter telomeres were at a higher risk of developing coronary artery disease than individuals with longer telomeres (odds ratio: 3. 315; 95% CI: 1. 662 to 6. 609; $P = 0.001$). Multivariate analysis showed that short telomere length and hypertension were independent risk factors for developing coronary artery disease. Our data suggest that mean leukocyte telomere length is a potential predictor of coronary artery disease and support the hypothesis that differences in biological aging can contribute to the risk and variability of developing hypertension and cardiovascular diseases.

In summary, our data support the concept that telomere dysfunction and DNA damage are interconnected pathways that are activated during human aging and diseases.

76

Overexpression of the Sarcoplasmic Reticulum Ca2^{+-} ATPase in Rat Heart after Myocardial Infarction

Fan P, Ma XJ, Yang B, Zhang C, Miao N, Hou YM, Roger J
Department of Cardiovascular Medicine, The First Teaching Hospital of Xinjiang Medical University, Urumqi City, Xinjiang 830054

Background Reduced expression of the sarcoplasmic reticulum Ca2^{+-} ATPase (SERCA2a) gene impairs the calcium-handling and contractile functions of the heart. We developed a SERCA2a gene transfer system using adenoviral vectors, and examined the short term effects of SERCA2a overexpression in a model of myocardial infarction (MI) in the rat, tested the electrophysiological responses of overexpressing SERCA2a immediately after coronary occlusion, studied the electrical mapping of rat hearts post-myocardial infarction.

Methods and results A transmural myocardial infarction was created by ligation of the left anterior descending coronary artery in rats. An adenoviral vector containing the SERCA2a gene was directed injected into a rat heart by the ischemic area delivery after MI. The transduction efficiency was about 70%. TWO weeks after transduction, echocardiogram and electrophysiological measurements revealed that the SERCA2a gene transfer had significantly protected against left ventricular (LV) dilation, and had improved contractile function of the left ventricle, decreased the threshold for ventricular arrhythmias. The SERCA2a gene was successfully integrated into the host heart, induced favorable molecular remodeling, prevented LV geometrical remodeling, and improved the survival rate.

Conclusions These results suggest that a strategy to compensate for reduced SERCA2a gene expression by adenoviral vectors can serves as a positive isotropic, lucitropic, and cardioprotective therapy for post-MI heart failure. These beneficial effects on electrical remodeling post MI need to be examined with long term expression of SERCA2a using adeno-associated vectors.

77

By using MEA, study for Alternation of electrophysiology in Rat Hearts after Myocardial Infarction by Overexpression of the Sarcoplasmic Reticulum $Ca2^{+-}$ ATPase

Ma XJ, Fan P, Roger J, Yang B, Song JG, Miao N, Zhang C, Liu ZJ, Hou YM

Laboratory of Arrhythmia, The First Affiliated Hospital of Xinjiang Medical University, Liyu Road 1#, Urumqi, Xinjiang 830054, China

Objective To study the therapy effect of adeno viral gene transfer of sarcoplasm in reticulum $Ca2^{+-}$ ATPase2a (SERCA2a) on arrhythmia after acute myocardial infarction in 2 weeks and the possible mechanism of the therapy effect.

Methods The rats were divided into three groups: control group SERCA2a group and saline group. Acute myocardial infarction rats were obtained by ligating left anterior descending coronary artery. 0.9% sodium chloride solution, recombinant adenovirus carrying SERCA2a gene, were respectively delivered to the heart of AMI rats in two groups by directed injection around the ischemic area. Electrocardiograph was tested immediately after surgery. Two weeks after gene transfer, electrocardiograph were tested again, the QRS interval R-R interval QT interval and arrhymic incidence rate of the two groups were analyzed. Field potential was detected by microelectrode arrays two weeks after transgene.

Results Two weeks after gene transfer, survival rate of the model rats is 60%. ECG show: arrhythmic incidence rate in control group, saline group and SERCA2a group are 36%, 30% and 0. Compare to the control group, QT interval and R-R interval are prolongated in saline group, but QT interval and QRS interval are shortened in SERCA2a group ($P < 0.05$). MEA show that in two weeks, the dispersion of the field potential duration is longer in saline group than it in SERCA2a group ($P < 0.05$).

Conclusions Adenoviral gene transfer of SERCA2a can reduce the incidence of arrhythmia after acute myocardial infarction. MEA is an ideal method to study the concordance of the myocardial in different part of whole heart.

Cardiovascular Imaging

1

Diagnostic Value of Stress-rest Myocardial Perfusion Imaging in Detection of Coronary Disease in Elderly Patients

Han PP, Tian YQ, Fang W, Yang MF, Shen R, Wei HX, Guo XH, He ZX
Department of Nuclear Medicine, Cardiovascular Institute and Fu Wai Hospital, CAMS and PUMC, Beijing 100037, China

Objective Coronary artery disease is one of the most common causes of death in elderly people. The aim of this study was to evaluate the diagnostic value of nuclear stress-rest myocardial perfusion imaging (MPI) in the detection of coronary disease in elderly patients.
Methods 205 elderly patients (≧ 60 years old, average of 67 ± 5) suspected of coronary disease, underwent both stress-rest myocardial perfusion imaging (185 with exercise stress and 20 with adenosine stress) and coronary angiography (CAG) in two weeks. The patients who had had a percutaneous coronary intervention (PCI) or coronary artery bypass grafting (CABG) were excluded. Coronary angiography was used as a "golden standard" to evaluate the sensitivity, specificity and accuracy of the stress-rest myocardial perfusion imaging.
Results Among 205 patients, there were 57 patients with an abnormal CAG result and 148 patients with a normal result. There were 30 one-vessel, 19 two-vessel, and 8 three-vessel stenoses. 36 patients with abnormal CAG results had positive stress-rest MPI, while 135 patients with normal CAG results had negative MPI. The sensitivity, specificity, accuracy, positive and negative predictive value of stress MPI are 63% (36/57), 91% (135/148), 83% (171/205), 73% (36/49) and 87% (135/156) in patient level, respectively. The diagnostic sensitivities of stress-rest MPI for detection of one-, two-, and three-vessel stenosis are 57% (17/30)、58% (11/19) and 100% (8/8), respectively. 185 patients who underwent exercise stress MPI were divided into 2 groups according to whether the patients reached the target heart rate or not. There were 53 patients (29%) in Group 1 who reached the target heart rate and 132 patients (71%) in Group 2 who did not. The sensitivity of Group 1 was higher than that of Group 2, but with no statistically significant difference [81% (13/16) VS. 58% (22/38), $\chi 2$ = 2.69, P = 0.1]. When coronary stenosis ≥75% was used as a standard in coronary angiography, there were 42 patients with an abnormal CAG in which 30 patients had a positive MPI. The sensitivity, specificity and accuracy of MPI are 71% (30/42), 88% (144/163) and 85% (174/205), respectively.
Conclusions Stress-rest myocardial perfusion imaging is a good method for detecting coronary disease in elderly people. The sensitivity of exercise stress MPI would be high when the target heart rate is reached.

2

Diagnosis of Left Ventricular Noncompaction by Cardiac Magnetic Resonance Imaging and the Differential Diagnosis with Left Ventricular Hypertrabeculation

Zhao SH, Yu JC, Jiang SL, Wang LM, Lu MJ, Ling J, Zhang Y, Yan CW
Cardiovascular Institute and Fu Wai Hospital, Chinese Academy of Medical Science, Beijing 100037, China

Objective The study was designed to assess LVNC with cardiovascular magnetic resonance (CMR) imaging and to explore the differential diagnosis between LVNC and hypertrabeculation.

Methods Twenty-five patients with LVNC, thirty-nine with dilated cardiomyopathy (DCM), sixteen with aortic stenosis, fifteen with aortic regurgitation, nineteen with hypertension, and twenty-two healthy volunteers were collected in the study. Cardiac magnetic resonance imaging was performed to evaluate noncompaction or hypertrabeculation of the left ventricle in diastole. The 17-segment model was used dividing the left ventricle (LV) into six basal, six midventricular, four distal segments, and the apex.

Results Hypertrabeculated segments were most detected in LVNC patients and the affected segments in each patients meant (10 ±2) segments. Each patient with LVNC was unexceptionally associated with apical noncompaction that was seldom found in other patients. The intermediate piece and the distal piece of lateral walls were the most vulnerable segments in all the patients. However, the basal and the middle septum were not detected affected. The ratio of non-compacted segments to compacted segments was 3.3 ±0.6. The proportion of non-compacted segments in patients with LVNC was the highest compared with other patients ($P < 0.05$). Receiver operating characteristics (ROC) analysis identified that when >2.5 was used as the cut-off value of the ratio of non-compacted segments to compacted segments, the sensitivity and the specificity of distinguishing LVNC from hypertrabeculation were 96% and 94.87%, respectively. The segments with the ratio of >2.5 in the LVNC patients were 4 ±2 segments. However, only 8 of 39 patients with DCM had only one segment with the ratio of >2.5.

Conclusions MRI is an excellent imaging modality to diagnose LVNC and to distinguish LVNC from hypertrabeculation. It is more feasible to regard the cut-off value of >2.5 than >2.3 to diagnose LVNC.

3

Echocardiographic Assessments after Double Root Translocation Procedures

Li YQ, Li SJ, Li P, Hu SS

Department of Echocardiography, Fu Wai Hospital, Chinese Academe of Medical Science & Peking Union Medical College, Beijing 100037, China

Objective To assess the function and hymodinamic performance of the reconstructed hearts after our newly developed double root translocation procedures (DRT) for patients with transposition of the great arteries, ventricular septal defect, and pulmonary stenosis by echocardiography.

Methods Between 2004 and 2008, thorough transthoracic echocardiography was performed in 39 postoperative patients underwent DRT procedure before discharged.

Results The morphology of left ventricular outflow track was normal in all cases. The flow velocities were normal in both ventricular outflow tracks. There was no aortic regurgitation in all cases; Only 2 cases were detected with more than moderate in degree pulmonary regurgitation. And biventricular function well in all cases.

Conclusions DRT procedure restored normal intracardiac anatomy with excellent early hemodynamic and ventricular performance. It is a true anatomic and physiological repair.

4

Clinical Application of Stress-rest Myocardial perfusion Imaging in 50-75% Coronary Stenosis

Han PP, Tian YQ, Fany W, Yang MF, Shen R, Wei HX, Guo XH, He ZX

Department of Nuclear Medicine, Cardiovascular Institute and Fu Wai Hospital, CAMS and PUMC, Beijing 100037, China

Objective It's hard to decide whether a percutaneous coronary intervention is needed when the coronary angiography (CAG) shows a stenosis of 50-75%. The aim of this study is to discuss the clinical application of stress-rest myocardial perfusion imaging (MPI) in such cases.

Methods 105 patients with coronary stenoses of 50-75% demonstrated by coronary angiography, underwent stress-rest myocardial perfusion imaging in 2 weeks. The relationship between the result of MPI and therapy was analyzed.

Results 71 (68%) patients underwent CAG before MPI, while others (34, 32%) underwent MPI first. Coronary angiography showed 147 stenotic coronary arteries of 50-75%, among which there were 86 LADs, 26 LCXs, 34 RCAs and 1 LM. There were 73 one-vessel, 22 two-vessel, and 10 three-vessel stenoses. Stress-rest myocardial perfusion imaging found 21 myocardial ischemia caused by 25 stenotic arteries (10 LADs, 7 LCXs, and 8RCA). The patients were divided into two groups according to the result of MPI: Group 1 with negative MPI (84/105, 80%) and Group 2 with positive MPI (21/105, 20%). In Group 1, all patients had medical treatment while in Group 2 15 patients had medical treatment and 6 patients had percutaneous coronary interventions. There was a statistically significant difference between the two groups ($\chi^2 = 20.4$, $P < 0.001$).

Conclusions In cases of 50-75% coronary stenoses, stress-rest myocardial perfusion imaging could evaluate whether the vascular lesions cause myocardial ischemia as well as the extent of ischemic myocardium, and help clinicians choose a appropriate therapy.

5

Ultrasonic Diagnosis of Diaphragm Paralysis after Paediatric Cardiac Operations

Li YQ, Li SJ, Lv XD
Department of Echocardiography, Fu Wai Hospital, Chinese Academe of Medical Science & Peking Union Medical College, Beijing 100037, China

Objective Retrospective study to analyse ultrasonic diagnosis of diaphragm paralysis after paediatric cardiac operation.

Methods Between May 2005 and May 2009, thirty-nine children after open heart operations were diagnosed diaphragm paralysis by bedside two-dimensional and M mode ultrasonography. Their average operation age is 2 ± 11months (5 day to 3-year and 5month).

Results Thirty-one children had immobility of hemidiaphragm (akinesia) and irregular flutter was encountered in the other eight. Twenty-six children got right hemi-diaphragm paralysis and the other thirteen got left side. After diaghram plication procedures, all children recovered smoothly and discharged.

Conclusions Bedside ultrasonography is accuracy, safe, and convenient in children with diaphragm paralysis after cardiac operations, and should be the first choice for diagnosis.

6

Echocardiographic Middle Term Follow-up of the Arterial Switch Operation for Transposition of the Great Arteries

Li YQ, Li SJ, Li P, Pan XB, Zhang YJ, Hu SS
Department of Echocardiography, Fu Wai Hospital, Chinese Academe of Medical Science & Peking Union Medical College, Beijing 100037, China

Objective Middle term follow-up by echocardiography to access the heart structure and function in patients with transposition of the great arteries (TGA) and Taussig-Bing malformation undergoing arterial switch operation (ASO).

Methods One hundred and fifty patients were reviewed, among them there were 120 male and 30 female. The mean age was 11.71 ± 26.3 months (3-57months). The operative time is from January 2004 and December 2007. The follow-up was finished between July and December 2008. The mean follow-up periods were 27.66 ± 14.6 months. Thorough echocardiography exam were performed in all patients.

Results Satisfying echo views were achieved in all patients. Neo-AVI were ; moderate-to-severe PAS; pulmonary hypertension.

Conclusions Echocardiographic results of Middle term follow-up support that ASO remains the optimal choice for the treatment of various forms of TGA.

7

Time-resolved Contrast-enhanced 3D MR Angiography Using Parallel Imaging with View Sharing (TREAT)-comparing with Breath-hold Single Phase High Spatial 3D Contrast Magnetic Resonance Angiography

Lu M, Zhao S, Jiang S, Zhang Y
Cardiovascular Institute and Fu Wai Hospital, Chinese Academy of Medical Science, Beijing 100037, China

Objective To assess the diagnostic value of time-resolved breath-hold contrast material-enhanced three-dimensional magnetic resonance (MR) angiography of the great vessels and its branches-comparing with breath-hold single phase high spatial 3D contrast magnetic resonance angiography.

Methods 32 patients underwent time-resolved MR angiography (TR-MRA, acquisition time per data set, 2-4 seconds) and single-phase high-spatial-resolution MR angiography (SH-MRA, acquisition time, 16-18 seconds) with a 1.5-T magnetic resonance imaging scanner (Avanto, Siemens). 12 of 32 underwent contrast material enhancement CT angiography, 20 of 32 underwent conventional digital subtraction angiography, 18 of 32 were treated by interventional or operation procedure. No bolus timing study was performed for TR-MRA and a bolus test with a power injector was used to calculate the optimal scan delay time for conventional SH-MRA. The space resolution was 1.7 mm × 1.2 mm × (2.5-4.0) mm for TR-MRA and 2.0 mm × 1.3 mm × 1.0 mm for SH-MRA. Image quality (artifacts, venous overlap on arterial phase images) and vascular diseases were assessed.

Results The mean total room time in the MRI unit was 27 minutes ranging from 15-41 minutes. MRA showed 8 patients with pulmonary embolism, 10 with aortic dissection including 4 with Stanford A and 6 with Stanford B, 4 with aneurysm and 10 with artery stenosis and occlusion disease including 5 with Takayasu arteritis and 5 with atherosclerotic lesion. Time-resolved MR angiographic images were characterized by less severe artifacts, less overlap of enhancing veins compared with single-phase MR angiographic images ($P < 0.05$). The mean sensitivity and specificity were 100% and 93.8% for detection of vessel disease, respectively. The technique also proved to be reliable for demonstration of venous disease.

Conclusions Time-resolved MR angiography is a convenient and effective sequence to perform and allow simultaneous evaluation of arterial and venous disease.

8

Dynamic MRI of Ferumoxide-labeled Bone Mesenchymal Stem Cells after Transplantation in the Heart

Liu Q, Zhao SH, Lu MJ

Cardiovascular Institute and Fu Wai Hospital, Chinese Academy of Medical Sciences, Beijing 100037, China

Objective To investigate the potential ability of magnetic resonance imaging (MRI) in tracking magnetically labeled mesenchymal stem cells (MR-MSCs) in a swine myocardial infarction (MI) model.

Methods Adult Chinese mini pigs ($n = 6$) were subjected to open-chest experimental MI. Their autogeneic bone marrow-derived mesenchymal stem cells (MSCs) was cultured and doubly labled with ferumoxides and DAPI. At the 14th day after MI, labeled MSCs were injected intramyocardially into peri-infarct zone and normal myocardium. At the 14th day after MSCs transplantation, the size and location of the myocardial infarction were assessed by using delayed-enhancement MRI (DE-MRI). The contrast and the volume of the MR-MSCs hypointense lesion from the FGRE images were acquired. At 24 and 3 weeks after injection, the contrast was determined using the difference in signal intensity between the hypointense and normal myocardium divided by signal intensity of the normal region. After humane euthanasia, the heart was excised and histology corresponding to MRI slices that demonstrated MR-MSCs lesions was performed.

Results Images of MSCs injection sites at 24 hours after injection appeared as ovoid hypoenhancing lesions with sharp borders. At 24 h after injection, the contrast [(67.00 ± 5.48)% vs. (61.92 ± 7.76)%, $P = 0.1158$) and the size [(0.56 ± 0.24) cm2 vs. (0.52 ± 0.25) cm2, $P = 0.7044$)] of the lesions showed no statistical difference between in peri-infarct zone and in normal myocardium. At 3 weeks after injection, the contrast of the lesions decreased and the size of the lesions diminished both in peri-infarct zone and in normal myocardium. Moreover, the contrast of the lesions in peri-infarct zone decreased rapidly than that in normal myocardium (26.88 ± 7.27 vs. 15.00 ± 4.51, $P = 0.0003$). Post mortem analysis showed that fluorescently labeled MSCs were demonstrated on histological sections. There were much more dense fluorescently labled MSCs per high power fields in injection sites of normal myocardium than in injection sites of peri-infarct zone (106 ± 25/HPF vs. 143 ± 31/HPF, $P = 0.0293$). At 3 weeks after transplantation, the capillary density in MSCs injection sites of the peri-infarct zone was significantly more than that in control sites (13.40 ± 4.00/HPF vs. 9.40 ± 3.10/HPF, $P = 0.0229$).

Conclusions Magnetic resonance imaging of MSCs is feasible and represents a method for noninvasively tracking the quantity and location of intramyocardial delivery after MI. But to semi-quantitatively analyze the development of transplanted MSCs by MRI is not dependable.

9

Quantitative Analysis of Lung Perfusion in Patients with Idiopathic Pulmonary Arterial Hypertension

Liu C, Fang W, He JG, Wang F, Xiong CM, Ni XH, Liu ZH, Tion YQ, He ZX
Department of Nuclear Medicine, Cardiovascular Institute & Fu Wai Hospital, Chinese Academy of Medical Sciences and Peking Union Medical College, Beijing 100037, China

Objective The aim of this study was to assess the value of lung perfusion scan in quantitative analysis of idiopathic pulmonary arterial hypertension (IPAH).
Methods Both lung perfusion scans and right heart catheterization were performed in thirty patients with IPAH. Lung perfusion images were analyzed and Perfusion index (P index) was obtained using quantitative software provided by NIH. Twelve age-matched control subjects were also underwent lung perfusion scans for drawing PAR curve. A Pearson correlation coefficient was determined between the P index and hemodynamic parameters. The patients were divided into three groups. The differences of P index among the groups were assessed by Student's t test.
Results The P index was significantly correlated with mPAP and TPR ($r = 0.541$ for mPAP, $P < 0.01$ and $r = 0573$ for TPR, $P < 0.01$). Significant differences of P index were showed in three groups divided by three typical characters in lung perfusion scan (Student's t test, t value: -2.83, -5.68, -2.65, all $P < 0.05$). The mPAP and TPR showed no significant differences for these 3 groups.
Conclusions The P index is a useful indicator for quantifying the non-uniform distributions of lung perfusion scan. Quantitative assessment of lung perfusion could provide useful information about the severity of IPAH.

10

Morphologic and Functional Evaluation of Complicated Congenital Heart Disease by Magnetic Resonance Imaging: Comparing with Echocardiography and X ray Cardio-Angiography

Lu MJ, Zhao S, Jiang S, Zhang Y, Liu Y
Cardiovascular Institute and Fu Wai Hospital, Beijing 100037

Objective To evaluate the diagnostic value of magnetic resonance imaging (MRI) in complicated congenital heart disease, comparing with echocardiography and X ray cardio-angiography.
Methods 20 patients with complicated congenital heart disease (male 12, female 8, mean age 17.8 y, ranging from 6-46 y) underwent MR examination. A wireless vector ECG-gating was used for triggering; all the sequences were applied with breath hold or free breathing. Turbo spin echo and multiple gradient echo sequences including FLASH (fast low angle shot) and TrueFISP (true fast imaging with steady-state precession.) with TSENSE (adaptive sensitivity encoding incorporating temporal filtering) and TREAT (time resolved echo-shared technique) were used to evaluate the morphology, function, flow status of the heart. MR findings were compared with the results of echocardiography and X ray cardio-angiography.
Results All the examination were accomplished successfully and diagnostic MR images were obtained satisfactory. The mean total scan time was 38 min ranging from 29-55 min. According to the main malformation diagnosed by MRI, double-outlet of right ventricle (DORV) were 12 cases, single ventricle were 3 cases, function-corrected transposition of great arteries were 2 cases, endocardial cushion defect, interruption of aortic arch and absent of right pulmonary artery combined with patent ductus arteriosus was 1 case, respectively. The total coincidence was 95.0% comparing with cardio-angiography, while the echocardiography was 75.0%. It is difficult for X-ray cardio-angiography to evaluate the atrio-rentriculor valve in 25% cases, while MR can clearly and precisely show the number, morphology and function of the valves in all cases. There is 20% of the cases that traditional X-ray cardio-angiography can not demonstrate the connection of ventricular-great arteries, or the main pulmonary artery and its main branches because of anatomy overlapping, tolerance of the patients and skill of catheterization, while MR provide important complementarities for these cases.
Conclusions Combined with new robust techniques, MRI can provide a comprehensive evaluation of complicated congenital heart disease including morphology, function, and flow and so on. With some characteristics of both echocardiography and X-ray angiography, in some aspects MRI is even better than X-ray angiography and can offer important supplemental information.

11

Evaluation of Global Cardiac Function Using Multiple Imaging Modalities in Patients with Chronic Myocardial Infarction: a Comparison Study with Echocardiography, Gated-SPECT, Catherterization and Cardiovascular Magnetic Resonance

Lu MJ, Zhao SH, Jiang SL, Liu S, Hu SS
Cardiovascular Institute and Fu Wai Hospital

To analyse and compare cardiac function using multiple imaging modalities including echocardiography, electrocardiographically gated single-photon emission tomography (SPECT), X-ray angiography, and cardiovascular magnetic resonance (CMR).

Methods 20 patients (age 59.5 ± 10y) with chronic myocardial infarction underwent echocardiography, SPECT, X-ray angiography and CMR within 2 weeks were retrospectively reviewed. The left ventricular volumetric data from different imaging modalities were compared with CMR.

Results LVEDV and LVEF obtained by X-ray angiography mismatched with those data obtained by MRI, with higher readings in X-ray angiography; the LVESV obtained by the above two methods were correlated well ($r = 0.62$, $p = 0.014$). LVEDV, LVESV and LVEF obtained by gated SPECT had the closest results to those obtained by MRI ($r = 0.65$, $r = 0.66$, $r = 0.64$, p values were 0.002, 0.002 and 0.043 respectively). LVEDV, LVESV and LVEF obtained by 3D-echocardiography had moderate correlation with MRI ($r = 0.61$, $r = 0.62$, $r = 0.62$, p values were 0.036, 0.014 and 0.007 respectively).

Conclusions MRI can accurately detect left ventricular volume and function for patients with old myocardial infarction. The left ventricular volume and function tested by gated SPECT and 3D-echocardiography were correlated well with MRI, while the left ventricular volumes and functions between X-ray angiography and MRI differed significantly.

12

Evaluation of Left Ventricular Dyssynchrony in Patients with Acute Myocardial Infarction using Two-dimensional Speckle Tracking Echocardiography

Ma CY, Li XY, Ren WD, Liu S, Zhao SJ
Department of Cardiovascular function
Department of cardiology, First hospital, China Medical University, Shenyang 110001, China

Objective To evaluate the left ventricular (LV) systolic dyssynchrony after the acute myocardial infarction (AMI) in patients with a narrow QRS complex using two-dimensional speckle tracking echocardiography (STE).

Methods STE were performed in 65 patients within 72 hours of AMI and compared with 60 age-and sex-matched healthy volunteers. The peak longitudinal strain (LSpeak) was measured at LV myocardium. LV dyssynchrony was defined as an interval ≥130 ms for the absolute difference in time to peak radial strain for the anteroseptal wall versus the posterior wall (TAS-POST). Size of myocardial infarction (MIS) were confirmed by wall-motion score index (WMSI). All the parameters were compared between the two groups.

Results The LSpeak and LV ejection fraction (LVEF) were lower, and WMSI and TAS-POST were larger in AMI patients compared with controls. 42 patients had developed LV dyssynchrony (64.62%), and there were strong correlation between LV dyssynchrony (TAS-POST) and LSpeak, LVEF, and WMSI (MIS). The MIS was the most independent predictor for systolic dyssynchrony.

Conclusions AMI with narrow QRS can induce LV dyssynchrony, which was mainly determined by MIS. And STE is a reliable technique for accurate evaluation of LV synchrony.

13

Diagnostic Efficacy of Lung Perfusion Scan Interpreted by PISAPED Criteria for Pulmonary Embolism: Comparison with CTPA

Wang F, He ZX, Fang W, Tian YQ, Yang MF, Shen R
Department of Nuclear Medicine, Cardiovascular Institute and Fu Wai Hospital, Chinese Academy of Medical Sciences & Peking Union Medical College, 167, Bei Li Shi Lu, Beijing 100037.

Objective To compare perfusion scan with CTPA in the diagnosis of PE.

Methods One hundred and four consecutive patients with suspected PE were enrolled. All patients underwent lung perfusion scan, CTPA and chest radiography. Lung perfusion scan was interpreted by PISAPED criteria. Final diagnosis was made using a composite reference test.

Results PE was finally diagnosed in 55 of the 104 patients. After excluding three patients (2.9%) with non-diagnostic CTPA from analysis, the sensitivity, specificity, positive predictive value and negative predictive value were 92.6%, 83.0%, 86.2% and 90.7% respectively for lung perfusion scan, and 96.3%, 93.6%, 94.5% and 95.7% respectively for CTPA. The agreement rate between the two modalities was 89.1% (kappa = 0.78, $p < 0.05$). In the segment based analysis, a total of 1664 segments were evaluated. The agreement rate between lung perfusion scan and CTPA was 79.7% (kappa = 0.58 $p < 0.05$).

Conclusions Lung perfusion scan interpreted by PISAPED criteria is as accurate as CTPA, and the two modalities both show high efficacy in diagnosing PE. The agreement between lung perfusion scan and CTPA was intermediate on segment-by-segment basis.

14

Diagnostic and Prognostic Value of Gated SPECT in Patients with Chronic Heart Failure

Wang F, He ZX, Fang W, Tian YQ, Yang MF, Shen R
Department of Nuclear Medicine, Cardiovascular Institute and Fu Wai Hospital, Chinese Academy of Medical Sciences & Peking Union Medical College. 167, Bei Li Shi Lu, Beijing 100037.

Objective To evaluate the diagnostic and prognostic value of quantitative rest electrocardiogram-gated single photon emission computed tomography (SPECT) with 99mTc-sestamibi in patients with chronic heart failure (CHF).

Methods One hundred and twenty (male, 94, female, 26, mean age, 56 ± 16 years) consecutive patients who had CHF were enrolled prospectively between August 2007 and October 2008. All patients underwent rest gated SPECT myocardial perfusion imaging. The mean follow-up time was 236 ± 94 days. The study endpoints were defined as cardiac death, or acute coronary syndrome (ACS), or CHF requiring hospitalization, or clinical need for cardiac surgery. Gated SPECT images were analyzed by Quantitative Gated SPECT (QGS) and Quantitative Perfusion SPECT (QPS).

Results Among the 120 patients with CHF, 39 patients were ischemic CHF, 81 patients were non-ischemic CHF. The mean left ventricular ejection fraction (LVEF) was 25.7% ± 12.2% and the mean summed rest score (SRS) was 10.2 ± 10.4 for all patients on gated SPECT. SRS of the patients with ischemic CHF were significantly higher than the patients with non-ischemic CHF (19.0 ± 12.5 vs. 6.0 ± 5.5, t test, $p < 0.05$). During follow-up, there were three cases of cardiac death, four cases of ACS, 23 cases of hospitalization for CHF, and nine cases of cardiac surgery. Cox regression demonstrated that SRS ≥ 9 (RR = 2.86, $p < 0.05$) and defect extent ≥ 14% (RR = 2.71, $p < 0.05$) were independent predictors of cardiac events.

Conclusions Gated SPECT has potential diagnostic utility for ischemic CHF, and important value for prognosis of CHF.

15

Comparative Study of Echocardiography and Surgical Results, Pathology in 242 Patients with Ruptured Mitral Chordae Tendineae

Wu W, Lou X, Wang L, Wang H, Sun X, Jiang Y, Huo S, Tu L
Cardiovascular Institute and Fu Wai Hospital, Chinese Academy of Medical Sciences & Peking Union Medical College, Beijing 100037, China,

Objective To study the character and regularity of ruptured mitral chordae tendineae (RMCT) in echocardiography and to analyze their relations among echocardiography, surgical results and pathology. The clinical, hemodynamic, surgical, and pathologic findings in 242 patients who required mitral valvular surgery and who had a preoperative diagnosis of RMCT were reviewed.
Methods Echocardiographic, pathologic and surgical studies were performed in 242 consecutive inpatients with ruptured mitral chordae tendineae of Fu Wai Hospital from 2002 to 2008. Thoracic (TTE) and transesophageal echocardiography (TEE) were used to evaluate mitral valve, chordae tendineae, the diameter of heart, heart function, pulmonary artery pressure and pericardial effusion etc.
Results Analyses of Echocardiography in the 242 RMCT patients demonstrated that most of patients had flail mitral valve, moderate to sever mitral regurgitation, dilated heart chamber, mild to moderate pulmonary artery hypertension and good heart function. Posterior leaflets (148 patients) were more frequently affected than anterior leaflets (81 patients), both chordae tendineae ruptured was rare. Furthermore, partial RCMT (218 patients) were more frequently occurrence than total RCMT (24 patients). Compared with surgical results, the diagnostic accordance rate of RMCT was 96.7% in TTE and 100% in TEE; the diagnostic accordance rate of posterior or anterior RMCT was 92.5% and total and partial RMCT was 89.3% by TTE. Surgical procedure of RMCT was depended on the location of ruptured chordae tendineae ($P < 0.01$), but there was no relationships between surgical procedure and total or partial RMCT ($P > 0.05$). The main cause of RMCT was primary valvular heart disease, and the following were infective endocarditis, coronary heart disease, congenital heart defect etc. Surgical and pathologic examination revealed the characters of RMCT were mucoid degeneration, fibrous degeneration, chronic inflammation etc.
Conclusions Echocardiography for diagnosing RMCT is a reliable method with high diagnostic accordance rate. We could guide surgical procedure and judge pathological types according to the echocardiograghic characters of RMCT.

16

Abnormal Drainage of the Inferior Vena Cava into the Left Atrium Accompanying with Partial Anomalous Pulmonary Venous Drainage

Wu Y, Liao CX, Shan ZG
Huazhong University of Science and Technology, Tongji Hospital, Tongji Medical College, Wuhan City, Hubei Province, No. 1095 Jiefang Road

Objective Report a case about diagnosis and treatment of abnormal drainage of the inferior vena cava into the left atrium accompanying with partial anomalous pulmonary venous drainage
Methods The diagnosis was confirmed by using color Doppler flow echocardiography and contrast echocardiography. A pericardium patch was inserted so as to divert flow to the proper atrium.
Results The surgery was successful and the patient got rehabilitation discharge 8 days later.
Conclusions Abnormal drainage of the inferior vena cava into the left atrium accompanying with partial anomalous pulmonary venous drainage is rare and is easy to be misdiagnosed, then, color Doppler flow echocardiography and contrast echocardiography are necessary to establish the diagnosis

17

The Electrocardiograms Change of Adenosine Technetium-99m Sestamibi Myocardial Perfusion Imaging in Chinese Population

Xie BQ, Tian YQ, Zhang XL, Shen R, Fang W, Yang MF, He ZX
Department of Nuclear Medicine, Cardiovascular Institute & Fu Wai Hospital, Chinese Academy of Medical Sciences and Peking Union Medical College, Beijing 100037, China

Objective To evaluate the changes of electrocardiograms of adenosine infusion in conjunction with Technetium-99m sestamibi (MIBI) myocardial perfusion single-photon emission computed tomography (SPECT) in Chinese population.

Methods From May 01, 2008 to November 31, 2008, a total of 676 consecutive Chinese patients (240 male, 436 female; mean age, 58 ± 29; range, 29-87 years) with known or suspected coronary artery disease referred for radionuclide perfusion imaging who were unable to perform exercise stress at Fu Wai Hospital (Beijing, China) were investigated. Adenosine was infused at a constant rate of 140 $\mu g \cdot kg^{-1}$ per min over 6 min (total dose 0. 8 mg · kg-1 body weight). After 3 min of infusion, Technetium-99m sestamibi (925 MBq) was administratered intravenously in all patients and the infusion continued for an additional 3 min. Systolic and diastolic blood pressure, heart rate were recorded at baseline, during each min of infusion, at the time of administration of the radiotracer and for at least 3 min after adenosine infusion. A 6-lead electrocardiograms (ECGs) were continuously monitored before, during, and after infusion. Patients with poorly tolerated side effects, significant ST-segment depression or severe atrioventricular block had the adenosine infusion terminated, depending on the severity of the effects. Technetium-99m MIBI myocardial perfusion SPECT was performed 1. 5 h after the completion of adenosine infusion, and rest images were obtained another day if there was a decrease considered abnormal.

Results Baseline characteristics: HR (bpm) 79, PQ interval (ms) 153, QRS 85ms, QT 375ms, arrhythmia existed in 125 (18%) patients: premature beats in 94 (75%), LBBB in 6 (5%), RBBB in 13 (10%), atrial fibrillation in 8 (6%), atrial flutter in 3 (2%), first-degree AVB in1 (1%). Post-stress characteristics : HR (bpm) 96, PQ interval (ms) 167, QRS 85ms, QT 366ms, arrhythmia average occurred after 3 minutes of infusion: Atrial fibrillation, atrial flutter, atrial premature beats, premature ventricular beats, junctional rhythm and paroxysmal supraventricular tachycardia were observed respectively in 11 (4%), 2 (0. 7%), 137 (49%), 113 (40%), 21 (7%) and 4 (1%) patients, first, second and third-degree AVB occurred in 15 (5%), 33 (12%) and 1 patients. Most AV blocks and premature beats were resolved spontaneously after the termination of infusion. Adenosine infusion was terminated in 81 patients (12%) because of poorly tolerated side effects. There were no deaths or acute myocardial infarction.

Conclusions The incidence of arrhythmia induced by adenosine infusion is high (42% in this study), but most resolved soon after termination of adenosine infusion without special treatment. Therefore, Technetium-99m MIBI myocardial perfusion SPECT with adenosine is a safe pharmacologic stress test for Chinese patients.

18

Comparison of MRI Features of Left Ventricular Noncom action and Dilated Cardiomyopathy

Zhao SH, Yu JC, Jiang SL, Wang LM, Lu MJ, Ling J, Zhang Y, Yan CW, Liu Q, Chen HB
Cardiovascular Institute and Fu Wai Hospital, Chinese Academy of Medical Science, Beijing 100037, China

Objective The study was designed to characterize the MR features that could be useful for differentiating left ventricular noncompaction (LVNC) and dilated cardiomypathy (DCM).

Methods In the study, 25 patients with LVNC and 21 patients with DCM proved by pathologic histology after heart transplantation were analyzed with magnetic resonance imaging. Using the 17-segment model, segments of affected myocardium, severity, and myocardial function were assessed.

Results Compared with LVNC patients, enlargement of left atrium and ventricle was more eminent in patients with DCM. And the LV ejection fraction (EF) was lower in patients with DCM than in patients with LVNC. Non-compated segments were more detected in patients with LVNC than in those with DCM (9 ± 1) segments vs. (5 ± 2) segments, $P < 0.05$). Each patient with LVNC was unexceptionally associated with apical noncompaction that was not found in DCM patients. The intermediate piece and the distal piece of lateral walls including the 11th, the 12th and the 16th segments were the most vulnerable segments in all the patients. However, the basal and the middle septum including the 2nd, 3rd, 8th and 9th segments were not affected. The ratio of non-compacted segments thickness to compacted segments thickness was 3.3 ± 0.6, which was higher than that of patients with DCM ($P < 0.05$).

Conclusions CMR can differentiate between LVNC and DCM accurately.

19

MRI in Diagnosis of Constrictive Pericarditis Retrospective Study for 12 Cases Confirmed by Surgery

Zhao SH[1], Feng GS[2], Jiang SL[1], Lu MJ[1], Zhang Y[1], Yan CW[1], Wei YQ, Ling J

1, Department of Radiology[2], Cardiovascular Institute and Fu Wai Hospital, Chinese Academy of Medical Science, Beijing 100037, China

2, Department of Radiology[1], Union Hospital, Tongji Medical College, Huazhong University of Science and Technology, Wuhan 430030, China.

Objective To determine the value of MRI in diagnosis of constrictive pericarditis (CP).

Materials and **Methods** Twelve patients (8 male, 4 female) underwent MRI scan with ECG-gated SE, cine-MRI and contrast-enhanced delayed MRI. Morphology of pericardium and heart were observed. All cases were confirmed by pericardiotomy. 20 healthy subjects were used for control group.

Results All cases showed irregularly thickened pericardium of (5.08 ± 1.73) mm. Widespread thickening was detected in 5 cases, and local thickening occurred in 7 cases. Bi-atrial enlargement with relatively normal bi-ventricular cavity and enlarged inferior vena cava were noted. The left atrial diameters and the right atrial diameters of the CP patients were (36.20 ± 10.96) mm and (49.79 ± 8.74) mm, respectively, which were larger than those of the control group. In all the patients with CP, the right ventricles appeared distorted, and 8 cases showed severe deformation. Ventricular coupling was displayed clearly by cine-MRI in 10 cases. No prominent regurgitation at mitral and tricuspid valves was observed. Pericardial enhancement was found only in one patient with CP.

Conclusions MRI can not only reveal irregularly thickened pericardium, secondary enlargement of atria and inferior vena cava, but also show abnormal swinging ventricular septum. As such, MRI is considered as an ideal imaging modality for constrictive pericarditis.

20

MRI Quantification in Patients with Restrictive Cardiomyopathy and Constrictive Pericarditis

Zhao SH, Jiang SL, Cheng HB, Lu MJ, Yan CW, Zhang Y, Ling JJ, Hou B, Feng GS*

Cardiovascular Institute and Fu Wai Hospital, Chinese Academy and Medical Science, Peking Union Medical College, Beijing 100037, China

*** Department of Radiology1, Union Hospital, Tongji Medical College, Huazhong University of Science and Technology, Wuhan 430030, China.**

Objective Magnetic resonance imaging (MRI) was one of the efficient modalifies to diagnose restrictive cardiomyopathy (RCM) and constrictive pericarditis (CP). The purpose of this study was to evaluate the value of MRI in differentiating RCM from constrictive CP.

Methods The patients population included 116 patients with RCM (RCM group), 50 patients with CP (CP group), and 55 healthy volunteer served as control group. All patients had objective evidence of impaired cardiac filling and other cardiovascular diseases were ruled out. The diagnosis of RCM was based on impaired cardiac filling in combination with the absence of pericardial thickening on MRI. The diagnosis of CP was based on impaired cardiac filling in combination with the presence of pericardial thickening (>4 mm) on MRI. Quantitative measurement included bi-atrial diameters and bi-ventricular diameters, pericardial thickness, ventricular septal (IVS) thickness and left ventricular free wall thickness. Qualitative assessment was visually performed.

Results Bi-atrial diameters, ventricular septal (IVS) thickness, left ventricular free wall thickness and right ventricular diastolic diameters of RCM group were larger than those of the CP group or the control group ($P < 0.05$). The left ventricular diastolic diameters and the IVS thickness of the CP group were smaller than those of the control group ($P < 0.05$). The mean pericardial thickness in CP group was (6.09 ±

2. 31) mm. S-shaped IVS and buffeting was detected in CP group by cine-MRI. Mild mitral regurgitation occurred in 43% of RCM patients and 24% of CP patients. Moderate mitral regurgitation occurred in 21% of RCM patients and 6% of CP patients. Moderate tricuspid regurgitation occurred in 33% of RCM patients and 8% of CP patients. Severe tricuspid regurgitation occurred in 7% of RCM patients.
Conclusions MRI is a valuable imaging modality to differentiate RCM from CP.

21

The Noninvasive Cardiac Imaging Diagnostic: Agenda 2010

Paetsch I, Jin H, Gerds L, Fleck E
German Heart Institute Berlin

Over the past decade considerable progress has been made in the field of cardiac magnetic resonance imaging (MRI): today magnetic resonance imaging can provide not only accurate evaluation of cardiac anatomy and function but is widely used for the detection of myocardial ischemia (functional stress MR testing) and infarction (i. e. postcontrast "delayed enhancement" or scar imaging). For functional stress MR testing wall motion and first-pass contrast-enhanced myocardial perfusion imaging during infusion of pharmacological stressors can be used to detect even subtle areas of subendocardial ischemia, and recent studies have demonstrated the consistently high diagnostic accuracy of both stress MRI approaches (sensitivity/specificity of about 85%/85% and 90%/75%, respectively) for detecting significant coronary artery disease. Stress MR perfusion and wall motion studies are equally valuable for prognostication with negative stress MR studies resulting in a very low cardiac event rate ($<1\%$ cardiac deaths and nonfatal myocardial infarction) over the two year period following stress testing.
Direct visualization of the epicardial coronary arteries with free-breathing, whole-heart coronary MR angiography was more recently introduced and enables depiction of all three major coronary arteries within a single three-dimensional acquisition. In addition, the field of vascular wall imaging of peripheral and coronary arteries is rapidly evolving and can be expected to become an integral part of clinical routine to further improve risk stratification and prognostication. Besides vascular and functional imaging of the heart, cardiac MRI is an objective and reproducible means for diagnosing and monitoring hypertrophic, arrhythmogenic, dilated, and restrictive cardiomyopathies and myocardial texture characterization with MRI has been found to provide relevant prognostic information, particularly in hypertrophic cardiomyopathy. Moreover, tissue characterization using edema visualization with T2-weighted and postcontrast "delayed enhancement" imaging is extremely useful to detect and follow-up inflammatory disease states of myocardium and pericardium.
Ultimately, with additional refinements in MRI techniques and the establishment of standardized clinical protocols, cardiac MRI will play a pivotal role in managing patients with primary cardiomyopathies and ischemic heart disease.

22

Clinical Application of 3DRA Imaging and new Catheter-Technique for AF Ablation

Jin H, Gerds L, Paetsch I, Fleck E
German Heart Institute Berlin

Catheter ablation of atrial fibrillation (AF) has become an important therapeutic option in patients with drug-refractory AF. It has been discovered that the complexity and variability of left atrium (LA) and pulmonary vein (PV) impose a great barrier in our quest for higher success and lower complication rates recently, a new high-speed rotational angiographic technique has been developed for interventional cardiology, and has been introduced into the field of electrophysiology to visualize LA-PV anatomy. The 3-dimensional rotational angiogram (3DRA) is performed to reconstruct LA during the ablation of AF and to integrate the 3DRA by superimposition into the life X-ray fluoroscopy images. It is very helpful to have a 3-dimensional image that can give us anatomy in high detail for better understanding the given situation. The better we know the anatomy, the better we get oriented, and we can lessen the overall exposure to X-rays. Traditional radiofrequency ablation is performed in a single-tip, point-by-point ablation process. This technique requires a high degree of operator skill and procedures are lengthy. There are a significant number of complications in this technique, such as thrombo-embolism, PV stenosis, atrio-esophageal fistulae. Innovative new catheter technologies (Cryoballoon technology, Mesh-Ablator and PVAC) are being developed to make isolation safer, easier and quicker. The new technologies are a promising approach because it is relatively easy to perform and with lower complications. For example, it has been shown that cryoenergy does not lead to PV stenosis, has never been associated with atrioesophageal fistula, and has a lower thrombogenicity and so on. But there are lesions of the phrenicus nerve happening, most of those are reversible within 1-3 month. The new single ablation catheter (cryo-balloon, Mesh-Ablator and PVAC) equipped with 3DRA may be effective in the near future, fast and safely used for recording and for ablation at the LA-PV junction to create electrical isolation of PVs. (examples will be demonstrated).

23

Contrast Echo Cardiography: Current Status 2009

Armstrong WF
Director of Echocardiography Lab Internal Medicine, Cardiovascular Division, University of Michigan Medical Center

Contrast echocardiography has been used clinically and investigativally for over 30 years. Its initial applications were for chamber and border definition. At present, contrast echocardiography is utilized for detection of shunts with saline contrast echocardiography and for enhanced border detection with specialized ultrasound contrast agents. The specialized ultrasound contrast agents have also shown tremendous promise for evaluation of myocardial perfusion. The clinical utility of contrast for border detection has been clearly established in numerous studies. Contrast for ventricular left opacification results in enhanced accuracy of chamber dimensions and detection of left and right ventricular dysfunction. Its greatest incremental impact appears to be in Intensive Care Unit patients where it often results in a change in clinical management. Several recent, large studies have demonstrated the excellent safety record of contrast for left ventricular border detection. Sophisticated analyses of bioeffects of these modern, ultrasound contrast agents have also been published in which the dose and ultrasound delivery mode and power can be directly related to thresholds of adverse effects of the capillary and myocardial level. These studies have demonstrated levels of contrast dosing and ultrasound detection methods below which bioeffects are nonexistent and above which bioeffects, including cell death and capillary rupture, have been noted. The ability to identify specific combinations of contrast dosing and ultrasound delivery at which myocardial damage can be created, raises the possibility of therapeutic options for these agents. A major thrust of the investigation with newer contrast agents has been determination of myocardial perfusion. Early studies utilized a mixture of hydrogen peroxide and blood to provide a contrast agent for myocardial perfusion. Modern studies typically utilize commercially available albumin or lipid microspheres. With scrupulous attention to detail, these techniques provide a quantitative method for assessing myocardial perfusion and determining myocardial infarction size. Unfortunately, they have been limited by lack of standardization of imaging algorithms and analysis techniques.

In summary, contrast echocardiography is a safe, clinically efficacious technique for detection of shunts and enhancing evaluation of left and right ventricular function and has shown tremendous promise for assessing myocardial perfusion. Finally, therapeutic aspects of these agents have also been demonstrated with respect to potential myocardial ablative procedures, thrombolysis and gene transfection.

24

Dynamic MRI of Ferumoxide-labeled Bone Mesenchymal Stem Cells after Transplantation in the Heart

Liu Q, Zhao SH, Lu MJ, Jiang SL, Yan CW, Zhang Y, Wei YJ, Meng XM, Wang LL
Cardiovascular Institute and Fu Wai Hospital, Chinese Academy of Medical Sciences and Peking Union Medical College, Beijing 100037, China

Objective It has been demonstrated that magnetic resonance imaging (MRI) can detect magnetically labeled mesenchymal stem cells (MR-MSCs) in vivo. This study was to investigate the potential ability of MRI in tracking MR-MSCs in a swine myocardial infarction (MI) model.
Methods Adult Chinese mini pigs (n = 6) were subjected to open-chest experimental MI. Their autogeneic bone marrow-derived MSCs was cultured and doubly labled with ferumoxides and DAPI. At the 14th day after MI, labeled MSCs were injected intramyocardially into peri-infarct zone and normal myocardium. At 24 and 3 weeks after injection, The contrast and the volume of the MR-MSCs hypointense lesion from MRI were acquired, the contrast was determined using the difference in signal intensity between the hypointense and normal myocardium divided by signal intensity of the normal region. After humane euthanasia, histology corresponding to MRI slices that demonstrated MR-MSCs lesions was performed.
Results Prussian Blue staining of ferumoxides-labeled MSCs revealed the presence of iron-containing vesicles in the cytoplasm. Images of MSCs

injection sites at 24 hours after injection appeared as ovoid hypoenhancing lesions with sharp borders. The contrast [(67.00 ± 5.48) % vs. (61.92 ± 7.76) %, P = 0.1158) and the size [(0.56 ± 0.24) cm^2 vs. (0.52 ± 0.25) cm^2, P = 0.7044)] of the lesions showed no statistical difference between in peri-infarct zone and in normal myocardium. At 3 weeks after injection, the contrast of the lesions decreased and the size of the lesions diminished both in peri-infarct zone and in normal myocardium. Moreover, the contrast of the lesions in peri-infarct zone decreased rapidly than that in normal myocardium (26.88 ± 7.27 vs. 15.00 ± 4.51, P = 0.0003). Post mortem analysis showed that fluorescently labeled MSCs were demonstrated on histological sections. There were much more dense fluorescently labled MSCs per high power fields in injection sites of normal myocardium than in injection sites of peri-infarct zone (106 ± 25/HPF vs. 143 ± 31/HPF, P = 0.0293).
Conclusions Magnetic resonance imaging of MSCs is feasible and represents a method for noninvasively tracking the quantity and location of intramyocardial delivery after MI.

25

Evaluation of 3-Dimension Vectrocardiography for Diagnosis of Left Ventricular Hypertrophy

Cui CY, Ke YN, Wang Y
Department of Cardiology, China-Japan Friendship Hospital, Beijing 100029, China

Objective With regular ECG, to evaluate for 3-Dimension vector cardiographic (3D-VCG) diagnosis criteria of left ventricular hypertrophy (LVH) diagnosis, comparing with regular ECG.
Methods The left ventricular mass index (LVMI) is measured by ultrasonic cardiography (UCG). The patients were divided into the LVH group and the control group according to LVMI. The LVMI of LVH is above 97 g/m^2 for the male or 86 g/m^2 for the female. The LVMI of control is below. Correlation between 3D-VCG and ECG was analyzed in two groups respectively. Sensitivity, specificity, positive accuracy, negative accuracy and diagnosis accuracy were calculated.
Results There was significant difference between those two methods in sensitivity ($P < 0.05$), while there was no significant difference in specificity ($P > 0.05$). Positive accuracy, negative accuracy and diagnosis accuracy, of 3D-VCG were significantly higher than regular ECG.
Conclusions 3D-VCG got more details information than regular ECG. 3D-VCG is more accurate than regular ECG to detect LVMI.

26

Seizing the Science of Ultrasound: Beyond Imaging and Into Physiology and Therapeutics

McPherson DD
University of Texas Health Science Center

Clinical diagnostic ultrasound has been with us for approximately five decades. The imaging aspects of ultrasound have significantly contributed to our knowledge of cardiovascular disease. However, the potential of ultrasound, in addition to its imaging capabilities, also lies in its biological effects. The physical effects of ultrasound can be classified into two principal groups: 1) thermal and 2) mechanical. The thermal effects of ultrasound are similar to those of other localized heat sources. The mechanical effects of ultrasound include: 1) acoustic radiation forces on a structure within the body at macroscopic and microscopic levels, resulting in exerted pressure and torque; 2) acoustically induced flow, or streaming; and 3) nucleation and pulsation of bubbles, or cavitation. The latter has been further utilized by developing therapeutic microbubbles, which encapsulate agents for targeted drug delivery and gene transfection into living cells upon exposure to ultrasound. This application stems from the finding that the permeability of cell walls for large molecules (drugs and genes) is increased in the presence of ultrasound and microbubbles.
This talk will go through some principles of the physical effects of ultrasound and uses, both in physiology and in therapeutics, to improve vascular flow and to utilize ultrasound to improve directed drug and gene delivery.
The importance is that many of these techniques can be additive to other imaging and therapeutic interventions to optimize pathophysiologic effect. These techniques are at the forefront of ultrasound research and are expanding the use of ultrasound beyond the area of diagnostic imaging.

27

Correlation between TCM Syndrome of CHD and CAG Results

Li FJ, Yang Y, Yang XC, Zeng H
WangJing Hospital, China Academy of Chinese Medical Sciences, Beijing 100102, China

Objective To observe the correlation between CHD (Coronary Heart Disease) Patterns and CAG (Coronary Arteriography) results, and observe the correlation between the Syndrome of spleen deficiency with phlegm turbidity and CAG results. CAG results were reflected by pathological artery distribution and arterial stricture degree.

Methods 81 patients who were diagnosed CHD by CAG were identified TCM (Traditional Chinese Medicine) patterns and syndromes, and then the data were analyzed with SAS 8.0 software.

Results The branch amount of pathological arteries in the group of blood stasis pattern is largest; arterial stricture degree in the group of cold-accumulation pattern is deepest; the coronary pathological changes of cases in the qi-stagnation pattern group and yin-deficiency pattern group are slighter; but there are not significant difference in the CHD patterns groups. Compared with the cases which did not show the syndrome of spleen deficiency with phlegm turbidity, the LCX (Left Circumflex Artery) and RCA (Right Coronary Artery) pathological changes are more serious among the cases which show the syndrome of spleen deficiency with phlegm turbidity, and this difference between the two syndrome groups is significant.

Conclusions Coronary pathological change and the clinical symptom of spleen deficiency with phlegm turbidity may exist the correlation of cause and effect.

28

Initial Utilization of Velocity Vector Imaging in The Investigation of Plaque Motion among Patients with Acute Ischemic Stroke

Liu Y, Zhang M, Xu MJ, Jiang GH, Zhang Y
Shandong University Qilu Hospital, Jinan, Shandong 250012, China

Objective To investigate plaque motion using velocity vector imaging (VVI) and to test the feasibility of VVI in the research on acute ischemic stroke.

Methods 106 consecutive participants were enrolled in our study, of which 57 were with acute ischemic stroke and 49 were without cerebrovascular history, symptom onset within 48 hours in acute ischemic stroke group. Then, two dimensional information was acquired using a linear-array 10-14 MHz transducer, with the frame rate controlled over 60Hz. After that, five ROIs on atheromatous plaques such as the distal base, the distal shoulder, the top, the proximal shoulder and the proximal base were tracked in each image clip using syngo VVI, out of the consideration that the behaviors of plaque deformation should differ in locations under the influence of hemodynamic forces, shear stress, plaque geometry, and vessel movement. During data analysis, the removable reference mark on B-mode image clips was put in the tissue across the lumen. Motion-related parameters such as tissue velocity, strain and strain rate were exported and later processed for the maximum, the minimum and the extreme variation. According where the reference mark was placed, a positive value of velocity means the tracked site is moving towards the lumen center, while a negative one has the opposite meaning. Strain and strain rate are positive during plaque extension and negative during contraction.

Results All the motion-related parameters were lower in acute ischemic stroke group compared to in asymptomatic group, but only the maximum of velocity and maximum of strain showed a significance ($P < 0.01$ and $P < 0.05$, respectively).

Conclusions Vector velocity imaging is an angle-independent visual and quantitative method for the assessment of carotid plaque motion. The velocity of plaque contraction is slower in patients with acute ischemic stroke than in asymptomatic people. The maximum of strain is lower in patients with acute ischemic stroke than in asymptomatic people.

29

Ultrasonic Evaluation of the Effective Ejection Fraction in the Left Ventricular for Patients with Mitral Regurgitation

Cai LH, Wu GL
Dept. of Ultrasound, First People's Hospital of Anqing, Anhui 246003, China

Objective The invalid stroke volume of mitral regurgitation (MR) should be measured in the ultrasonography for patients with MR, which can help provide a comparatively accurate observed value of the effective ejection fraction (EF) in the left ventricular.
Methods 95 cases of patients with MR aged from 32 to 81 were observed, including 46 male patients and 49 female patients, with the average age of 64.5. All of the patients were diagnosed rheumatic heart disease, dilated cardiomyopathy, coronary heart disease, degenerative mitral valve or mitral valve prolapse, with different levels of mitral regurgitation (MR). A small number of reflux was observed in 30 cases of them. 33 cases of the others were in the volume of reflux and the 32 cases left were observed with a large number of reflux. Ultrasonic Doppler method diagnostic equipment of Medison 8000Live, Toshiba SSA-660, with probe frequency of 2.0-5.0 MHz were used in the research. Conventional echocardiography was taken for the patients. Simpson method was used to observe and measure the left ventricular end diastolic volume (VD4), the left ventricular end systolic volume (VS4), and the conventional left ventricular ejection fraction (LVEF4). The mitral regurgitation capacity (VMR) was calculated according to the mitral regurgitation beam. Based on the steps above, the effective left ventricular ejection fraction (ELVEF) was calculated. The formula goes as the following: $ELVEF = (VD4 - VS4 - VMR)/VD4 \times 100\%$. Then the LVEF and ELVEF of patients with different level of reflux were compared.
Results Compared to the normal value of LVEF, the effective LVEF of patients with a small number of reflux decreased by $3.6 \pm 1.3\%$ ($P > 0.05$) on average; patients with the volume of reflux decreased by $10.4 \pm 2.5\%$ ($P < 0.05$) on average; and patients with a large number of reflux decreased by $13.7 \pm 3.2\%$ ($P < 0.05$) on average. There is little statistical significance in the difference between the effective LVEF of patients with a small number of reflux and the normal value of LVEF, while there is certain statistical significance in those differences of patients with the volume of reflux and patients with a large number of reflux.
Conclusions The clinicists mainly evaluate the ultrasonic EF in LV of patients when they carry out their observation and treatment for patients with heart diseases, especially for patients with heart failure. The EF of Patients with mitral regurgitation (MR) is sometimes over-evaluated, which will result in the inconsistency between the observed EF value and the clinical symptoms of the patients. The research explained in this paper concluded that the ultrasonic evaluation of the effective ejection fraction (EF) in the left ventricular (LV) for patients with mitral regurgitation (MR) is helpful for the regulation of the over-evaluated LVEF. The significance of regulation is comparatively obvious among the patients with the volume of reflux and those with a large number of reflux. The accurate evaluation of MR is crucial for the evaluation of effective EF. Ultrasonography through esophagus can increase the accuracy of the evaluation, especially for patients with eccentric mitral regurgitation. The evaluation can take advantage of other evaluating methods, such as the formula of ELVEF calculation, observation of the frequency spectrum of dp/dt, segmental evaluation of EF value, the examination of cardiac muscle function and so on. Other factors should also be taken into account. The evaluation of the LV function is one of the criterions of the Quality Management Reform for Monotypic Disease. The ultrasonography for patients with MR should provide the accurate observed value of the effective ejection fraction so that it can be consulted by clinicists, which is helpful for them to give correct suggestions for the prophylaxis and treatment of heart failure, reducing and preventing medical tangle.

Clinical Cardiology

1

The Effect of Difference Time Taking Aspirin, Clopidogrel on Platelet Aggregation in Patients with Acute Coronary Syndrome

Li Z, Liu F, Cui W, Xie RQ, Yang XC, Ren XJ, Liu J
Department of Cardiology, The Second Hospital of Hebei Medical University and Institute of Cardiocerebrovascular Disease of Hebei Province, Shijiazhuang 050000, China

Objective To study the effect of the different time taking medicine on the circadian rhythm changes in platelet aggregation of the patients with coronary heart disease, and to choose the more effective time taking medicine.
Methods 30 patients with acute coronary syndrome were divided into, day-time and night-time medication group, when Plasma concentration reached steady state, platelet aggregation was assessed at 5 time points in one day with a mobile four-channel whole blood impedance aggregometer. The platelet aggregation was induced by ADP and arachidonic acid. Then the two groups exchanged and platelet aggregation was assessed in the same way.
Results Arachidonic acid-induced platelet aggregation after taking medication during the day was highest at 10:00 when compared to values at 0:00, but these changes did not achieve statistical significance($P > 0.05$). After night-time medication, platelet aggregation was significantly highest at 20:00 when compared to values at 10:00($P < 0.05$). ADP-induced platelet aggregation after taking medication during the day was highest at 10:00 when compared to values at 16:00 and after night-time medication, ADP-induced platelet aggregation was highest at 20:00 when compared to values at 10:00, but these changes did not achieve statistical significance ($P > 0.05$). when compared two groups at individual time points, platelet aggregation induced by two inducers was significantly highest at 10:00 in day-time group when compared to values in night-time group ($P < 0.05$).
Conclusions There was a visual tendency towards differentiated diurnal platelet response to aspirin and clopidogrel. Taking aspirin and clopidogrel during the evening was superior to intaking during the day.

2

Assessment of the Effect of Bosentan in the Treatment of Pulmonary Hypertension Early After Congenital Cardiac Surgery in Infants

Ling Y, Shen XD, Guo SX
The Department of Cardiac Surgery, Fu Wai Hospital, Beijing 100037, China

Objective To assess the effect of endotherine-1 dual-receptor blockade bosentan in treatment of pulmonary hypertension (PH) early after the operation of congenital heart diseases in infants.
Methods Children with moderate to severe pulmonary hypertension, and pediatric NYHA cardiac functional class III to IV, who discharged from mechanical ventilation and without obvious lung infection early after the congenital cardiac operation, were selected. Bosentan 3-4 mg/kg.

day were given orally. The pulmonary artery systolic pressure (PASP), left and right heart function were assessed by echocardiography, and modified Ross pediatric heart failure index (mRPHFI) before and 24-48 hours after the Bosentan therapy were compared.

Results 16 infants, 12 boys, 4 girls, aged 13.7 ± 18.4 (3-63) months were selected. The averaged weights were 6.9 ± 3.0 (4.2-13.3) kg. The operations included 7 cases of arterial switch and ventricular septal defect repair, 2 cases of double outlet right ventricular with intra-ventricular baffles repair, ventricular septal defect repair, correction of total abnormal pulmonary venous connection, and atrioventricular septal defect respectively, and one case of correction of right pulmonary artery originated from ascending aorta. 15/17 of them were with severe PAH, 2 cases were already treatment with sildenafil 1-2 mg/kg. day, and 2 cases needed continuing milrinone therapy intravenously to maintain stable Hemodynamic before given bosentan. The average dosages of bosentan were 3.2 ± 0.8 (1.9-4.2) mg/kg. day. After the Bosentan therapy, the PASP decreased from 76 ± 16 mmHg to 47 ± 14 mmHg (P = 0.00001), only in one patient the PASP decreased less than 30%, who turned to sildenafil treatment later. The left ventricular (LV) end-diastolic diameter increased (24.0 ± 4.4 mm vs. 25.3 ± 3.4 mm, P = 0.02), the right ventricular (RV) end-diastolic diameter decreased (22.4 ± 3.4 mm vs. 20.1 ± 3.6 mm, P = 0.02), and the ration of them (eccentricity index) increased markedly (1.08 ± 0.20 vs1.28 ± 0.18, P = 0.005). The LV cardiac index and RV area change fraction increased significantly (3.41 ± 0.78 L/min · m^2 to 3.81 ± 0.90/min · m^2, P = 0.04, and 0.44 ± 0.13 vs. 0.57 ± 0.06, P = 0.007). The myocardial performance index of RV by tissue Doppler image reduced from 0.75 ± 0.22 to 0.52 ± 0.20 (P = 0.04). The mRPHFI decrease from 6.9 ± 1.9 to 2.3 ± 1.3 (P = 0.00001). The average duration of bosentan administration lasted for 1.7 ± 1.3 (1-6) months. Most of them stopped the therapy one month after the treatment because of the gradually normalized pulmonary pressure. Two patients remained severe PAH six months after the operation, when the Bosentan were discontinued. The liver transaminase was all in normal range during the therapy.

Conclusions These initial data suggested that bosentan can effectively reduce the perioperative PAH, improve the left and right heart function rapidly in infants after congenital heart operation. Short-term bosentan treatment in very young, low-weighted children is safe.

3

The position of Antiplatelet therapy in secondary prevention of Vascular Diseases

Liu JM

Fuwai-Oxford Collaborative Centre for Cardiovascular Health, Cardiovascular Institute and Fu Wai Hospital, CAMS and PUMC, Beijing 100037, China

Study demonstrates that patients who are at high risk because they already have occlusive vascular diseases, long-term antiplatelet therapy with aspirin reduce the yearly risk of serious vascular events by about a quartel, 2. The Latest meta-analysis from Antithrombotic Trialists' Collaboration (ATT) also shows that the absolute benefits of aspirin in secondary prevention outweigh the risks with no heterogeneity between men and women3. The details are followed.

In primary prevention, although aspirin allocation yielded a 12% proportional reduction in serious vascular events per year (about absolute benefit 0.7/1000), the net effect on stroke and vascular death were not significant, and aspirin allocation increased major gastrointestinal and extracranial bleeds. Conversely, in secondary prevention, aspirin allocation yielded a 19% proportional reduction in serious vascular events (about net benefit 15/1000), 20% proportional reduction in major coronary event, 20% reduction in total stroke with non-significant increase in haemorrhagic stroke, 9% reduction in vascular death. Aspirin allocation increased major extracranial bleeds with less number (23 aspirin vs. 6 control).

Above all, it isn't recommended that aspirin is given to large health people. However, for secondary prevention, the benefits from aspirin substantially exceed the risks. So, if no contraindication, all patients with occlusive vascular diseases should be given aspirin for long-term. In china, at present, aspirin in secondary prevention is much more optimal4, however, there are a lot of confusion in primary prevention, it should be clarified. It is believed that this latest meta-analysis will help to the use of aspirin not only in secondary prevention, but also in primary prevention.

4

Prognostic Significance of the Serum sodium level in Patients with ST-elevation myocardial infarction

Liu Y, Yang YM, Zhu J, Liang Y, Yu LT
Chinese Academy of Medical Sciences and Peking Union Medical College, Department of Emergency, Fu Wai Hospital, Beijing 100037, China

Objective The prognostic value of serum sodium in patients with ST-elevation myocardial infarction (STEMI) has not been well defined.
Methods We analyzed 7461 STEMI patients with at least one time serum sodium measurement in the first 24 hours of hospitalization from the CREATE-ECLA trial database. The study population was categorized into three groups based on the lowest level of the serum sodium measurements: ≥135 mmol/L, 130 to134 mmol/L and < 130 mmol/L. Baseline characteristics and 30-day outcomes including mortality and other adverse cardiac events were analyzed and compared among the three groups.
Results 45.8% of the total patients developed hyponatraemia in the first 24 h and 10.9% of the patients with the lowest sodium level < 130 mmol/l. Patients in the two lower serum sodium groups were associated with more adverse baseline clinical characteristics, especially the serum sodium < 130 mmol/l patients. The 30-day mortality (16.8% versus 10.2%, P < 0.001), cardiogenic shock (10.4% versus 6.2%, P < 0.001), heart failure (23.8% versus 18.0%, P = 0.001) and life-threating arrhythmia (13.1% versus 9.0%, P < 0.001) rates were all increased in patients with sodium < 130 mmol/l compared to the patients with normonatraemia, but patients with serum sodium 130-134 mmol/l were not (P > 0.05 for the above events compared with normonatraemic group). After multivariable-adjusted analysis, the serum sodium < 130 mmol/l remains a strong and independent predictor of mortality (OR 1.44, 95% CI 1.14-1.82, P = 0.002) and the above other events. Moreover, the effect of neurohormonal activation inhibitors (ACE inhibitor and β-blocker) treatment on mortality reduction is more pronounced in patients with the serum sodium < 130 mmol/l.
Conclusions The serum sodium level < 130 mmol/l in STEMI patients during the first 24 h after admission is an independent predictor of 30-day mortality and major cardiac complications.

5

Prevalence, Management and Stroke Prevention for Non-vavular Atrial Fibrillation Patients with Hypertension

Liu Y, Yang YM, Zhu J
Chinese Academy of Medical Sciences and Peking Union Medical College, Department of Emergency, Fu Wai Hospital, Beijing 100037, China

Objective Hypertension is the most common and important risk factors for atrial fibrillation (AF) and also the independent predictor of stroke for AF patients. This study sought to determine the prevalence, management and stroke prevention pattern for Chinese non-vavular AF patients with hypertension.
Methods Consecutive patients with documented diagnosis of non-vavular AF or atrial flutter at the time of emergency department visit were recruited from January to May 2009 in 15 hospitals of 9 cities (10 tertiary and 5 secondary hospitals from 9 provinces) in China. Baseline demographics, medical history of hypertension and other risk factors for AF, management pattern including anti-hypertensive and anti-thrombotic therapy were recorded.
Results 1. A total of 501 emergency department visited patients with non-vavular AF or atrial flutter were recruited and 298 patients (58.2%) with a history of hypertension. The AF patients with hypertension were older (72 years vs. 67 years, p < 0.001) and more likely to be female (57.5% vs. 42.3%, p < 0.001) compared with patients without hypertension. The AF risk factors including coronary artery disease, diabetes mellitus, sleep apnea, left ventricular hypertrophy and left ventricular systolic dysfunction were more common among hypertension patients. 2. The average blood pressure for AF patients with hypertension were 141/85 mmHg compared with 122/76 mmHg for non-hypertension patients. 88.5% of the hypertension patients were pharmacologically treated with β-blocker (44.4%), calcium channel blocker (35.9%), diuretics (31.9%), ACE inhibitor (23.1%) and ARB (22.4%). 3. The stroke/TIA rates were significantly higher among hypertension patients compared with patients without hypertension (21.7% vs. 10.3%, p < 0.001). Hypertension patients were also associated with higher CHADS2 (Congestive heart failure, Hypertension, Age > 75 years, Diabetes mellitus, and Stroke/TIA) stroke risk score, the proportion of

score 3-6, 2, 1 for hypertension patients were38.3%, 30.0%, 31.7% versus for non-hypertensions respectively ($p < 0.001$).4. Anticoagulation by warfarin were underused in both patients with and without hypertension (9.5% vs. 9.8%, $p > 0.05$).

Conclusions A high proportion of Chinese AF patients showed hypertension, they were associated with more AF risk factors and higher stroke rates. Most of the hypertension patients were medically treated to reach the blood pressure within the normal range. Despite higher risk of thrombotic stroke, warfarin was significantly underused for AF patients with hypertension.

6

Central Aortic Blood Pressure as a Marker of Arteriosclerotic Vascular Damage and Cardiovascular Risk

Liu ZD, Lu FH, Zhao YX, Wang SJ, Jin SK, Sun SW

Cardio-Cerebrovascular Control and Research Center, Shandong Academy of Medical Sciences, 18877, Jingshi Road, Jinan, Shandong 250062, China

Objective To investigate the association between noninvasively determined central aortic blood pressures and arterial stiffness.

Methods In a cross-sectional study, structural and functional arterial properties were assessed using ultrasound and applanation tonometry in 2114 subjects.

Results Brachial pulse pressure, central arterial systolic pressure, and central arterial pulse pressure was significant higher in men compared to that in women ($p < 0.01$, respectively). Aortic augmentation index in men (25.3 ± 4.7%) was higher than in women (23.8 ± 3.4%), however there was no significant difference ($p = 0.067$). With increasing in age, both brachial blood pressure and central artery blood pressure level elevated. Brachial and central artery systolic blood pressure and pulse pressure were at higher level ($p < 0.05$, $p < 0.01$, respectively), as age increasing every ten-year. Central artery systolic blood pressure and pulse pressure increased faster than brachial systolic blood pressure and pulse pressure. Brachial systolic blood pressure and pulse pressure were higher than that in central artery in subjects at <30, 30-40, 40-49, 50-59 ($p < 0.01$, respectively) and 60-69 years ($p < 0.05$) age-stage, but they were at similar level of blood pressure at >70years age-stage. There were no significant differences in augmentation index of subjects who were at every age-stage, however, there were significant differences compared subjects at higher age-stage (50-59, 60-69, >70 years) with subjects at lower age-stage (<30, 30-39 years) ($p <$ 0.05, 0.01, 0.001, respectively). Central artery systolic blood pressure and pulse pressure was strongly correlated with age, BMI, TCH, TG, FBS, brachial blood pressure, mean and maximum IMT, stiffness β and plaque score ($p < 0.001$, respectively), and moderately with HDLc and creatinine ($p < 0.01$, respectively). Augmentation index was strongly correlated with age, TG, FBS, brachial blood pressure, central artery blood pressure, mean IMT, stiffness β and plaque score ($p < 0.001$, respectively). Parameters analyzed included age, BMI, brachial systolic blood pressure, brachial pulse pressure, augmentation index, mean and maximum IMT, and stiffness β, which were shown significant correlation with central artery systolic blood pressure and pulse pressure, TCH and FBS moderately correlated with central artery systolic blood pressure and pulse pressure.

Conclusions Noninvasively determined central aortic systolic and pulse pressure strongly related to parameters reflecting atherosclerosis. Increased central aortic blood pressures may be a simultaneous risk factor for atherosclerotic cardiovascular disease.

7

Therapeutic Value of Continuous Veno-venous Hemofiltration Administration in Treating Fulminant Myocarditis: A Retrospective Study

Ma M, Hui J, Cheng XJ

The First affiliated Hospital of Soochow University, Suzhou, Jiangsu 215006.

Objective To evaluate the therapeutic effects of continuous veno-venous hemofiltration (CVVH) in treating fulminant myocarditis (FM).

Results We retrospectively analyzed 8 cases of FM patients in our institution from March 2005 to December 2008 and reviewed our experience in treating them with CVVH. Using the paired t-test, we compared the following clinical variables between prior to and post CVVH: patient's vital signs, serum chemistry, cardiac enzyme profile, ECG, echocardiography, critical conditions, special treatments including intra-aortic balloon pump (IABP) and pacemaker, and hemofiltration parameters including initiation time, filtration speed and volume and sustaining time.

Furthermore, we summarized the clinical and hemofiltration parameters of the deceased patients and compared to survivors. We found CVVH treatment significantly ameliorated patients' condition with most of the studied clinical variables skewing within a normal range. In addition, the application of CVVH was started earlier and sustained longer in survivors than those who died.

Conclusions Early and prolonged use of CVVH is associated with increased survival rate in FM. CVVH is a potential choice of treatment for FM when other supportive treatment is not available and should be used early and sustained for at least 40 hours.

8

Nt-proBNP reflects the Cardiac Index better than LVEF and LVEDd in Patient with Acutely Decompensate Heart Failure

Mao Y, Zhang J, Wang GG, Zhu J, Yang YJ

Cardiovascular Institute and Fu Wai Hospital, Chinese Academy of Medical Sciences and Peking Union Medical College, Beijing 100037, China

Objective To investigate the correlation between invasive and non-invasive parameters of cardiac function parameters' and cardiac index, to determine their consequence to the hemodynamic of acutely decompensated heart failure.

Methods This study recruited 34 acutely decompensated chronic heart failure patients (NYHA III-IV, LVEF <40%, and a PCWP≥15 mm Hg) from Sept 2007 to Sept 2008, who agreed to accept Swan-Gans catheter inspection. Nt-proBNP, LVEF and LVEDd were tested within 8 hours before implanting the catheter. MPAP、PCWP、SVRI and CI were recorded in the process of Swan-Gans catheter examination.

Results 1, the parameters of heart function for 34 patients are as below MPAP: 34. 59 ±10. 80 mmHg, PCWP: 24. 68 ±9. 36 CmH2O, SVRI: 1480. 18 ±363. 43 dynes. s/cm5. M2, CI: 2. 28 ±0. 57 L/min · m^2, Nt-proBNP: 2537. 79 ±1256. 16 ng/L, LVEF: 26. 35 ±7. 36, LVEDd: 71. 79 ±10. 35 mm; 2, MPAP、PCWP and SVRI were all correlated with CI (r = -0. 358, -0. 309, -0. 576, P <0. 05); 3, Nt-proBNP was correlated with CI (r = -0. 356, P <0. 05), but LVEF and LVEDd was not; 4, Only MPAP was correlated with PCWP (r = 0. 822, P < 0. 05), the other parameters were not (P >0. 05).

Conclusions For the acutely decompensated heart failure patients, invasive hemodynamic parameters were correlated with CI strongly. While in the non-invasive heart functional parameters, Only Nt-proBNP was significantly correlated with CI, and LVEF, LVEDd was not. Nt-proBNP presented more importance in evaluating the hemodynamic of the acutely decompensated heart failure patients.

9

Effects of Combination Therapy to Improve Vascular Damage in Elderly Patients with Essential Hypertension

Sun SW, Lu FH, Jin SK, Sun Y

Cardiovascular Disease Control and Research Center, Shandong Academy of Medical Sciences, Jinan 250062, Shandong, China

Objective Hypertension frequently requires combination therapy to obtain efficient control and to prevent cardiovascular and cerevascular diseases effectively. This study was conducted to determine which combination treatment is better in improving vascular damage and BP controlling in combination of amlodipine and aminoacridine or telmisartan.

Methods 256 elderly patients with essential hypertension were randomly assigned to receive combination of amlodipine and aminoacridine (A group) or combination of amlodipine and telmisartan (B group) (The initial amlodipine dose was 2. 5mg/day, aminoacridine dose was 1/2 table/day, telmisartan dose was 40mg/day, adjusting to blood pressure, amlodipine dose could be add to 5. 0mg/day, aminoacridine add to 1 table/day, telmisartan add to 80mg/day.) For 12 months treatment, Pulse-wave velocity [PWV] and ankle-brachial pressure index [ABI], intima-media thickness (IMT) of carotid arteries were determined before and 12 months after the start of treatments.

Results 129 cases were assigned to combination of amlodipine and aminoacridine (A group) and 127 cases to combination of amlodipine and telmisartan (B group); 1 case in a group was lost for severe hypotension. PWV values after 12 months of treatment in two groups were significantly decreased compared to previous values (1840 ±332 cm/s to 1638 ±285cm/s, P <. 001 A group; 1851 ±320 cm/s to 1482 ±292 cm/s, P <. 001, B group), whereas ABI values and IMT were unchanged. After 12 months, mean (SD) SBP and DBP were significantly decreased from baseline in both groups (P <. 001), the changes in SBP at month 12 did not differ significantly between the two groups, the changes in DBP differ significantly between the two groups. The control rate between two group were not differ significantly (82.3% vs. 83.1%, $P > 0.05$). In addition, these were significant differ between two group in the changes in PWV ($P < 0.05$). Reduction in PWV by B group correlated significantly only with reduction in DBP ($P < 0.05$) and remained signicantly even after controlling for reduction in DBP. Reduction in PWV by A group correlated significantly with reduction in DBP and SBP and was not signicant after controlling for reduction in DBP and SBP.

Conclusions These results showed that treatment with combination of amlodipine and aminoacridine or combination of amlodipine and telmisartan functionally improve the stiffened arteries of elderly patients with essential hypertension, whereas treatment with combination of amlodipine and telmisartan is to be independent of its effects on BPs. The SBP and DBP control rate accounted for over 80% in two groups, and combination of amlodipine and telmisartan were superior to other group in DBP lowering.

10

Infective Endocarditic: Analysis of Pathogenic Bacterium and the Clinical Feature in Prosthetic Valve and Native Valve

Sun XL, Guan J, Wang GG

Department of Cardiology, Fu Wai Hospital, CAMS&PUMC, Beijing 100037

Objective To analysis the clinical characteristic and pathogenic bacterium of infective endocarditic (IE), and to compare the pathogenic microorganism and vegetation localization between the prosthetic valves endocarditic (PVE) and the native valve endocarditic (NVE).

Methods The data were collected from in-patient who fulfilled Duke Criteria for IE from May 2005 to May 2008 in Fu Wai hospital. The demographics, clinical data were analyzed retrospectively.

Results One hundred and one patients with IE suffered from congenital heart disease, 77 patients suffered from non-rheumatic valvular heart disease, and 62 patients suffered from rheumatic heart disease. Two hundred and eighteen patients (82%) with vegetation were identified, and the most common vegetation localization was aortic valve, mitral valve, and aortic plus mitral valve in turn. Bacterial cultures were positive in 49.5 percent of patients. The proportion of Gram-Negative bacillus and Fungi had risen in pathogen of IE. Detection rate of vegetation was lower in PVE group ($P < 0.01$), however the positive rate of bacterial cultures was higher ($P < 0.01$). Streptococcus, coagulase negative staphylococcus, gram-negative bacteria showed significant difference between the two groups ($P < 0.05$). The spectrum of microorganism was different between the early and the late PVE. The in-hospital mortality rate of PVE is higher than NVE.

Conclusions The spectrum of disease and pathogenic bacterium of IE has changed obviously during the past years. Early diagnosis, promptly bacterial cultures and transesophageal echocardiography, the effectively usage of antibacterial, and actively prevention of nosocomial infection seem to be effective.

11

The Value of NT-proBNP at Admission in Predicting In-Hospital Mortality in Decompensated Heart Failure Due to Valvulur Heart Disease

Wei BQ, Zhang J, Yang YJ

Department of heart failure care unit, Cardiovascular Institute and Fu Wai Hospital, Chinese Academy of Medical Sciences and Peking Union Medical College, Beijing 100037, China

Objective This study aimed to evaluate the value of plasma NT-proBNP at admission in predicting in-hospital mortality in patients with decompensated heart failure due to valvulur heart disease.

Methods Plasma NT-proBNP levels were measured in patients with decompensated heart failure due to valvulur heart disease within 24 hours after admission with ELISA method. The NT-proBNP levels were compared between dying non-survival patients in hospital and survival patients at discharge. ROC analyses were performed to evaluate if plasma NT-proBNP at admission was a predictor for in-hospital mortality and identify the optimal NT-proBNP cut-point for predicting in-hospital mortality. A binary logistic regress analyses was used to evaluate if NT-proBNP was an independent predictor for in-hospital mortality.

Results Total of 293 patients with decompensated heart failure due to valvulur heart disease was enrolled in his study, the number of NYHA classes Ⅱ, Ⅲ, and Ⅳ was 31 cases, 161 cases and 101 cases respectively. 24 cases of the 293 patients died in hospital. The plasma NT-proBNP levels of these cases were much higher than that of survivals [4995.9 (3436.7, 6799.6) pmol/L vs. 1597.8 (777.7, 3537.9) pmol/L, $P<0.01$]. ROC analysis of plasma NT-proBNP to predict in-hospital mortality had an area under the curve (AUC) of 0.815 (95% CI: 0.735-0.896, $P<0.01$), the optimal plasma NT-proBNP cut-point for predicting in-hospital mortality was 3500 pmol/L, with a sensitivity of 75.0%, a specificity of 74.3%, an accuracy of 74.4%, a positive predictive value of 20.7% and a negative predictive value of 97.1%. Patients whose NT-proBNP levels were equal or more than 3500 fmol/ml had a much higher in-hospital mortality (20.7%), compared with that (2.9%) in those with NT-proBNP levels less than 3500 pmol/L ($P<0.01$). Binary logistic regress analyses demonstrated that, in factors such as age, sex, body mass index, systolic blood pressure, diastolic blood pressure, heart rate, NYHA class, serum creatinine levels, plasma NT-proBNP levels, atrial fibrillation, anemia, pneumonia, abnormal liver function and high bilirubinemia, plasma NT-proBNP at admission and pneumonia were selected as independent predictors for in-hospital mortality in patients with decompensated heart failure due to valvulur heart disease ($P<0.05$ or 0.01). And plasma NT-proBNP at admission was the strongest predictor for in-hospital mortality.

Conclusions Plasma NT-proBNP level at admission was an independent predictor for in-hospital mortality in patients with decompensated heart failure due to valvulur heart disease. The optimal NT-proBNP cut-point for predicting in-hospital mortality was 3500fmol/ml.

12

Clinical Analysis of 21 cases of Isolated Pulmonary Takayasu's Arteritis

Xiong CM, Liu ZH, He JG, Ni XH, Cheng XS
Pulmonary Vascular Disease Center, Cardiovascular Institute and Fu Wai Hospital, Chinese Academy Medical Science and Peking Union Medical College, Beijing 100037

Objective To summarize the clinical characterizations of isolated pulmonary Takayasu's arteritis.

Methods The clinical features, the sites of pulmonary artery involvement and the level of pulmonary hypertension were analyzed retrospectively in 21 patients.

Results In our series of patients, the most was in female, the ratio of male and female was 1: 4.3, Palpitation and dyspnea on exertion were the most frequent symptoms. Erythrocyte sedimentation rate (ESR) and C-reaction protein (CRP) were elevated in 7 patients (33.3%) and 9 patients (42.9%) respectively. Bilateral pulmonary arteries involvement were observed in 16 patients (76.2%). The trunk and branches of right pulmonary artery were involved in 19 patients (90.5%), the trunk and branches of left pulmonary artery were involved in 18 patients (85.7%). Nineteen patients (90.5%) were associated with pulmonary artery hypertension, sixteen of which had mildly and severely elevated in pulmonary artery pressure levels. Misdiagnosis was found in 14 patients (66.7%).

Conclusions Isolated pulmonary Takayasu's arteritis is not rare. Early diagnosis and treatment can slow development of pulmonary hypertension. There is poor prognosis in patients with severe pulmonary hypertension.

13

Pulmonary Hypertension Associated with Hereditary Hemorrhagic Telangiectasia: 8 cases Report and Literature Review

Xiong CM, Liu ZH, He JG, Ni XH, Cheng XS
Pulmonary Vascular Disease Center, Cardiovascular Institute and Fu Wai Hospital, Chinese Academy Medical Science and Peking Union Medical College, Beijing 100037

Objective To improve identification of Pulmonary hypertension associated with hereditary hemorrhagic telangiectasia.

Methods Case analysis and literature review.

Results There were 6 female and 2 male patients with average age of 40 years old. the ratio of male and female was 1: 3, All patients met diagnostic criteria of hereditary hemorrhagic telangiectasia. Palpitation and dyspnea on exertion were frequent symptom. Except clinical manifestation of HHT, 8 patients were associated with severe pulmonary artery hytertension with average pulmonary arterial systolic pressure of

92 mmHg. All patients were misdiagnosis for idiopathic pulmonary arterial hytertension.
Conclusions Pulmonary hypertension associated with hereditary hemorrhagic telangiectasia is not common, it has been often misdiagnosed.

14

The Perindopril and Carvedilol Treatment on Coronary Heart Disease Complicated with Diastolic Heart Failure

Yan J
Dehui City, Jilin Province People's Hospital

Objective To evaluate the effects of perindopril and carvedilol on patients with coronary heart disease complicated with diastolic heart failure.
Methods We selected 16 cases with coronary heart disease in line with the diagnostic criteria of diastolic heart failure without contraindication for application of perindopril and carvedilol. The patients received the basic conventional treatments, such as drugs to improve coronary circulation, nutrition drugs for cardiomyocytes and appropriate amount of diuretics. All patients were prescribed perindopril and carvedilol tablets. Started from small doses and adjusted the dose weekly until the target dose or maximum tolerated dose was reached. After the maximum tolerated dose was determined for the patients and the patients were in stable condition, the patients were then discharged and continued the medication of perindopril and carvedilol tablets for 6 months. Finally, the cardiac function before and after the medication was evaluated. The cardiac function improved significantly in 8 cases after the treatment, 6 cases were effective, 2 cases were ineffective, the total effective rate was 87.5%. Before and after treatment, systolic blood pressure were 138 ± 16 mmHg and 122 ± 12 mmHg; diastolic blood pressure were 76 ± 8 mmHg and 67 ± 6 mmHg; heart rate were 94 ± 11 beats/min and 72 ± 7 beats/min; 6-minute walk test distance were 231 ± 123 meters and 392 ± 138 meters. Compared to the values before treatment, heart rate, 6-minute walk test distance were significantly improved ($P < 0.01$).
Conclusions The effects of perindopril and carvedilol tablets on treatment of coronary heart disease complicated with diastolic heart failure were significant.

15

Continuous Renal Replacement Therapy Combines with Reducing The Heart Preload to Treat the Severe Acute Left Heart Failure After Cardiovascular Operations

Yang R, Yu CT, Chang Q
Cardiovascular Institute and Fu Wai Hospital, Chinese Academy Medical Science and Peking Union Medical College, Beijing 100037

Objective This study was to reduce the heart preload and the heart acting to promote heart function restoration.
Methods Six patients with severe acute left heart failure were enrolled (LVEF < 30%, pulmonary artery wedge presses (PAWP) > 20 mmHg). Four kinds positive inotropic drugs were used to maintain circulation stability. CRRT and mild hypothermia (34℃) were applied to reduce the preload of the heart, and the mean arterial pressure was 68 mmHg.
Results After 6-day of CRRT, the left heart function was improved. The core temperature was rewarmed to 36.5℃, and the MAP were increased to > 80 mmHg. Five of the patients discharged from hospital and one died.
Conclusions The application of CRRT accompanied the therapeutic mild hypothermia can reduce the preload of the heart and improve the left heart function after cardiovascular operations. It is a new method for treatment the severe left heart failure.

16

Clinical Outcome of Patients with Diabetes Mellitus and Acute Myocardial Infarction Treated with Drug-Eluting Stents

Yang SL, Liu HL, Zhang H, Jin LM, Liu Y, Luo JP, Ma DX
Department of Cardiology, the General Hospital of Chinese People's Armed Police Forces, Beijing 100039, China

Objective The prognosis of patients with acute myocardial infarction (AMI) and diabetes mellitus treated with percutaneous coronary intervention (PCI) and drug-eluting stent (DES) implantation is unknown.
Methods We compared the 12-month outcomes of 46 diabetic patients with AMI after successful PCI who underwent DES implantation with that of 45 patients with diabetes and AMI previously treated with bare-metal stents (BMS). Death, myocardial infarction and repeat PCI or coronary artery bypass surgery were considered as a combined primary endpoint.
Results At 1-year follow up, the primary endpoint occurred in 2.2% ($n = 1$) of patients treated with DES and 8.9% ($n = 4$) of the patients treated with BMS ($p < 0.01$). One patient in the DES group and 2 patients in the BMS group died during follow up ($p > 0.05$). Logistic regression analysis identified DES (odds ratio [OR] = 9.6, $p < 0.01$), total occlusion (odds ratio [OR] = 8.1, $p < 0.01$) and final minimal lumen diameter (odds ratio [OR] = 10.1, $p < 0.01$) as independent correlates for major adverse cardiac events (MACE) at follow up.
Conclusions In patients with acute myocardial infarction and diabetes mellitus, DES were superior to bare-metal stents in reducing the MACE and should be considered a preferred treatment strategy for patients with diabetes and AMI undergoing PCI.

17

Efficacy of 9-month Intervention on Prehypertensives Assessed by 24-hour Ambulatory Blood Pressure Monitoring

Yao GT, Lu FH, Liu ZD
Shandong Academy of Medical Sciences, Jinan 250062, China

Objective To investigate the significance of antihypertensive drug treatment with the combination of lifestyle intervention in different treatment groups of patients with prehypertension by evaluating the change of 24-hour Ambulatory Blood Pressure Monitoring (ABPM) before and after the 9-month test.
Methods According to "Guide to Prevention and Treatment of Hypertension in China (2005 revision)" Repeated casual blood pressure (CBP) measurement in line with the mean blood pressure 120-139/80-89 mmHg for prehypertension was recommended. 236 cases with prehypertensives in normal subjects were sieved out who were randomly divided into 3 groups: Non-intervention group (A group) 66 cases, Simple lifestyle intervention group (B group) 87 cases, Lifestyle intervention and oral telmisartan group (C group) 83 cases. All the subjects were performed 24 h ABPM before and after the 9-month test. Lifestyle intervention: Emphasized the importance of rational diet, salt restriction, exercise, especially advised smoking cessation, drinking limitation, weight control to those who used to the lifestyles and issued them the healthy lifestyle guide. Telmisartan treatment: After 2 weeks of the introduction period, telmisartan, 40mg, po, qd.
Results 1) The level of blood pressure: 24 h SBP increased by 4.59 ± 3.27 mmHg, 24 h DBP by 2.60 ± 1.63 mmHg in group A ($P < 0.05$); 24 hSBP decreased by 4.7 ± 3.15 mmHg, 24 h DBP by 2.21 ± 1.59 mmHg in group B ($P < 0.05$); 24 hSBP decreased by 19.74 ± 9.32 mmHg, 24 h DBP by 10.62 ± 5.38 mmHg in group C ($P < 0.05$). Compared to group A and B, 24 h SBP and 24 h DBP in groupC decreased remarkably ($P < 0.01$). There was a significant difference between group A and B ($P < 0.05$). 2) Before and after test, SBPF was $12.53 \pm 6.52\%$ and $12.21 \pm 5.99\%$, DBPF $11.33 \pm 3.25\%$ and $11.27 \pm 3.07\%$ in group A, SBPF was $12.41 \pm 6.64\%$ and $12.98 \pm 6.52\%$, DBPF $11.67 \pm 3.72\%$ and $11.75 \pm 3.69\%$ in group B. There was a significant difference between group A and B ($P < 0.05$). SBPF was 12.58% and 14.58%, DBPF 11.22% and 15.57% in group C ($P < 0.01$). The ratio of non-dipper BP in group C declined from 25.3% to 20.48% ($P < 0.05$). The ratio of non-dipper BP was not significant changed in group A and B ($P > 0.05$). 3) Before and after test, variation coefficient of 24 h SBP was 18.22 ± 4.87 and 18.54 ± 5.02, 24 h DBP 15.34 ± 2.28 and 15.86 ± 2.46 in group A; 24 h SBP17.39 ± 4.90 and 16.91 ± 4.29, 24 h DBP15.11 ± 2.35 and 14.58 ± 1.96 in group B; 24 h SBP17.26 ± 4.75 and 15.24 ± 4.29, 24 h DBP 13.17 ± 2.12 and 10.04 ± 1.85 in group C. 4) T/P in SBP was 67.2%, in DBP was 80.1%. It was more effective to the control of DBP than SBP.
Conclusions Lifestyle intervention can reduce the level of blood pressure, prevent from the increasing of blood pressure level, but have limited

impact on blood pressure rhythm. It is safe and effective that lifestyle intervention and oral telmisartan treatment for the control of blood pressure especially DBP in 24 h in patients with prehypertensives, and it has a great significance for the improvement of circadian rhythm.

18

The Clinic Research of Myocardial Contrast Echocardiography in Evaluating Blood Supply of Left Ventricular Aneurysm Walls and the Severity of Coronary Artery Stenosis

Yao KC, Li WX, Hou SS
Department of Ultrasound, Air force General Hospital, Beijing 100142

Objective To explore perfusion characteristics of the blood supply of left ventricular aneurysm walls by myocardial contrast echocardiography and to study its relationship with coronary artery stenosis.

Methods Twenty-one cases of aneurysm with old myocardial infarction had echocardiography and myocardial contrast echocardiography examinations by using Philips iE33 color ultrasound. The Philips iE33 ultrasound has the most advanced real-time myocardial contrast imaging analysis procedures and related software. All patients had coronary artery stenosis disease confirmed by coronary angiography and consented all exams. After finished conventional echocardiography, the intravenous access was established in all patients. Clearly showed the aneurysm, 2ml SonoVue was injected rapidly through his left elbow using bolus intravenous injection. SonoVue is widely used in clinical cardiac imaging and has a good effect. After injection, aneurysm and surrounding normal myocardial wall of the myocardial perfusion was continuous real-time observed.

Results Conventional echocardiography showed that 21 cases had apical aneurysm, the size was (2.4 ± 1.2) cm, and there was no thrombosis in the aneurysm cavity, and 12 myocardial segments show unclear (12/63). Coronary angiography showed 9 cases had 2 coronary arteries stenosis, and other 12 had 3 coronary arteries stenosis. After myocardial contrast echocardiography examinations, the endometrial and segments of myocardial wall were showed clearly. The effects of myocardial contrast were divided into four types. Type I: 13 cases had uniform perfusion imaging, but the perfusion was more osteoporosis than the normal myocardium, 9 cases with 2 coronary artery diseases and other with 3 coronary artery diseases. In addition to left anterior descending artery, the stenosis of other coronary arteries was less than 50%. Type II: six patients had sparse imaging, excepting left anterior descending artery, the stenosis was less than 75%. Type III: one had weak image and his coronary artery stenosis was more than 75%, the left anterior descending artery was almost entirely occlusion. Type IV: one patient with cardiac insufficiency was no perfusion, and his left anterior descending artery was almost entirely occlusion and the stenosis of coronary artery was more than 90%.

Conclusions The myocardial imaging of aneurysm is closely related to the degree and the number of coronary artery stenosis. The myocardial contrast echocardiography can not only clearly display myocardial segments and endometrial of myocardial walls, but also provide the objective and precise diagnose information for the blood supply of left ventricular aneurysm walls, at the same time, can offer valuable clinical reference for the aneurysm therapy.

19

Percutaneous Transluminal Septal Myocardial Ablation in Hypertrophic Obstructive Cardiomyopathy

Yuan JS, Qiao SB, You SJ, Gao RL, Duan FJ, Tian YQ, Yang WX, Hu FH, Chen JL
Department of Cardiology, Cardiovascular Institute and Fu Wai Hospital, Chinese Academy of Medical Sciences and Peking Union Medical College, Beijing 100037, China

Objective Evaluating the acute effect of Percutaneous transluminal septal myocardial ablation (PTSMA) as a treatment for hypertrophic obstructive cardiomyopathy (HOCM).

Methods PTSMA was performed in-122 patients with symptomatic HOCM. All patients had echocardiography performed before the procedure, three to seven days and six months after the procedure.

Results Procedure success was achieved in 99 patients, success rate was 81.1%. The average left ventricular outflow tract (LVOT) gradient was 95.96 ± 37.65 mmHg before the procedure, 51.68 ± 34.93 mmHg three to seven days post-PTSMA ($p < 0.001$) and 48.39 ± 39.13 mmHg six month post-PTSMA ($p<0.001$). The thickness of inter ventricular septum (IVS) was 21.95 ±4.88 mm before the procedure, 20.91 ± 4.60 mm three to seven days post-PTSMA ($p<0.05$) and 16.94 ±4.18 mm six month post-PTSMA ($p<0.05$). In 3 patient (2.45%) occurred ventricular fibrillation, but recovered well thereafter. Right bundle branch block occurred at a rate of 47.5% (58 in 122 patients). Balloon-induced dissections of the LAD did not occur. Acute mitral regurgitation also did not occur. Transitory trifascicular blocks occurred at a rate of 58.2% (71 in 122 patients). Only one patient (0.82%) underwent permanent pacemaker implantation due to permanent trifascicular block. Two patients (1.63%) died. One was because of alcohol leakage down the Left anterior decencending coronary artery, another occurred drug-induced liver injury.

Conclusions PTSMA is an effective non-surgical procedure for symptomatic patients with HOCM with low risk and significant hemodynamic and echocardiographic improvement.

20

Clinical Prognostic Value of Low Diastolic Blood Pressure Hypertension in Patients with Coronary Artery Disease

Zhao X, Han YL, Zhang XY, Tong M, Xu FZ
Department of Cardiology, Shenyang General Hospital of Military, Shenyang, Liaoning 110016, China.

Objective To evaluate the clinical prognostic value of low diastolic blood pressure hypertension (200 mmHg > systolic blood pressure > 140 mmHg and diastolic blood pressure < 60 mmHg) in patients with coronary artery disease.

Methods Patients with CAD in our hospital from July 2006 to December 2008 were included in this study. All selected patients were not treated with drug and diet control. Patients were divided into low diastolic pressure hypertension group ($n=48$) and control group (normal diastolic pressure, $n=48$) which were analyzed on total mortality and the risk for major adverse cardiac events (MACE, including death, recurrent MI, recurrent angina, heart failure, readmission for any reason) in inhospital, 30 days and 3 months after discharge from the hospital.

Results The 3-months mortality of low diastolic pressure hypertension group and control group was 1.3% and 0.7% and 3-month incidence of MACE was 17.9and 7.1% respectively. Multivariate logistic regression analyses showed that the low diastolic pressure hypertension predicted 30-day ($r=0.2090$, $P<0.01$) and 3-month ($r=0.2391$, $P<0.01$) mortality and 30-day ($r=0.266$, $P<0.05$) and 3-month ($r=0.2011$, $P<0.05$) incidence of MACE independent of traditional risk factors such as age, gender, family heredity, hypercholesterolemia, diabetes, smoking and LVEF.

Conclusions Low diastolic pressure hypertension is a good predictor for early mortality and MACE incidence in CAD patients.

21

Predictors of Stress-Hyperglycemia and Short-term Prognostic Impact on Acute Myocardial Infarction

Zhao ZY[1], Liu B[2], Wang XM[1], Song GY, Pei HJ[1], Chen JL[1], Yang YJ[1], Gao RL[1], Wu YJ[1]
1Center for Diagnosis and Treatment of Coronary Heart Disease
2Department of Biostatistics Division, Cardiovascular Institute and Fu Wai Hospital, CAMS and PUMC, Bejing 100037, China

Objective To evaluate the predictive factors and prognostic impact for stress-hyperglycemia phenomenon after ST segment elevation acute myocardial infarction (AMI) during primary percutaneous coronary intervention (PCI) era.

Methods From august 2005 to apirl 2009, a total of 329 patients without diabetes were admitted to FuWai-Hospital within 12 hours after the onset of ST segment elevation AMI. Plasma glucose was measured in the second day. Stress-hyperglycemia was defined as the fast glucose in the second day ≥7.0 mmol/L. Factors related to stress-hyperglycemia were analyzed by logistic regression model. The risk of death and major adverse cardiovascular events (MACE) were analyzed by multivariate Cox proportional hazard regression model in-hospital.

Results Stress-hyperglycemia occurred in 121 out of 329 patients. Older age [(64 ± 12.3) vs. (58 ± 12.1), $P<0.001$], women[(33.1% vs. 13.9%, $P<0.001$)], killip class ≥ II [(52.9% vs. 16.0%, $P<0.001$)], blood glucose level[(9.11 ±3.27) vs. (5.38 ±0.44), $P<0.001$], the incidence of death (16.5% vs. 3.8%, $P<0.001$) and MACE (20.7% vs. 6.7%, $P<0.001$) were significantly higher in stress-hyperglycemia patients than that in patients without hyperglycemia. Logistic regression analysis showed that patients with older age[odds ratio (OR) 1.024, 95% confidence interval (CI) 1.001to 1.047, $p=0.043$], women[OR 3.013, 95% CI 1.617 to 5.616, $p=0.001$], more killip class[OR 2. 161, 95% CI 1. 532to 3. 048, p < 0. 001] were independent predictors of stress hyperglycemia. Multivariate Cox proportional hazard regression model showed that stress-hyperglycemia was independent predictors of in-hospital mortality [OR 2. 459, 95% CI 1. 022 to 5. 921, p = 0. 045] and MACE[OR 1. 994, 95% CI 1. 022 to 5. 921, p = 0. 047].

Conclusions Older age, women, more killip class were independent predictors of stress-hyperglycemia with AMI. Stress-hyperglycemia after AMI was an independent predictor of in-hospital MACE and mortality.

22

Gender and Age Difference in Trends of Acute Myocardial Infarction Events: a 15 years (1999-2008) Single Center Report

Zheng X, Li JJ, Yang YJ
Coronary heart diseases center, Cardiovascular Institute and Fu Wai Cardiovascular Hospital, CAMS and PUMC, Beijing 100037, China

Objective To analyze the gender and age difference in trends of acute myocardial infarction (AMI) events over the 15-year period (1994-2008).

Methods The medical records with the diagnosis of coronary heart disease and acute myocardial infarction in Fu Wai cardiovascular hospital during 1994-2008 were reviewed. The proportion of female patients, mean age and peak onset age were calculated according to time period, first and recurrent events and gender.

Results During 1994-2008, 11859 patients with AMI including 9737 first and 2122 recurrent cases were admitted to Fu Wai hospital. The number of cases per year has been increasing over the years (P < 0. 001). In the first and recurrent cases, the proportion of female patients was 21. 9% and 20. 4%, respectively. The proportion of female patients over years was similar. Among the first cases, the mean age of all males was 56. 40 ± 12. 00 years, with a decreasing linear trend over years (P < 0. 01). The mean age of males was 60. 58 ± 10. 09 years in 1994 and 55. 26 ± 11. 54 years in 2008. And the peak onset age declined from 55-64 years to 45-54years. The mean age of females in first cases was 65. 68 ± 10. 25 years, without significantly change over the years (P > 0. 05). And the peak onset age has increased from 55-64 years to 65-74years. In recurrent cases, the mean age of males was 62. 80 ± 11. 66 years, with a decreasing linear trend over years (P < 0. 05). While the mean age of females was 70. 18 ± 8. 77 years, with an increasing linear trend over years as well (P < 0. 05).

Conclusions During last 15 years, the number of patients with AMI admitted to Fu Wai hospital has been increasing. In first onset cases, the onset age of males has been decreasing over years, while the onset age of females remained stable relatively. In recurrent onset cases, the onset age of males was with a decreasing trend over years, while that of females was with an increasing trend. In both first and recurrent cases, the proportion of females remained unchanged.

23

Hemodynamic Effects and Safety of Non-ionic Contrast Medium Bolus Injection During Pulmonary Angiography in Patients with Pulmonary Hypertension

Zhang HL, Wang Y, Luo Q, Zhao ZH, Zhao Q, Xiong CM, Ni XH, He JG, Liu ZH
Center for Pulmonary Vascular Disease, Fu Wai Hospital, Chinese Academy of Medical Sciences, Peking Union Medical College
Center for Pulmonary Vascular Disease, Fu Wai Hospital, Beilishi Road 167, Xicheng District, Beijing 100037, China.

Objective To investigate the changes of right heart hemodynamic parameters and incidence of complications in patients with pulmonary hypertension (PH) who had undergone pulmonary angiography with non-ionic contrast medium.

Methods All patients who underwent pulmonary angiography for pulmonary hypertension were consecutively enrolled in Center for Pulmonary Vascular Diseases, Fu Wai Hospital between Jan 2008 and Jun 2009. Pulmonary angiography was performed with a 6-French pigtail catheter through standard right femoral vein or right jugular vein access with the placement of a 6-or 7-French vascular sheath. Main pulmonary artery angiography on posterior-anterior position were routinely performed, additional selective right or left pulmonary artery angiography and subselective injections were performed at the discretion of the attending physician. Contrast medium injection rates ranged from 12-to 17-ml/second, and volumes for contrast medium ranged from 30 to 45 mL when performing main pulmonary artery angiography, and 20 to 35 mL for right or left pulmonary artery angiography per injection. All patients received non-ionic contrast medium, with 82 (86.4%) receiving Iopromide and the remainder receiving Iopamidol. Before and after diagnostic angiography, heart rate, right atrial pressure, right ventricular systolic, diastolic and end of diastolic pressure, pulmonary arterial systolic and diastolic pressure, and mean pulmonary arterial pressure and complications were obtained.

Results Ninety-seven patients had undergone pulmonary angiography, in which two patients were exclude because they had normal pulmonary arterial pressure. There were 38 men (40%) and 57 women (60%) with a mean age of 37.47 ± 12.45 years. The pulmonary hypertensions were idiopathic in forty patients (42.1%), chromic thromboembolic in 25 (26.3%), associated with connective tissue disease, congenital heart disease and other causes in 16 (16.8%), 11 (11.6%) and 3 (3.2%) respectively. They had a mean pulmonary arterial pressure of 60.35 ± 17.92 mmHg, and the mean volume of contrast medium was 75.73 ± 29.82 ml (range 30-150 ml). After pulmonary angiography, heart rate mildly decreased (86.40 ± 14.73 beats per minute vs. 84.33 ± 13.61 beats per minute, P = 0.004); right atrial pressure, right ventricular diastolic pressure and pulmonary arterial systolic pressure slightly increased (10.26 ± 6.60 mmHg vs. 11.89 ± 6.49 mmHg, P = 0.001; 5.23 ± 5.79 mmHg vs. 7.38 ± 7.05 mmHg, P = 0.004; 95.00 ± 25.23 mmHg vs. 97.87 ± 26.13 mmHg, P = 0.002, respectively); right ventricular end of diastolic pressure tended to increase, but did not reach the significance level (14.59 ± 7.30 mmHg vs. 16.49 ± 10.50 mmHg, P = 0.054). Right ventricular systolic pressure, pulmonary arterial diastolic pressure and mean pulmonary arterial pressure were not significantly different before and after pulmonary angiography. However, after controlling for volume of contrast medium, only right ventricular diastolic pressure slightly increased (5.23 ± 5.79 mmHg vs. 7.38 ± 7.05 mmHg, P = 0.045). Seven patients (7.37%) experienced complications, none of them were fatal. When accessing right femoral vein, one patient experienced breathless, bradycardia and hypotension, which were disappeared after giving nasal cannular oxygen, atropine 0.5 mg and dopamine 3 mg. When passing the pigtail catheter through right ventricle, four patients had premature ventricular contractions, and one patient had supraventricular tachycardia; after administrated amiodaronum 150 mg, the supraventricular tachycardia turned to normal sinus rhythm. And one patients had severe cough when injection of contrast medium, which resolved spontaneously.

Conclusions Pulmonary angiography with 30-150 ml non-ionic contrast medium at an injection speed of 12-to 17-ml/second in patients with pulmonary hypertension is safe. It has little effect on heart rate and right heart hemodynamic paramiters except right ventricular diastolic pressure slightly increases and the complication is low.

24

Homocysteine-lowering And Cardiovascular Disease: Is The Door Closing Now

Clarke R

The B-Vitamin Treatment Trialists' Collaboration, Clinical trial Service Unit, University of Oxford, Oxford, United Kingdom

Elevated plasma total homocysteine levels have been associated with risk of cardiovascular disease in observational studies, but the efficacy and safety of supplementation with B-vitamins to lower homocysteine levels is still uncertain. The B-Vitamin Treatment Trialists' Collaboration was set up to combine individual participant data from all randomized trials assessing the effects of lowering homocysteine levels with B-vitamins on risk of vascular and non-vascular outcomes. Among the 11 large-scale trials involving more than 1000 participants treated with folic acid or placebo for at least one year, data were available on 37, 485 participants in 8 trials completed before 2009 for the 1st cycle of this collaboration. The primary analysis assessed the effects on major vascular events (MVE), stroke, major coronary events (MCE), any incident cancer and cause-specific mortality. Additional analyses assessed the effects on vascular and cancer outcomes in sub-groups defined by age, sex, population level of fortification and pre-treatment levels of folate and homocysteine and duration of treatment. On average, the meta-analysis assessed the effects of lowering homocysteine levels by 24% for 5 years. Allocation to B-vitamins had no beneficial effects on vascular outcomes with hazard ratios (95% confidence intervals) of 1.01 (0.97 to 1.06) for major vascular events, 1.03 (0.96 to 1.09) for major coronary events and 0.96 (0.87 to 1.06) for stroke, with no benefits in sub-groups by sex, age, folate status or duration of treatment. Allocation to B-vitamins had no significant effect on cancer (1.06 [0.99 to 1.14]) overall, or in any pre-specified sub-groups, or on total mortality (1.02 [0.97 to 1.08]). Supplementation with B-vitamins did not reduce the risk of cardiovascular events or mortality, nor did it have any effect on cancer. These results do not support the routine use of B-vitamins for the prevention of cardiovascular diseases.

25

Primary and Secondary Prevention of Cardiovascular Diseases in the Community. Facts and Fiction.

Fodor JG
University of Ottawa Heart Institute, Ottawa, Ontario, Canada.

Since the 1970s there has been a steady and rapid decline in the cardiovascular (CVD) mortality of males and females in western Europe and North America (WEST). No such similar decline has been observed in low and medium income countries (EAST).
To achieve a successful control of CVDs in EAST, the determinants of success in the WEST should be assessed.
It is generally believed that smoking cessation, healthy diet and exercise are keys to community oriented preventive strategies. The beneficial effect of smoking cessation on reduction of CVD mortality is well established. Smoking was reduced in most countries of the WEST (e. g. in the UK) from 45% in 1974 to 22% in 2006.
However, evidence linking changes in nutrition or physical activity to CVD prevention is weak.
On the other hand, control of hypertension by aggressive pharmacological therapy and intensive professional and public education has proven successful, particularly in Canada and the U. S. Acute coronary care, percutaneous interventions, thrombolytic and antiplatelet therapy have resulted in an approximate 50% reduction of stroke and coronary heart disease mortality.
A successful CVD prevention policy in low and middle income countries should be based on strategies of proven efficacy and effectiveness. The first priority of public health policies should be the control of hypertension and anti-smoking measures.

26

Fifteen Most Important Randomized Trials/Advances in Interventional Cardiology 2008/2009

Ellis SG
Section Head, Invasive Cardiology, Cleveland Clinic Foundation

Interventional cardiology continues to be one of the medical subspecialties that best supports their practice of evidence base medicine. The field continues to evolve rapidly. This report will summarize the results of 15 studies reported in 2008 or 2009 expected to directly impact daily practice. These include HORIZONS (demonstrating the clinical benefit of bivälirudin in ST-segment elevation myocardial infarction), FINESSE (demonstrating overall lack of benefit of two facilitated approaches for patients undergoing delayed primary PCI), TAPAS and subsequent meta-analysis (demonstrating the benefit of simple aspiration thrombectomy for patients with STEMI), SYNTAX (helping to clarify the respective roles of bypass surgery and intervention with patients with multi-vessel disease) the mega-meta analysis of DES vs. Bare Metal Stent (supporting the general use of DES in many subgroups of patients), ENDEAVOR IV, SPIRIT III, SORTOUT III and ZEST (all providing further information on the use of second generation drug-eluting stents), TRITON-TIMI 38 (establishing the benefit of Prasugrel across multiple populations, but also raising issues about risk) and PARTNER and WATCHMAN (establishing or seeking to establish the role of new percutaneous therapies for patients with aortic stenosis and atrial fibrillation respectively). In general, derived information from these studies suggests continuing rapid evolution of the field.

27

Premature Deaths Attributable to Blood Pressure in China

Jiang H, Gu DF, Chen J, Wu XG, Kelly TN, Huang JF, Chen JC, Chen CS, Bazzano LA, Reynolds K, Whelton PK, Klag MJ
Tulane University School of Public Health and Tropical Medicine and School of Medicine, New Orleans, LA, USA;
Cardiovascular Institute and Fu Wai Hospital, Chinese Academy of Medical Sciences and Peking Union Medical College, and National Center for Cardiovascular Disease, Beijing, China;
Kaiser Permanente Southern California, Pasadena, CA;
Loyola University Medical Center, Maywood, IL, USA;
Johns Hopkins Bloomberg School of Public Health, Baltimore, MD, USA.

Background Hypertension is a major global-health challenge because of its high prevalence and concomitant risks of cardiovascular disease. We estimated premature deaths attributable to elevated blood pressure in China.

Methods We conducted a prospective cohort study in a nationally representative sample of 169, 871 Chinese adults aged 40 years and older. Blood pressure and other risk factors were measured at a baseline examination in 1991 and follow-up evaluation was conducted in 1999-2000. Premature death was defined as mortality before 72 in men and 75 years in women. The numbers of total and premature deaths attributable to blood pressure were calculated using population-attributable risk, mortality, and the population size of China in 2005.

Findings Hypertension and pre-hypertension were significantly associated with increased all-cause and cardiovascular mortality. We estimated that in 2005, a total of 2. 33 million cardiovascular deaths (95% confidence interval, 2. 21-2. 45) were attributable to elevated blood pressure in China: 2. 11 million (2. 03-2. 20) in hypertensives and 0. 22 million (0. 19-0. 25) in pre-hypertensives. In addition, a total of 1. 27 million premature cardiovascular deaths (95% confidence interval, 1. 18-1. 36) were attributable to elevated blood pressure in China: 1. 15 million (1. 08-1. 22) in hypertensives and 0. 12 million (0. 10-0. 14) in pre-hypertensives. The majority of blood pressure-related deaths were from cerebrovascular diseases, 1. 86 million (1. 76-1. 96) total deaths and 1. 08 million (1. 00-1. 15) premature deaths.

Interpretation Elevated blood pressure is the leading preventable risk factor for premature mortality in the Chinese general population. The prevention and control of this condition should receive top public-health priority in China.

28

Redefining Myocardial Infarction for the Twenty-first Century

Alpert JS
Professor of Medicine, Department of Medicine, University of Arizona Health Science Center, Tucson, Arizona; Editor-in-Chief, American Journal of Medicine

Progress in the identification and quantification of biochemical markers of myocardial injury has led to a redefinition of myocardial infarction (MI). The World Health Organization previously defined acute MI as a combination of at least two of the following three components: symptoms consistent with an acute MI, ECG changes diagnostic of an acute MI, and a temporal pattern of enzyme rise and fall consistent with myocardial cell death. The enzyme that was employed in this traditional definition was creatine kinase (CK) and its MB subfraction. Unfortunately, CK and CKMB measurements failed to identify a subgroup of patients with an acute coronary syndrome (ACS) who were at increased risk for morbidity and mortality. Troponins are molecules that are integral parts of the myocardial contractile machinery. An elevated blood troponin level has been shown to be a more specific and sensitive marker for myocardial injury than CK or CKMB. Indeed, blood troponin determinations can detect minute quantities of necrotic myocardium. Revision of the current WHO definition for acute myocardial infarction (AMI) occurred in 2001. This redefinition made blood troponin determination a critical component in the identification of myocardial cell death. The new definition of acute MI now includes patients with ACS and elevated blood troponin levels despite normal blood determinations for CK and CKMB. It is important to identify these patients because they experience a reduction in risk of morbidity and mortality with specific therapy. The clear association of troponin elevation with increased mortality along with the availability of therapy that diminishes this risk has led to the current redefinition of acute myocardial infarction. The new definition identifies this previously unidentified and undertreated high risk population. The original definition report, published simultaneously in the European Heart Journal and Journal of the American College of Cardiology in 2000, reviewed the reasoning and the data that led to the new definition of acute MI. Since previously unidentified, small myocardial infarcts are now being detected, the new definition of MI has many implications including changes in therapy, epidemiology, and public policy. New research, performed over the years since the original definition was published made it imperative to update the definition of MI. An international task force concluded work on the universal definition of MI which was simultaneously published in the European Heart Journal, Circulation, and the Journal of the American College of Cardiology. The new universal definition still uses blood troponin values as a gold standard for identifying ischemic myocardial infarction. Changes from the document of 2000 include a new categorization of patients with MI into 5 subclasses including a sudden death category. Non-invasive imaging for the diagnosis of MI is covered in much greater detail in the new document. This lecture will discuss the changes in the global definition of myocardial infarction that have been incorporated into the 2007 document.

29

Assessing the Effects of Novel Treatments for Pulmonary Arterial Hypertension on Pulmonary Vascular and Cardiac Remodeling

Wilkins M
Experimental Medicine and Toxicology, Imperial College London, Hammersmith Hospital

The current treatments for pulmonary arterial hypertension (PAH) target pulmonary vascular tone and attempt to address an imbalance in circulating and locally produced vasoconstrictors and vasodilators; namely restoring prostacyclin and cyclic GMP activity and inhibiting endothelin. New treatments for PAH are directed more at the structural vascular changes that characterize the condition. There is also greater interest in improving right ventricular function. This poses a challenge to the early assessment of efficacy-the important stage in drug development when decisions are made about investments in large scale clinical trials. First, drugs that act to reduce pulmonary vascular resistance by altering vascular structure and address cardiac remodeling might be expected to take longer to demonstrate evidence of benefit than drugs that act on vascular tone. Second, there is the problem of measuring changes in vascular structure in vivo. Cardiac magnetic resonance (CMR) is an excellent tool for assessing right ventricular mass and function and is increasingly used in clinical trials. Novel biomarkers are required to signal structural changes in blood vessels in response to a drug. Imaging tools may offer a solution, particularly techniques used to answer questions on drug efficacy in oncology studies.

30

Assessment on the Effect of Standardization Management for Hypertension in the Community in Huai'an City

Pan EC, Hu W, Xiang QY, Wang ZW
Huai'an Center for Disease Control and Prevention, Huai'an 223001, China

Objective To assess the effect of standardization management for hypertension in the community in Huai'an City.
Methods In the community, 28777 cases of hypertension were screened and managed according to the uniform protocol by the trained physician.
Results After a standardization management, the average systolic blood pressure and diastolic blood pressure went down by16.56 mmHg and 8.97 mmHg, respectively. The awareness rate, the treatment rate, control rate and treatment control rate of hypertension increased from 83.53%, 66.20%, 3.93% and 4.42% to 100%, 99.40%, 38.73% and 41.81% with statistical significant difference ($p < 0.01$), respectively. The proportion of level 2 and level 3 of high blood pressure dropped from 50.01% to 10.94%; by repeated measure analysis in 2822 cases, the average blood pressure had a downtrend with the more management frequency.
Conclusions The results of this study indicated that the community based standard management for hypertension was an effective way to modify unhealthy lifestyle, enhance medication compliance and control of blood pressure, reduce complications and improve the quality of life in the community.

31

Why Do We Need Gendermedicine

Mahmoodzadeh S, Vera RZ
Institute for Gender in Medicine, Charite University Medicine, Berlin, Germany.

It is still largely unrecognized that gender differences in frequent diseases play a great role in clinical medicine. Knowledge on very important sex and gender differences is still rather poor. Women get older than men, and the manifestations of many diseases differ between both genders, as do outcomes after therapeutic interventions. Myocardial infarction and coronary bypass surgery both have a greater lethality in young women than in young men, stroke is becoming increasingly frequent in younger women, heart failure presents as systolic failure in men and diastolic failure in women and the tako-tsubo cardiomyopathy affects almost only women. Autoimmune diseases and depression are more frequent in women than in men and diabetes is a greater risk factor in women than in men. Prevention, diagnostic and treatment strategies and access to health care and management also differ between women and men. In many of these fields, women do worse.

It is largely unknown that women do have a higher likelihood to die from cardiovascular disease and stroke than men. Major sex-dependent risk factors for cardiovascular disease include hypertension, aging, obesity and diabetes. Hypertension is more frequent in women. Obesity and diabetes lead to more severe increase of cardiovascular risk in women. At the vascular level, interactions between free radicals and the protective NO system plays a role. In addition, less intensive treatment and less careful diagnosis are obvious. The latter was just documented by the Euro Heart Survey published in 2006. Therapeutic cardiovascular interventions carry a greater risk in women. Particularly younger women have a higher mortality after coronary artery bypass surgery compared with men of the same age group and risk factor profile. Pacemakers, mechanical circulatory support, heart and kidney transplantation is differently used among women and men and has different outcomes. Psychosocial risk factors do play a greater risk in women compared with men.

Drug associated side effects occur more frequently in women and this is true in all disciplines of internal medicine. In drug development and use, sex differences in body composition, liver enzymes and kidney function are frequently neglected. Most drugs are developed in young male mice. However female animals differ in most cardiovascular stress tests significantly from the male animals. Effects of estrogen may provide benefit to premenopausal women and the loss of these protective mechanisms may render the heart and other organs of postmenopausal women more vulnerable. In addition, sex-specific gene expression and proteins and interaction with hormones may contribute to differences in women and men. Gender medicine offers a great chance to treat both genders specifically and therefore better; it helps women and men.

32

Clinical Practice on Warfarin Personalized Medicine

Zhong XB
Department of Pharmacology, Toxicology, and Therapeutics, University of Kansas Medical Center, 3901 Rainbow Boulevard, Kansas City, Kansas 66160, USA

Warfarin is the most widely prescribed anticoagulant because of its effectiveness for preventing thrombosis and embolism. However, warfarin is also one of the leading drugs to cause adverse events because of its narrow ranges of therapeutic index and toxicity. Accurately dosing warfarin both initially and for maintenance is a big challenging in clinical practice. Recent studies on genome-wide scan for common genetic variants and on clinical pharmacogenetic analysis with a large sample size indicate that common variants in VKORC1 and CYP2C9 genes along with other non-genetic factors correlate significantly with warfarin dosing. I will discuss how to apply the pharmacogenetic information on clinical practice of warfarin for personalized medicine. Furthermore, I will discuss recent findings on epigenetic regulation of VKORC1 gene expression in human liver and discuss approaches to identify epigenetic mechanisms related to pharmacoepigenetics of warfarin in future basic and clinical research.

33

L-Carnitine and Cardiovascular Disease-from Basic Science to Clinical Applications

Bai YY, Sun L, Liu JH, Sun RT
The Key Laboratory for Clinical Cardiovascular Genetics & Sino-German Laboratory for Molecular Medicine, Cardiovascular Institute & Fu Wai hospital, Chinese Academy of Medical Sciences & Peking Union Medical College, Beijing, China.
Hypertension Division, Cardiovascular Institute & Fu Wai hospital, Chinese Academy of Medical Sciences & Peking Union Medical College, Beijing, China.
National center for Pharmaceutical Screening, Institute of Materia Medica Chinese Academy of Medical Sciences & Peking Union Medical College, Beijing, China.

Background Acute and chronic L-carnitine application exerts protective effects in a number of cardiac diseases. These favorable effects are attributed to improvements of the energy metabolism and have been found both in animal experiments and in man. The aim of this systematic review is to investigate the effect of oral L-carnitine substitution on cardiovascular diseases.
Methods We systematically searched PubMed, Cochrane Library, Embase, reviews, and reference lists of relevant papers. The search strategy paired the term "levocarnitine OR L-carnitine" with the following: "coronary heart disease", "myocardial infarction", "heart failure", "peripheral artery disease", "cardiovascular disease" and "trial". All trials were included if they addressed the research question and provided outcome data for intervention and control subjects. Two reviewers independently assessed trials. Differences were resolved by consensus. Treatment effects were summarized as weighted mean differences (WMD) with 95% confidence intervals by using random or mixed effects model.
Results In small short-term studies, L-carnitine acts as an antianginal agent that reduces ST segment depression and left ventricular end-diastolic pressure. In a meta-analysis of four studies, compared with placebo, a significant attenuation of left ventricular dilation in the first year after acute myocardial infarction was observed in patients treated with L-carnitine (end-diastolic volumes[EDV]: WMD 8.16ml, 95% confidence interval-10.44 to-5.88, $P<0.001$; end-systolic volumes[ESV]: WMD 3.97 ml, 95% confidence interval-4.72 to-3.21, $P<0.001$). No significant differences were observed in left ventricular ejection fraction changes over time in the two groups (WMD 0.26%, 95% confidence interval-0.59 to 1.11, $P=0.551$). It was also showed that treatment with L-carnitine produced statistically significant increases in maximal walking distance and initial claudication distance in patients with peripheral vascular disease.
Conclusions L-Carnitine supplementation may be important to any therapeutic strategy designed to benefit patients suffering from ischemic heart disease, heart failure, and peripheral vascular disease. Future studies in this area are of clinical importance.

34

Clinical, Biochemical and Angiographic Characteristics of Patients with Early Onset Coronary Heart Disease in Chinese

Chen GL, Liu LW, Xie S, Liu H, Liu YQ, Li YS
Key Laboratory of clinical Trial Research in Cardiovascular Drug Ministry of Health, Cardiovascular Institute and Fu Wai Hospital Peking Union Medical College and Chinese Academy of Medical Science, Beijing 100037, China

Objective The purpose of this study was to investigate Clinical, angiographic, and biochemical features in patients with early onset coronary heart disease.
Methods 76 consecutive patients with clinical onset of coronary heart (CHD) disease at age ≤45 years, 164 older patients with clinical onset of disease at ≥55 years and 45 age matched healthy subjects were enrolled in the study. All patients had documented coronary artery disease by angiography. Angiographic features, clinical risk factors and biochemical features were compared between these groups.
Results Compared with healthy subjects, early onset CHD patients showed more prevalence in hypertension (43.4 vs. 15.6% $p<0.01$), diabetes (26.3 vs. 8.9% $p<0.05$), smoking (71.1 vs. 44.4%; $p<0.01$) and Family history of coronary artery disease (34.2 vs. 13.3%; $p<0.05$). Mean plasma total cholesterol and low density cholesterol level was $4.95 \pm 1.95$and 2.81 ± 0.96 mmol/L in early onset CHD patients and $4.68 \pm 0.97$and 2.60 ± 0.97 mmol/L in late onset CHD patients ($p=NS$). Younger patients, however, had lower high-density lipoprotein cholesterol (0.96 ± 0.18 mmol/L and 1.16 ± 0.26 mmol/L; $p<0.01$), lower Apia-I levels (571.95 ± 82.35 mg/L and 873.95 ±

203. 37 mg/L; $p < 0.01$), higher plasma triglyceride levels (2. 26 ± 1. 29 mmol/L vs. 1. 76 ± 0. 77 mmol/L; $p < 0.05$), higher lipoprotein (a) levels (151. 82 ± 169. 56mg/L and 79. 83 ± 49. 15mg/L; $p < 0.01$), higher high-sensitive CRP (1. 88 ± 2. 03 mmol/L vs. 0. 69 ± 0. 74 mmol/L; $p < 0.05$), Mean uric acid level was 320. 16 ± 77. 37 umol/L vs. 305. 30 ± 84. 74 umol/L (p = NS) in early and late onset CHD group.

Compared with late onset CHD group, 42. 1% patients presented with acute myocardial infarction ($p < 0.001$), but the number of coronary artery involved, severity of coronary artery stenosis and Gensini score did not show significant difference ($P > 0.05$). As to the clinical and biochemical risk factor only prevalence of hypertension (43. 3 vs 59. 8% $p < 0.05$), HDL level (0. 96 ± 0. 18 mmol/L and 1. 10 ± 0. 27 mmol/L; $p < 0.01$), higher high-sensitive CRP (1. 88 ± 2. 03 mmol/L vs. 2. 99 ± 3. 28 mmol/L; $p < 0.05$) showed significant different.

Conclusions Our findings reconfirmed that hypertension, diabetes, heavily smoking, family history, high plasma triglyceride, low HDL cholesterol levels and Apia-I are associated with early onset coronary artery disease. Of them Apia-I may be a valuable alternative marker for evaluating CHD. Coronary angiography showed no obvious angiography characteristics compared with late onset CHD.

35

Characteristics of the 24 h Ambulatory Blood Pressure in the Patients with Renal Artery Stenosis

Chen PP, Jiang XJ, Huang JF
Hypertension Center, Cardiovascular Institute and Fu Wai Hospital, PUMC and CAMS, Beijing 100037, China

Objective To investigate the characteristics of the 24 h ambulatory blood pressure in the patients with renal artery stenosis.

Methods A total of 123 patients (80 males and 43 females) with renal artery stenosis (RAS) were recruited from outpatients and patients hospitalized in Fu Wai hospital & Cardiovascular Institute (Beijing, China), whose mean age was 43. 9 ± 18. 0 years. All patients were identified by renal arteriography and had no history of interventional therapy. The 24 h ambulatory blood pressure monitoring (ABPM) and blood pressure at clinic were obtained from each patient.

Results The mean systolic pressures in the clinic, the 24 h, daytime and nighttime increased significantly (155. 50 ± 27. 11 mmHg, 137. 08 ± 20. 82 mmHg, 140. 02 ± 21. 02 mmHg, 131. 33 ± 21. 94 mmHg, respectively). The decline rate of the ambulatory systolic blood pressures in the nighttime was 6. 21%. The mean diastolic pressures were 92. 10 ± 21. 22 mmHg, 81. 39 ± 15. 34 mmHg, 83. 68 ± 15. 34 mmHg and 76. 87 ± 15. 63 mmHg, respectively, and the decline rate of the ambulatory diastolic blood pressures in the nighttime was 8. 14%. 78% of the patients with renal artery stenosis had less than a 10% decline in BP at night, which was referred to as non-dippers. The 24 h, daytime and nighttime diastolic pressures in male patients were higher than that in female. The 24 h and daytime systolic pressures and the 24 h, daytime and nighttime diastolic pressures in patients with age < 45 were higher than those in patients with age ≥ 45 ($P < 0.05$). The daytime and nighttime systolic pressure loads were 47. 54% and 65. 10%, while the loads of diastolic pressure were 35. 21% and 42. 48%, respectively for those patients.

Conclusions The study showed that patients with renal artery stenosis had high ambulatory systolic pressures. The altered diurnal rhythm of BP, and increased systolic and diastolic blood pressure loads revealed the existence of target organ damage in those patients. The results of ABPM could provide evidence for antihypertensive and interventional therapy and evaluate the effect of treatment.

36

Influence of Statins in Coronary Flow Reserve of Patients with Slow Coronary Flow

Fan Y, Yang SS, Huang YL
Department of Cardiac Medicine, First Affiliated Hospital, Haerbin Medical University, Haerbin, Heilongjiang, 150001

Objective To investigate changes of coronary flow reserve (CFR) of patients with slow coronary flow and effects of statins in CFR.

Methods 91 patients with chest pain and slow coronary flow but normal coronary angiography were involved, and they were divided into two groups, statin group and no statin group. Treatments of atrovastatin 20mg were given to statin group for 8 weeks. 26 healthy subjects with normal angiography and negative exercise ECG test served as controls. Blood cholesterol was measured. Doppler measurements of distal left anterior descending (LAD) were recorded at rest and hyperemia state by adenosine infusion (140 $\mu g \cdot kg^{-1} \cdot min^{-1}$), and CFR was calculated by the ratio of maximal hyperemia and baseline peak diastolic coronary flow velocity (hCFV and bCFV) before and after treatment of atrovastatin 20 mg.

Results 1. After treatment of Atrovastatin, statin group had lower total cholesterol and LDL-C than no statin group and control group [total cholesterol (3.83 ± 0.80) mmol · L^{-1} vs. (5.30 ± 1.18) mmol · L^{-1} vs. (5.32 ± 1.17) mmol · L^{-1}, P < 0.05; LDL-C (2.26 ± 0.64) mmol · L^{-1} vs. (3.28 ± 0.85) mmol · L^{-1} vs. (3.30 ± 0.82) mmol · L^{-1}, P < 0.05]. 2. CFR in those patients of statin group and no statin group was lower than that of control group before treatment (2.32 ± 0.30 vs. 2.25 ± 0.33 vs. 3.15 ± 0.34, P < 0.05). Compared with no statin group and statin group before treatment, statin group after treatment had lower bCFV [(26.06 ± 3.22) cm · s^{-1} vs. (29.02 ± 3.36) cm · s^{-1} and (26.06 ± 3.22) cm · s^{-1} vs. (28.43 ± 3.40) cm · s^{-1}, P < 0.05], higher hCFV [(77.63 ± 8.96) cm · s^{-1} vs. (65.17 ± 7.22) cm · s^{-1} and 77.63 ± 8.96) cm · s^{-1} vs. (64.58 ± 6.26) cm · s^{-1}, P < 0.05] and higher CFR (3.07 ± 0.29 vs. 2.28 ± 0.35 and 3.07 ± 0.29 vs. 2.32 ± 0.30, P < 0.05), Furthermore, bCFV, hCFV and CFR in statin group was similar to that of controls (P > 0.05).

Conclusions Patients with slow coronary flow had lower CFR. Treatment of atrovastatin 20mg for 8 weeks could improve CFR while lowering cholesterol.

37

Comparative Study of Clinical Characteristics Between Impaired with Normal Left Ventricle Function of Patients with Triple Coronary Artery Disease

Gao Z, Yang YJ, Xu B, Qiao SB, Gao RL

Cardiovascular Institute and Fu Wai Hospital, CAMS 100037

Background Ischemic cardiomyopathy is one of the fatal courses of coronary heart disease; its clinical characteristics still need to be identified.

Methods From April 2004 to April 2007, 4494 consecutive patients with triple coronary artery disease identified by coronary angiogram (> 70% stenosis of each vessel) in our center were divided into two groups according to left ventricle ejection fraction (LVEF) (N group: n = 4129, LVEF > 40%; L group: n = 365, LVEF ≤ 40%).

Results Patients in L group was younger (60.6 ± 9.72 vs. 65.2 ± 10.7 years; p < 0.001). There were more previous myocardial infarction (MI) and diabetes and less hypertension and hyperlipidemia in L group (83.3% vs. 47.0%; p < 0.001, 34.0% vs. 28.0%; p = 0.018, 57.5% vs. 62.0%; p = 0.005 and 27.7% vs. 37.9%; p < 0.001, respectively). Logistic regression analysis indicated that the age, previous MI, diabetes, previous percutaneous coronary intervention (PCI) and hyperlipidemia were independent indexes to left ventricle function of triple vessel disease (HR: 0.988, 95% CI: 0.977-0.999, HR: 5.825, 95% CI: 4.371-7.762, HR: 1.422, 95% CI: 1.122-1.803, HR: 0.694, 95% CI: 0.504-0.955 and HR: 0.704, 95% CI: 0.549-0.902, respectively).

Conclusions Results from this one center, large sample study showed clinical characteristics of ischemic cardiomyopathy previous, MI and diabetes might contribute to its impaired left ventricular function, and PCI might prevent it.

38

Profound Thrombocytopenia Induced by Clopidogrel with a Long-term Safe Administration Before

Guo LY, Li JJ, Yuan JQ, Qin XW, Zheng X, Mu CW, Hua YH

Department of Cardiology, Fu Wai Hospital, Chinese Academy of Medical Sciences, Peking Union Medical College, Beijing 100037, People's Republic of China.

Clopidogrel, in combination with aspirin, is commonly used for the prevention of thrombosis in patients who have received coronary artery stents. Moreover, it shows an excellent safety and tolerability as well as its efficacy since its marketing. However, there were still cases of clopidogrel-associated serious adverse effects reported, including thrombocytopenia and severe allergic reaction (including cutaneous reactions and angioedema). Here we reported a rare case with profound thrombocytopenia after clopidogrel administration once again for another coronary stent. It reminds us that thrombocytopenia might be induced by clopidogrel even with a safe history of long-term administration before.

39

The Clinical Meaning of Mixed Venous Oxygen Saturation after Acute Myocardial Infarction

Han RJ, Sun K
Central Hospital of Baotou, Inner Mongolia

Objective To observe the Clinical meanings of mixed venous oxygen saturation (SvO2) in patients after acute myocardial infarction (AMI).
Methods 160 patients with AMI were included. The cases were divided into two groups according to the SvO2: SvO2 >60% (group A n = 80) and SvO2 ≤60% (group B n = 80); SvO2 and cardiac index (CI) were measured after four weeks; Left ventricular end-systolic volume (LVESV), End-diastolic Volume (LVEDV) and Left Ventricular Ejection Fraction (LVEF) were measured by PHILIPS color Doppler flow imaging system; Record the incidence of adverse events of patients.
Results The general situation in the two groups, including gender, age, and complications (diabetes, hypertension); the differences were not statistically significant ($P > 0.05$).

40

Morphological Characteristics of Left Ventriculography in Patients with Hypertrophic Cardiomyopathy

He C, Yuan JQ, Gao RL
Coronary Heart disease Division, Cardiovascular Institute and Fu Wai Hospital, CAMS and PUMC, Beijing 100037, China

Objective To determine the morphological characteristics of hypertrophic cardiomyopathy (HCM) by left ventriculography from a right anterior oblique projection, 74 patients were analyzed 14 patients with obstructive HCM (HOCM), 60 patients with no obstructive HCM (HNCM).
Methods 74 patients with hypertrophic cardiomyopathy were diagnosed with ventriculography and ultrasonography. The left ventricular outflow tract pressure gradient ≥30 mmHg was defined as HOCM, while the gradient ≤30 mmHg was defined as HNCM. Statistical analysis was performed using R software methods for small samples.
Results (1) in 74 patients, 14 cases (18.9%) were HOCM (6 cases of SAM, 3 cases of coronary heart disease), 60 cases (81.1%) were HNCM (11 cases of coronary heart disease). (2) Ultrasonography: septal wall thickness was 13.1 ± 4.8 mm, posterior wall thickness was 10.4 ± 2.7 mm, LV end-diastolic inner diameter (LVEDD) was 47.8 ± 5.1 mm, LA anterior posterior diameter was 36.2 ± 5.00 mm. (3) left ventriculography: LV end-diastolic volume indexes (LVEDV) was 124.4 ± 31.8 ml, LV end-systolic volume indexes (LVESV) was 27.7 ± 12 ml, ejection fraction was 78% ± 7%. (4) Morphological characteristics: In 14 cases of HOCM 5 cases normal, 9 cases abnormal. In 60cases of HNCM, 27 cases normal, 33 cases abnormal.
Conclusions (1) there is no significant difference between two groups in LVEDD, LVEDV, LVESV, (2) there is no significant difference between two groups in EF, both of them are higher than normal. (55%-65%) (3) There is no significant difference between two groups in LV morphological characteristics.

41

The 6 Month Mortality After Acute Myocardial Infarction in Women and Men

Hu FH, Yang YJ
Cardiovascular Institute and Fu Wai Hospital, CAMS and PUMC, Beijing 100037, China

Objective To be assessing the clinical, and angiographic features, procedural characteristics and in-hospital results of women suffering AMI and comparing their results with those of a group of men throughout the same period.
Methods Consecutive patients (n = 723) presenting to coronary care between Jan 2005 and Apr 2008 with acute ST segment elevation myocardial infarction (AMI) were recruited. Details of the presentation and management were obtained from the medical notes. The primary endpoint

was three month all cause mortality.

Results Of these patients 30. 1% (218/723) were female. Mean age of women was (71. 3 ± 11. 5) and (63. 5 ± 12. 2) for men ($p < 0.001$). There was no difference between the sexes for delay in presentation or treatment or for ST elevation infarction site. Women had prior hypertension more than men (47. 2% 103/218 vs. 35. 0% 177/505, $p = 0.007$). Women were less likely to have diagnostic catheterisation (67. 8% 149/218 vs. 82. 1% 415/505 $p = 0.0009$). Both genders had similar coronary artery disease extent and frequencies of LV impairment (EF < 45%) and were equally likely to undergo revascularisation (75. 8% 113/149 vs. 80. 9% 336/415 p = NS). There was an excess 6 month mortality among women (9. 6% 21/218 vs. 4. 9% 25/505 in men $p = 0.007$). The rate that combination of death, MI and all ischemic drived revascularization was higher in women than that of in men (17. 2% 34/197 vs. 12. 9% 62/480, $P = 0.04$). Independent predictors of 3 month mortality by logistic regression analysis were age (OR 1. 08, 95% CI 1. 02-1. 12, $p < 0.001$) and LV impairment (OR 0. 29, 95% CI 0. 14-0. 57, $p < 0.001$).

Conclusions The rate of mortality in women post AMI 6 months is higher than that of men. It might be due to older age in women.

42

Relationship between Serum Visfatin Concentration and Coronary Artery Disease

Huang F, You S, Zeng HS

Huazhong University of Science and Technology, Tongji Hospital, Tongji Medical College of Wuhan City, Hubei, No. 1095 Jiefang Road.

Objective To investigate the plasma visfatin levels and explore the relationship between visfatin and coronary artery disease.

Methods 69 coronary heart disease (CHD) patients identified by coronary angiography were recruited and divided into 2 groups according to their coronary angiographic characteristics and clinical histories in this investigation: 37 of acute coronary syndrome patients; 32 of stable angina patients; 24 control subjects were recruited in this study. The serum visfatin concentration of the subjects was measured by ELASA method to determine the relationship between the serum visfatin concentration and coronary heart disease.

Resluts The serum visfatin concentrations in the CHD group (SAP and ACS) [(31. 01 ± 16. 66) mg/L, (46. 4 ± 19. 03) mg/L] were significantly higher than those in the control group [(18. 24 ± 6. 45) mg/L], ($p < 0.05$, $p < 0.01$). The different concentrations between ACS group and SAP group also showed significant difference in statistics, $P < 0.05$. Visfatin may be a singificant variance to the morbidity of CHD.

Conlusions The visfatin concentration of the CHD group is significantly higher than those of the control group. The lever of serum visfatin concentration may be an indicator for evaluation of CHD.

43

Analyses of Safety from 439 Endomyocardial Biopsy Procedures via the Right Internal Jugular Vein Approach

Huang J, Yang YJ, Feng L, Yin D

Cardiovascular Institute and Fu Wai Hospital, Chinese Academy of Medical Science and Peking Union Medical College, Beijing 100037, China

Objective Primary Indications for endomyocardial biopsy include heart transplant rejection surveillance and the evaluation of cardiomyopathy or arrhythmia for possible myocarditis. EMB procedures have not been gained widespread accepted because of concerns of possible complications associated with EMB procedures. Our single-center retrospective study analyzed the incidence of major and minor EMB procedure-related complications of 439 EMBs over a 4. 5-year period.

Methods From May, 2004 to Dec, 2008 with the use of a modified Cordis bioptome, 15 patients with cardiomyopathy and 1 patient with suspected cardiac tumors underwent 16 EMB procedures. 131 heart transplant recipients underwent 423 EMB procedures, and all EMB procedures via the right internal jugular vein approach and taking EMBs from the RV septum under fluoroscopic guidance without any additional echocardiographic control. Operators were allowed to perform EMB procedures alone independently if a minimum of 50 EMB procedures had been previously supervised by a senior operator. All patients underwent a 12-lead electrocardiogram (ECG), 12-hour continuous ambulatory ECG monitoring, chest x-ray and a transthoracic echocardiography before and after EMB procedures to obtain a detailed evaluation of the incidence of conduction abnormalities, arrhythmias, pericardial effusions and worsening valve insufficiency.

Results No major complications like cardiac tamponade, hemothorax and pneumothorax occurred. Minor complications such as conduction abnormalities including RBBB were temporary (lasting <24 hours after EMB procedures) in 2 cases (0.47%) and sustained (>24 hours) in 1 case (0.23%). There were no cases of A-V block, complex ventricular arrhythmias or episodes of atrial fibrillation. In addition, 4 (0.91%) cases of mild-moderate tricuspid regurgitation induced during the EMB procedure was diagnosed by echocardiography. All complications did not result in significant long-term consequences.

Conclusions The EMB procedure via the right internal jugular vein approach under fluoroscopic guidance has a very low complication rate when performed by experienced operators.

44

Curative Effect Observation of Qi-benefiting and Yang-waring, Blood-Activating and Water-Disinhibiting on the Treatment of Coronary Heart Disease Heart Failure

Jiang H, Liu M, Yu H

The second hospital of Baoding city in Hubei province

Objective We observed the curative effect of: Qi-benefiting and yang-waring, Blood-Activating and Water-Disinhibiting in therapy of coronary heart disease (CHD) heart failure.

Methods The one hundred patients were divided randomly into the treatment group and the control group, and both groups were underlayed routine therapy, but the treatment group treated with: Qi-benefiting and yang-waring, Blood-Activating and Water-Disinhibiting, Qili Qiangxin capsule and the control group treated with dummy respectively. The six minutes walking experiment, the heart function and the rehospitalization rate of patients were observed after six-month treatment.

Results The six minutes walking experiment and the heart function of the treatment group surpassed the control group, and rehospitalization rate of the treatment group were significantly lower than the control group.

Conclusions By use of: Qi-benefiting and yang-waring, Blood-Activating and Water-Disinhibiting, Qili Qiangxin Capsule, the heart faction of the CHD heart failure patients was improved, the six-minute walking distance was increased, and rehospitalization rate was decreased.

45

Normal Reference Range and Internal Quality Control for Serum Cardiac Troponin I Measurement

Kang JS, Wang KJ, Jing N

Cardiovascular Institute and Fu Wai Hospital, Chinese Academy of Medical Sciences and Peking Union Medical College, Beijing 100037, China

Objective This study investigated the serum cardiac troponin I (cTnI) concentrations of healthy people in Beijing, and established the upper limit of reference range of local laboratory. The quality control method was also determined to provide more dependable evidence for the diagnosis of myocardial infarction.

Methods The study enrolled 162 healthy people in Beijing, including 80 males and 82 females. The enrolled people were divided into 10 groups by gender and age (21-40, 41-50, 51-60, 61-70, >70). Using Access2 automatic immune analyzer, the 99 percentile values of serum cTnI in healthy people and the cTnI concentration under 10% day variation were determined. Then we compared the variations of different concentrations of quality control product and home-made mixed serum, and determined the blank detection limit of the analyzer by using the matching buffer of Access AccuTnI reagents as a blank. According to the light quantum value of the blank, the warning value of the blank detection limit was accounted as the mean plus 2 times of the standard deviation.

Results a. The cTnI levels of 162 cases of healthy people in Beijing were skewed distribution, and there was no significant difference among different age (P = 0. 262) or gender groups (P = 0. 468). The 99th percentile value was 0. 0487 ng/ml, corresponding to the intra-coefficient of variation of 8. 6% and day coefficient of variation of 16. 3%. Under 10% day coefficient of variation, the cTnI value was 0. 112 ng/ml. b. Thereis a good correlation between the home-made mixed serum and Beckman coulter quality control (r2 = 0. 958). The day coefficient of variation was 25% and 12. 2% when the cTnI value of home-made mixed serum was 0. 03 ng/ml and 0. 08 ng/ml, respectively. c. The warning value of blank detection limit was 0. 02 ng/ml. When higher than 0. 02 ng/ml, the detection values of buffer were positively correlated with sample concentrations (r = 0. 433 p = 0. 009).

Conclusions The upper limit of normal reference range in our study is slightly higher than that provided by manufacturers, which indicates that the reference range provided by manufacturers could not be quoted directly. It is capable to reflect the status of Access2 equipment and reagents well and is suitable for routine work to use the home-made mixed serum as the quality control and the matching buffer as a blank.

Cardiovascular Epidemiology

1

Preventive Cardiology: The Cardiometabolic Risk Initiative in China

Yue HW
International Keystone Healthcare Management Group, Bridgewater, USA 08807

Cardiometabolic health is a measure of a person's risk for diabetes and heart disease and is a good gauge of overall health. Cardiometabolic risk (CMR) is a construct that comprises a cluster of risk factors that are good indicators of a patient's overall for risk for type 2 Diabetes and Cardiovascular Disease (CVD).

Cardiometabolic risk factors include: overweigth/obesity, hypertension, high blood glucose, abnormal lipid metabolism, inflammation, hypercogulation, physical inactivity, smoking, age, race and ethnicity, gender and family history. Other risks factors are also important such like stress and nutrition deficiency.

Each of these risk factors pose a danger to good health, and the more the patients have, the greater their risk of type 2 Diabetes and CVD.

Cardiometabolic health is determined by a set of conditions known as Cardiometabolic risk (CMR) factors. Keeping an eye on these risk factors can help a person avoid diabetes and heart disease and live a longer, better life. CMR focuses clinical attention on the value of systematic evaluation, education, lifestyle behavior changes, disease prevention, and treatment. Assessing cardiometabolic risk gives clinicians a more comprehensive picture of a patients' health and potential risk for future disease and complications.

There are three levels of prevention/intervention based on the concept from WHO, and the key step is primary prevention/intervention, so we should focus on health management, not just sickness (disease) management. We should also take the disease as a whole and focus on the basic five for health, which are education, excise, nutrition, lifestyle and wellness. Therapeutic Lifestyle Change (TLC) and nutraceutical approach play the key role in the first line of preventing type 2 Diabetes and Cardiovascular Disease.

By comparison and combination of epidemiological studies and scientific statements/guidelines in US and China, the goal of the Cardiometabolic Risk Initiative will be stimulate substantial improvements in primary prevention and early detection through collaboration among key organizations; greater public awareness about healthy lifestyles; legislative action that results in more funding for and access to primary prevention programs and research; and reconsideration of the concept of the periodic medical checkup as an effective platform for prevention, early detection, and treatment. The Cardiometabolic Risk Initiative in China should be a national effort to encourage health care providers to focus on the prevention, recognition and treatment of all risk factors for type 2 Diabetes and heart disease. We should educate both the clinicians and public through continuing medical education (CME credit) and a variety of educational and public awareness activities.

2

Impact of smoking on Cardio Ankle Vascular Index

Li FJ, Yuan XC, Guo XY
WangJing Hospital of China Academy of Chinese Medical Sciences

Objective To observe the impact of smoking on the stiffness of the great arteries measured by Cardio Ankle Vascular Index (CAVI).

Methods 539 subjects aged 31-65 years without of stroke or coronary heart disease were recruited in this study, and were measured by the detectors of VaSeraTM VS-1000 angiosclerosis to assess impact of smoking on CAVI. Information on smoking, body weight and height and blood pressure was collected.

Results For stiffness of the great arteries, positive rate of 21. 7% (72/332) in smoking group was significantly higher than 5. 3% (11/207) in non-smoking group. By smoking index (number of daily cigarette × smoking years), 332 cases of smokers were divided into mild, moderate and severe smoker groups. CAVI values were significantly difference among the three different groups. There was a positive correlation between CAVI and smoking index, independent of age. Multiple linear regression analysis showed that the main impact factors of CAVI were smoking, age, body mass index and systolic blood pressure (SBP) in order.

Conclusions Smoking, age, BMI and SBP were main impact factors of CAVI. Of them, smoking, especially with large number cigarettes for a long-term was one of the most important independent risk factors to increase the stiffness of the main artery reflected through CAVI value.

3

Genetic Variants in the Renin-Angiotensin-Aldosterone System and Salt-Sensitivity of Blood Pressure

Kelly TN
Department of Epidemiology, Tulane University
New Orleans, Louisiana, USA

We conducted single marker and haplotype analyses to examine the association between renin-angiotensin-aldosterone system (RAAS) genes and salt-sensitivity of blood pressure (BP) among 1, 906 Chinese participants who took part in a 7-day low-sodium followed by a 7-day high-sodium dietary intervention. BP measurements were obtained at baseline and following each intervention using a random-zero sphygmomanometer. Diastolic BP (DBP) and mean arterial pressure (MAP) responses increased with the number of alleles of rs4524238 in angiotensin II receptor, type 1 (AGTR1) gene. For example, mean DBP responses (95% CI) among those with genotypes G/G, G/A, and A/A were-2. 53 (-2. 89, -2. 18), -3. 49 (-4. 13, -2. 86), and-5. 78 (-9. 51, -2. 06) mmHg, respectively, following low-sodium intervention (p = 0. 0008). Carriers of the rare and allele of rs5479 in the hydroxysteroid (11-beta) dehydrogenase 2 (HSD11B2) gene had a decreased DBP response to low-sodium (p-value = 0. 00004). Those with the C/A and C/C genotypes had DBP responses of-0. 70 (-6. 62, 5. 22) and-2. 71 (-4. 88, -0. 54) mmHg, respectively. X-chromosome renin-binding protein (RENBP) gene markers rs1557501 and rs2269372 were associated with systolic BP (SBP) response to low-sodium in men (p = 0. 00004 and 0. 0001, respectively). SBP responses (95% CI) were-6. 13 (-6. 68, -5. 58) versus-4. 07 (-4. 88, -3. 26) and-6. 04 (-6. 57, -5. 52) versus-3. 94 (-4. 90, -2. 99) mmHg among men with major compared to those with minor alleles of rs1557501 and rs2269372, respectively. Haplotype analyses of these genes supported our single marker findings. We identified genetic variants that were predictive of salt-sensitivity. These results may help identify individuals who will obtain maximum health benefit from low-sodium diet.

4

Incidence of Metabolic Syndrome Over 7 Years among Chinese Men and Women

Cao J, Chen JC, Li JX, Liu DH, Wu XG, Gu DF

Department of Evidence Based Medicine, Cardiovascular Institute and Fu Wai Hospital, Chinese Academy of Medical Sciences and Peking Union Medical College, Beijing 100037, China

Objective To determine the 7-year cumulative incidence of metabolic syndrome among Chinese adults, and its distribution by geographic region and urbanization.

Methods In 2000-2001, International Collaborative study of Cardiovascular Disease in ASIA (InterASIA) used a 4-stage stratified sampling method to select a nationally representative sample of the general population aged 35 to 74 years in China. A total of 15 838 persons aged 35-74 years completed the survey and examination. In 2007-2008, a follow-up survey was conducted among these same populations. Of the 10361 individuals who attended the follow-up survey, 593 subjects with missing data on clinic examination at baseline or follow-up, and 2055 subjects for having metabolic syndrome at baseline were excluded, leaving data from 7713 subjects (3878 men, 3835 women) for these incident analyses. Metabolic syndrome was defined according to the International Diabetes Federation (IDF) criteria.

Results During an average follow-up period of 7 years, we documented 1177 new cases of metabolic syndrome (incidence rate 15.3%). The age-specific incidence of metabolic syndrome among individuals aged 35 to 44 years, 45 to 54 years, 55 to 64 years, and 65 to 74 years was 14.1%, 15.4%, 17.0% and 17.2%, respectively. Over the follow-up period, 12.7% (n = 493) of men and17.8% (n = 684) of women developed incident metabolic syndrome, and the incidence was significantly higher in women than men at all age groups except the 35-44 years group. The incidence of metabolic syndrome was higher with higher baseline age group for women ($P < 0.01$). Male individuals aged 35-44 years and 65-74 years had higher incidence than the other two age groups. The incidence of metabolic syndrome among individuals in northern and southern china was 18.4% and 12.0% ($P < 0.001$), respectively, 16.3% and 14.3% ($P < 0.05$) for urban and rural areas, respectively.

Conclusions These data indicated that metabolic syndrome was quite prevalent in Chinese adults, and its incidence over 7 years was 15.3%. There is an urgent need to develop national strategies that focus on the prevention, detection and treatment of the metabolic syndrome as an important component for the prevention and control of cardiovascular disease in China.

5

The Serum Lipid Levels and the 8-year Trend in the Cohort of InterASIA in China

Chen JC, Cao J, Gu DF

Department of Evidence Based Medicine, Cardiovascular Institute and Fu Wai Hospital, Chinese Academy of Medical Sciences and Peking Union Medical College, Beijing 100037, China

Objective To investigate the levels of serum total and lipoprotein cholesterol, the distribution of characteristics and their trends from 2000 to 2008.

Methods In 2000 to 2001, serum total and lipoprotein cholesterol levels for urban and rural adult populations aged 35-74 years were examined from 10 provinces in China for InterASIA study. Follow up for those adults conducted during 2007 to 2008. Fasting plasma levels of total cholesterol (TC), triglyceride (TG) and high-density lipoprotein cholesterol (HDL-c) were determined with the enzyme methods in the central clinical laboratory. Serum TC, TG and HDL-c levels were classified on the basis of the guideline of prevention and treatment of dyslipidemia in Chinese adults, and were analyzed by different age groups, gender and regional groups.

Results This analysis included 9188 participants who had complete information with average age 56.5 years. Mean levels of TC, TG and HDL-c were 4.87, 1.66, and 1.38 mmol/L in the follow-up population, respectively. Mean levels of TC and HDL-c were higher in women than in men (TC: 4.99 versus 4.75 mmol/L, HDL-c: 1.43 versus 1.33 mmol/L, all $P < 0.001$), whereas the mean level of TG was higher in men than in women (1.71 vs 1.62 mmol/L, $P < 0.001$). Contrast to rural, the urban population had higher mean levels of TC (4.92 versus 4.83 mmol/L, $P < 0.001$), lower levels of HDL-c (1.34 vs. 1.42 mmol/L, $P < 0.001$), and without difference in mean TG level (1.68 vs.

1.64 mmol/L, P > 0.05) between urban and rural residents. Compared with the southern residents, the northern population had lower mean HDL-c levels (1.33 vs. 1.44 mmol/L, P < 0.001), but higher TG levels (1.74 versus 1.57 mmol/L, P < 0.001), similar TC level (4.86 vs. 4.89 mmol/L, P > 0.05). The age-standardized prevalence of borderline high TC (5.18 to 6.19 mmol/L) and hypercholesterolemia (≥6.22 mmol/L) were 24.6% and 7.1%, separately. Of the general population, 14.8% had borderline high TG (1.70 to 2.25 mmol/L) and 17.6% had hypertriglyceridemia (≥2.26 mmol/L). The age-standardized prevalence of low HDL cholesterol (< 1.04 mmol/L) was 14.4%. The prevalence of hypercholesterolemia in female and hypertriglyceridemia in male increased gradually with age (P < 0.001). Compared with the result of InterAsia study in 2000-2001, for adult aged 42-74 years old during 8 years, the average TG and HDL-c levels of male and female were increased (all P < 0.001), whereas TC levels of men and women decreased slightly (P < 0.001). Figure1. The serum lipid levels of population compared in same age groups (42-74 years old) between InterASIA study and its follow-up, from 2000-2008

Conclusions The TG levels appeared upward trend in this cohort population during follow-up. The prevalence of hypercholesterolemia and hypertriglyceridemia were still relatively high. It is important to strengthen public health education and health management for prevention and treatment of dyslipidemia in general population in China.

6

Polymorphisms in the ADD1 and GNB3 Genes and Blood Pressure in the Chinese Population

Chen SF, Lu XF, Gu DF
The GenSalt Collaborative Research Group

Objective Blood pressure (BP) is a complex trait that involves multiple common variants in different genes. The effects of the GNB3 C825T and ADD1 Gly460Trp (rs4961) polymorphisms on BP variance or hypertension have been investigated emphatically. This study aimed to examine the association between variations in ADD1 and GNB3 genes and systolic (SBP), diastolic (DBP), and mean arterial (MAP) blood pressure in Chinese population.

Methods A total of 3142 persons from 636 families from six field-centres in Hebei, Henan, Shandong (two sites), Shaanxi and Jiangsu provinces in rural north China were recruited. Three morning BP measurements were obtained on each of the 3-days of observation. Nine SNPs from the ADD1 gene and six SNPs from the GNB3 gene were chosen for genotyping based on linkage disequilibrium (LD) structure from HapMap data. SNP genotyping was performed using SNPlex assays on an automated DNA Sequencer. The mixed linear model was used to estimate the blood pressure level and 95% confidence interval of each genotype using the appropriate genetic model.

Results Of the fifteen genotyped SNPs, two monomorphic SNPs and one with a low genotyping call rate (53.1%) were excluded from the analysis. After Bonferroni correction, marker rs4963516 remained significantly associated with DBP (corrected p-values = 0.006, 0.007 and 0.002 in the codominant, additive and recessive genetic models, respectively) and MAP (corrected p-values = 0.02, 0.049 and 0.005 in the codominant, additive and recessive genetic models, respectively). Compared to carriers of the common A allele, CC homozygotes appeared to have higher DBP (75.81 ± 0.62 vs. 73.46 ± 0.25 mmHg, p = 0.0002, p corrected = 0.0024 corrected by the Bonferroni method) and MAP (91.87 ± 0.68 vs. 89.42 ± 0.28 mmHg, p = 0.0004, p corrected = 0.0048) after multivariable adjustment for age, gender, BMI, BP measurement room temperature and study site.

Conclusions These data support a role for the GNB3 gene in BP regulation in Chinese population. Future studies aimed at replicating these novel findings are warranted.

7

Homocysteine and Risk of Coronary Heart Disease and Stroke

Gao Y
Fuwai-Oxford Collaborative Centre for Cardiovascular Health, Cardiovascular Institute and Fu Wai Hospital, CAMS and PUMC, Beijing 100037, China

The relationship between homocysteine and vascular disease has been studied for more than 30 years. At the end of the 20th century, a large number of observation studies published. In 1995, Boushey meta-analysis1 which includes 17 none prospective studies draws a conclusion: A

5-mumol/L lower homocysterine level was associated with a 60% lower CHD risk; this result was exciting in that time. In 1998, Danesh & Lewington meta-analysis2 which includes 5 prospective studies draws a conclusion that a 5-mumol/L lower homocysterine level was associated with a 25% lower CHD risk. In 2002, the JAMA published "Homocysteine studies collaboration3", this study include 12 prospective studies which involve almost 2000 CHD events and 500 stroke events and 18 retrospective studies, after adjustment for other cardiovascular risk factors and correction for regression dilution, the conclusions from the prospective studies were that a 25% lower homocysteine was associated with about 10% lower CHD risk or 20% lower stroke risk.

Although the association between homocysteine and vascular disease appears to be weaker than it had previously been thought, however, if this expected result can be confirmed by large-scale randomized trial, the clinical value still was very important

In the beginning of 21st century, many large-scale randomized clinical trials were carried out. SEARCH trail4 published in 2007 involving a total of 12, 064 myocardial infarction participants who were randomly assigned to folic acid plus vitamin B12 and control group and a 3.8 umol/L (28%) reduction in blood homocysteine level between the two groups, after an average of 6.7 years of follow-up, the 3030 major vascular events were obtained, the conclusion of SEARCH shown that it was not significant difference between the two groups in major vascular events and mortality caused by vascular events or non-vascular events. Recently, a meta-analysis (BVTT) 5 will be published by the University of Oxford, at present the major results had been released on its Web site, this study included almost all of the current trails which has been published about homocysteine and risk of vascular disease, BVTT meta-analysis included CHAOS-2、HOST、WENBIT、VISP、NORVIT、WAFACS、HOPE-2 and SEARCH trails which involving a total of 37485 participants and obtaining major coronary events of 3973 cases and stroke events of 1528 cases and major vascular events of 9238 cases, and a 25% reduction in blood homocysteine levels between folic acid plus vitamin B12 and control group during a median of 5 years follow up, the final results shown that despite a 25% lowering in homosysteine levels for 5 years, B-vitamins had no beneficial effects on vascular risk and the sub-group analysis shown that it was not statistically significant in major vascular events whether or not grouped by gender or by age or by duration of follow-up or even by folic acid or homocysteine level.

In fact, no randomized trail published has clearly shown that lowering blood homocysteine reduces the risk of cardiovascular events so far; many researchers analyzed the reasons which may be related to each clinical trial to lack adequate statistical power to detect plausible effects due to relatively small numbers of vascular events or short duration of treatment. However, BVTT study was a summary of these individual clinical trials, it included such a large sample size and the number of events can be fully confirmed that lower homocysteine levels can not reduce the major vascular events risk. Therefore, in clinical practice the treatment and prevention incident of cardiovascular and cerebrovascular using folic acid and vitamin B12 should not be allowed to go on.

8

Effects of Statins in Patients with Chronic Kidney Disease

Ge L

Fuwai-Oxford Collaborative Center for Cardiovascular Health, Cardiovascular Institute and Fu Wai Hospital, CAMS and PUMC, Beijing 100037, China

Dyslipidaemia occurs frequently in chronic kidney disease (CKD) patients and contributes both to cardiovascular disease and worsening renal function. Data in people with chronic kidney disease have been conflicting; some studies in CKD patients have shown a clear relation between low density lipoprotein cholesterol and cardiovascular end points, whereas others have not.

In two meta-analyses, claims of improved renal outcomes have been made, encouraging broader adoption of statins in patients with pre-dialysis (stages I-IV) chronic kidney disease. Douglas et al reported the beneficial effects of statins in patients with overt proteinuria (protein excretion >300 mg/day) but not in those with microalbuminuria or normoalbuminuria. Similarly, Sandhu et al reported a slowing of the decline in glomerular filtration rate in patients with chronic kidney disease and concomitant cardiovascular disease (0.93 ml/min/year slower than in control patients), along with improvement in proteinuria. Neither of these reviews intended to analyse the effect of statins on lipid concentrations or mortality in patients with kidney disease specifically on the basis of the stage of kidney disease (pre-dialysis, dialysis, and transplantation). In three most recent meta-analyses, it showed that statins significantly reduced the risk of all-cause and cardiovascular mortality in CKD patients who are not receiving renal replacement, statins decreased cholesterol levels in dialysis patients similar but efficacy of decreasing the mortality rate in dialysis patients is still unclear. Statins significantly reduced hyperlipidaemia and tended to reduce cardiovascular events in kidney transplant recipients, but no effect has yet been demonstrated for mortality outcomes. Some large-scale trials involving the patients with chronic kidney disease showed no significant benefit of Statins therapy. In Die Deutsche Diabetes Dialyse Studie (the 4D study), 1225 patients with type 2 diabetes undergoing maintenance hemodialysis received either atorvastatin at a dose of 20 mg or placebo. Although the median LDL cholesterol level was reduced by 42% with atorvastatin, there was no significant reduction in the composite primary cardiovascular end point (relative risk, 0.92; 95% CI, 0.77 to 1.10). Some have attributed the lack of benefit to the very high cardiovascular risk among patients with type 2 diabetes and end-stage renal disease and to the futility of a single intervention. Fellstr? m et al. reported that there were no significant effects of rosuvastatin, at a dose of 10 mg per day, in 2776 patients undergoing hemodialysis, either on a composite end point (hazard ratio for the combined end point in the rosuvastatin group, 0.96; 95% CI, 0.84 to 1.11) or on its single components. The lack of a benefit of statin therapy in studies suggests that cardiovascular disease in patients undergoing hemodialysis differs from that in other patients.

Some trials examining cardiovascular outcomes in patients with chronic kidney disease have shown to reduce the incidence of cardiovascular events. These results contrast with the lack of benefit in patients undergoing hemodialysis seen in 4D and AURORA studies and raise the questions of whether statin therapy becomes ineffective with worsening renal disease and, if so, at which stage? These questions may be answered by the ongoing Study of Heart and Renal Protection (SHARP), which will complete in 2010.

9

Genetic Variants in the Renin-angiotensin System and Blood Pressure Reactions to the Cold Pressor Test

Hou LP, Li HF, Gu DF
Department of Evidence Based Medicine and Population Genetics, Cardiovascular Institute and Fu Wai Hospital, Chinese Academy of Medical Sciences and Peking Union Medical College, Beijing, China

Objective The purpose of this study was to examine the association between genetic variants in the renin-angiotensin system and blood pressure (BP) responses to cold pressor test (CPT).

Methods CPT was conducted among 2, 006 Han Chinese participants from rural north China. BP measurements were obtained before and after the CPT using a standard mercury sphygmomanometer according to a standard protocol. Six candidate genes in the RAS were selected based on their potential biological effect on BP regulation, and included AGT, REN, RENBP, ACE, AGTR1, and AGTR2. Sixty-seven SNPs in these candidate genes were chosen for genotyping based on linkage disequilibrium (LD) structure in the Chinese population, as determined by the Chinese HapMap, or based on previously reported associations with BP. The association between SNP genotypes and BP responses to CPT was assessed using a mixed linear model.

Results Of 67 SNPs genotyped in 6 genes, two were strongly associated with DBP responses to CPT ($P < 0.001$; false discovery rate ≤ 0.005): rs2006765 and rs943580 in the AGT gene. Compared with the C allele carriers of the rs2006765, the T/T homozygotes had a significantly decreased DBP responses to the CPT. For participants with the T/T genotype, percent DBP responses were 5.68 (4.25, 7.10), compared to corresponding responses of 9.17 (8.66, 9.68) among participants with the C/C + C/T genotype. In addition, there were dose-response relationships between the number of the minor A allele of SNP rs389566 in the AGTR1 gene and percent SBP responses to CPT although these relationships were not statistically significant after adjustment for multiple comparisons ($P = 0.005$; false discovery rate $= 0.151$).

Conclusions This study identified variants in the AGT and AGTR1 genes that may influence BP responses to CPT in a Han Chinese population. These results show that genetic variants in the RAS play an important role in BP responses to CPT.

10

Association between Atherosclerotic Risk Factors and Distribution of Cerebral Artery Stenosis

Liu ZZ, Si LP, Fang F, Zhang G, Wang RM, Kang XX
The Center for Laboratory Diagnosis, Beijing Tian Tan Hospital, Capital Medical University, Beijing 100050, China;
The neurology department, Beijing Tian Tan Hospital, Capital Medical University, Beijing 100050, China

Objective To investigate the association between atherosclerotic risk factors and distribution of cerebral artery stenosis.

Methods 438 adult patients with cerebral large-artery stenosis confirmed by angiography were divided into the alone intracranial stenosis, only extracranial stenosis and combined stenosis group. The difference of atherosclerotic risk factors among the three groups was analyzed.

Results The fibrinogen levels of the only extracranial stenosis and combined stenosis group were significantly higher than that of the alone intracranial stenosis group (all $P < 0.05$), but no significant difference was found between the only extracranial stenosis and combined stenosis group. The significant difference in the CRP levels was found only between the alone intracranial stenosis and combined stenosis group ($P < 0.05$). The other atherosclerotic risk factors were not associated with the distribution of cerebral artery stenosis.

Conclusions Inflammatory markers, rather than conventional risk factors, are associated with the distribution of cerebral artery stenosis.

11

The Effect of Total Cholesterol on Myocardial Infarction in Chinese Male Hypertension Population

Li JX, Cao J, Gu DF

Department of Evidence Based Medicine, Cardiovascular Institute and Fu Wai Hospital, Chinese Academy of Medical Sciences and Peking Union Medical College, Beijing 100037, China

Objective Total cholesterol (TC) is an important risk factor for myocardial infarction (MI), but the effect of TC on MI in Chinese male hypertension population has not been well documented. We conducted a prospective cohort study to determine the incidence and relative risk for MI across a wide range of TC levels in Chinese male hypertension population.

Methods A cohort of 5, 298 male employees aged 18-74 years recruited from Capital Steel and Iron Company in China in 1974-1980 was followed up for an average of 20.8 years. 122 incident MI cases were identified during the period of follow-up. Cox proportional hazards models were used to adjust for baseline variables, and compute hazard ratios of MI associated with level of TC. The population attributable risk was used to estimate the proportion of MI explained by TC level.

Results The incidence of MI among participants with elevated TC (baseline TC > = 5.17 mmol/L) and those with desirable TC (baseline TC < 5.17 mmol/L) in male non-hypertension population was 137.20 and 63.81 per 100, 000 person-years, respectively; and the corresponding incidence in male hypertension population was 279.80 and 130.96 per 100, 000 person-years, respectively. After adjustment for important covariables, 10.38, 16.71, and 23.80% of MI cases were attributable to hypertension, elevated TC, and hypertension plus elevated TC, respectively. In male hypertension population, the multivariate adjusted hazard ratios of MI were 1.21, 2.39, 3.38, and 3.95 for participants with TC level of 5.17-5.68, 5.69-6.20, 6.21-6.71, and > = 6.72 mmol/L, compared with those with TC < 5.17 mmol/L. The corresponding population attributable risks were 2.92, 9.20, 8.87, and 9.84%, respectively.

Conclusions Elevated TC was an important independent risk factor for MI both in male non-hypertension and in male hypertension population. There was a linear association between TC level and MI incidence in Chinese male hypertension population. Strategies that aim to prevent MI in China need to incorporate the prevention, treatment, and control of elevated TC, especially, in male hypertension population.

12

Aspirin in the Primary Prevention of Vascular Disease: Meta-Analysis from Randomised Trials

Li L

Fuwai-Oxford Collaborative Center for Cardiovascular Health

Cardiovascular Institute and Fu Wai Hospital, CAMS and PUMC, Beijing 100037, China

Low-dose aspirin is of definite and substantial net benefit for many patients with occlusive vascular disease. More than 50 million US adults take aspirin regularly for long-term prevention of cardiovascular disease. Meanwhile a lot of studies have assessed the benefits and risks in primary prevention. But the balance of beneficial effects and bleeding hazards in primary prevention is less clear.

To review the efficacy and safety of aspirin. Antithrombotic Trialists' Collaboration undertook meta-analyses of serious vascular events (myocardial infarction, stroke, or vascular death) and major bleeds in six primary prevention trials (95 000 individuals at low average risk, 660 000 person-years, 3 554 serious vascular events) that compared long-term aspirin versus control. Individual participant data were available for 6 primary prevention trials. Primary prevention trials were sought only if they recruited at least 1000 non-diabetic participants with at least 2 years of scheduled treatment. In the primary prevention trials, allocation to aspirin yielded an 18% proportional reduction in major coronary events, but only a small absolute reduction (0.28% vs. 0.34% per year; RR 0.82 [95% CI 0.75-0.90], $p < 0.0001$). Most of this decrease derived from a 23% proportional reduction in non-fatal myocardial infarction (0. 18% vs. 0. 23% per year; RR 0. 77 [99% CI 0. 67-0. 89], $p < 0.0001$), with no clear reduction in mortality from coronary heart disease (0. 11% vs. 0. 12% per year; RR 0. 95 [99% CI 0. 78-1. 15], $p = 0.5$), although the CI for the proportional reduction in mortality from coronary heart disease is wide. Aspirin had no net effect on strokes of known cause (haemorrhagic plus ischaemic), on strokes of unknown cause, or on the aggregate of all strokes. The main hazard of aspirin is haemorrhage and, apart from any effect on intracerebral haemorrhage, aspirin increased major gastrointestinal and other extracranial bleeds by about half in the primary prevention trials (0. 10% vs. 0. 07% per year; RR 1. 54 [1. 30-1. 82], $p < 0.0001$. The proportional reduction in major coronary events seemed to be similar in primary and secondary prevention (RR 0. 2 [95% CI 0. 75-0. 90] primary and RR 0. 80 [0. 73-0. 88] secondary), but the absolute benefit differed by an order of magnitude (absolute benefits 0. 06% per year primary and 1. 00% per year secondary). Poisson regression in 93, 918 individuals without known vascular disease at entry within the primary prevention trials indicated that age (per decade), male sex, diabetes, current smoking, and mean blood pressure (per 20 mm Hg) were each associated with about a two-fold increased risk of major coronary events, whereas total cholesterol (per 1 mmol/L) and body-mass index (per 5 kg/m^2) were much weakly associated with such events. The main risk factors for coronary events were also associated with haemorrhagic events, although for most the associations were slightly weaker for bleeding than for occlusive events. The absolute incidence of vascular events and of major extracranial bleeds varied substantially among participants in the primary prevention trials.

Hence, currently available trial results do not seem to justify general guidelines advocating the routine use of aspirin in all apparently healthy individuals.

13

Alcohol and Stroke

Li X, Li LM

Department of Epidemiology & Biostatistics, School of Public Health, Peking University Health Science Center, Beijing 100191

CVD, which causes lots of deaths and disables every year, is a common non-communicative chronic disease with great prevalence and recurrence. As a result of changes in life style and aging of population, CVD has become one of the most important health issues in China, especially among seniors.

Alcohol drinking is a life style risk factor of concern for NCDs. However, the lack of a world-wide standardized measure also creates some difficulty for the purposes of research, and the comparisons among findings as well. There are different definitions of "standard drink" (or "drink unit") in different countries. Nowadays, the official definition of it in the USA (14g pure alcohol) has become well accepted all over the world, and will also be used in this literature.

During the last two decades of the 20th century, there were many epidemiology studies on alcohol drinking as a causative factor of stroke. Sacco and colleagues found that the relationship between amount of alcohol and risk of first ever ischemic stroke could present as a "J" curve, which means compared with moderate drinkers (less than 3 standard drinks per day), both of nondrinkers and heavy drinkers have a higher risk. This finding has been repeated in some other researches with larger samples. On the other hand, drinking has been proved to be an unnegligible independent risk factor for hemorrhagic stroke, too. A meta-analysis pooling 41 researches reported the positive correlation between amount of alcohol and risk of hemorrhagic stroke, and heavy drink does increase the risk of ischemic stroke, but because of limitations of several researches, the protective effect of moderate stroke is still not sure. Besides these, irregular drunk were proved to be more harmful.

Among the mechanical studies of alcohol and stroke, the interaction and confounding are always challenges. For hemorrhagic stroke, a quite believable explanation is alcohol can raise artery blood pressure, and hypertension is believed to be a risk factor of hemorrhagic stroke. While, for ischemic stroke, the mechanism may be much more complicated. Firstly, atrial fibrillation and other kinds of arrhythmia, as well as cardiomyopathy, which may increase the risk of cardiogenic cerebral embolism, can occur after both acute and chronic alcohol ingestion. Secondly, alcohol may induce the imbalance of intracellular calcium and magnesium, and precipitates vascular smooth muscle cell damage. It's an important reason for vasoconstriction.

Does the protective effect of moderate drink really exist? How does this work? No affirmative answer can be given based on evidences by now. It has been found that drink can raise serum HDL, which may slower formation of atherosclerosis. That's a potential explaination why the risk of ischemic stroke is depressed. Otherwise, the hematological effects of alcohol may contribute to the risk for both ischemic and hemorrhagic strokes. Factors participating in fibrinolysis (plasminogen activator), hemostasis (platelet count and aggregability) and blood clotting (fibrinogen) could be influenced by alcohol. Briefly, small quantities of alcohol will promote fibrinalysis system, and hold coagulation back. Drinking habits also powerfully affect the risk, because it can modify several system related with onset of stroke, such as fibrinolytic and hemostatic activities. Periodic heavy drinking is perhaps the most detrimental drinking habit in this respect, because it causes great fluctuation in the effects, i. e. the initial effects are followed by rebound effects after discontinuation of drinking.

Heavy drink can definitely increase the risk of both hemorrhagic stroke and ischemic stroke, although the mechanic pathway is still in the "black box". The researches above suggest that risk of stroke can be reduced by controlling heave drinking, but there is not yet enough evidence to propose nondrinkers taking alcohol moderately

14

Prevalence of Overweight, and Its Relationship to Cardiovascular Risk in Urban of Taiyuan in China

Li YF, Xiao CS, Bian YF, Li H, Zhao WP, Liu GZ, Li JN, Li ML

Department of Cardiology, The Second Hospital of Shanxi Medical University, 382 Wuyi Road, Taiyuan 030001, PR China.

Objective Excess bodyweight is the sixth most important risk factor contributing to the overall burden of disease worldwide. This study was designed to investigate the epidemiologic features of overweight, and to evaluate the associations between overweight and coronary heart disease (CHD) in urban residents of Tiayuan, China.

Methods The study was conducted in Taiyuan, capital city of Shanxi province, from April to October 2008, with a cluster multistage and random sampling method. 4, 166 residents (1, 285 men, and 2, 881 women) aged ≥31 years were selected to participate in the study. Data on demographic and clinical characteristics and body weight, height were collected. According to World Health Organization (WHO) criteria, overweightis defined as a body mass index (BMI) ≥25 kg/m^2. CHD were defined using the WHO Multinational Monitoring of Trends and Determinants in Cardiovascular Diseases (MONICA) criteria. Sex-specific prevalence rates of overweight were calculated. Odds ratios (ORs) and their 95% CIs were obtained using logistic regression. All reported p values were two tailed.

Results The prevalence of overweight (BMI ≥25. 0 kg/m^2) was 47. 4% (45. 6% in men and 51. 5% in women) in urban residents in Taiyuan, China. BMI was strongly associated with a higher risk of CHD. Compared with subjects with normal bodyweight (BMI <25. 0 kg/m^2), overweight individuals had a high risk factor for CHD. The adjusted ORs for CHD was 1. 425 (95% CI: 1. 091-1. 860), after adjustment for gender, age, education, physical exercise, smoking status, and drinking status.

Conclusions Overweight is highly prevalent in urban of Taiyuan in China, and is an important risk factor for CHD.

15

Prevalence of Prehypertension and Its Relationship to other Risk Factors for Cardiovascular Disease in Urban of Taiyuan in China

Li YF, Xiao CS, Bian YF, Zhao WP, Liu GZ, Li JN, Li ML

Department of Cardiology, The Second Hospital of Shanxi Medical University, 382 Wuyi Road, Taiyuan 030001, PR China.

Objective To estimate the prevalence of prehypertension in urban residents of Taiyuan, China and evaluate the relationship between prehypertension and other risk factors for CVD.

Methods The study was conducted in Taiyuan, capital city of Shanxi province, from April to October 2008, through cluster multistage and random sampling method. 4, 166 subjects aged ≥31 years were recruited in the study. Blood pressure and information on history of hypertension for participants was obtained. Prehypertension was defined according to JNC-7. Univariate variance analyses were used for comparison of characteristics among normotensive, prehypertensive, and hypertensive groups. Odds ratios (ORs) for associations of prehypertension with CVD factors were calculated by logistic regression. Potential confounders were adjusted including gender, age, education, smoking, alcohol drinking, and physical exercise.

Results The prevalence of prehypertension in urban of Taiyuan was 23. 6%, compared to 42. 1% the prevalence of hypertension. Prehypertension is more common in men (26. 6%) than in women (22. 2%). Body mass index (BMI), waist to hip ratio, fasting glucose, low-density lipoprotein cholesterol (LDL-C), total cholesterol (TC), triglyceride (TG), and uric acid (UA) showed an increasing trend ($p < 0.001$)

from nromotensive, pre-hypertension to hypertensive. Prevalence of CVD risk factors such as obesity, diabetes mellitus, and dyslipidemia were significantly higher in the prehypertensive and hypertensive groups (p for trend, $p < 0.001$) compared to the normotensive group. The adjusted ORs of obesity, diabetes mellitus, and dyslipidemias were 2.407 (CI 1.69-3.43), 1.48 (CI 1.19-1.85), and 1.32 (CI 1.05-1.64) respectively for prehypertensive subjects, compared with normotensive subjects ($p = 0.016$ or, $p = 0.0001$ respectively).

Conclusions Prehypertension occurs in 23.6% of urban individuals in Taiyuan, China, and is associated with many other CVD risk factors. Lifestyle therapeutic modifications of those CVD risks in prehypertension subjects are strongly recommended in order to prevent them from cardiovascular diseases.

16

Prevalence of Metabolic Syndrome by Differing Criteria, and its Relationship to Cardiovascular Risk in Urban of Taiyuan in China

Li YF, Xiao CS, Bian YF, Zhao WP, Liu GZ, Li JN, Li ML

Department of Cardiology, The Second Hospital of Shanxi Medical University, 382 Wuyi Road, Taiyuan 030001, PR China.

Objective This study was designed to compare the prevalence of MetS in urban of Taiyuan in China according to revised National Cholesterol Education Program (NCEP) ATP III and International Diabetes Federation (IDF) definitions, and to evaluate its association with coronary heart disease (CHD) and stroke.

Methods 4, 166 subjects (1, 285 men, and 2, 881 women) aged ≥31 years were recruited from urban of Taiyuan, China in the period of April to October, 2008. Subjects were classified by the presence or absence of metabolic syndrome, which was defined by revised NCEP or IDF criteria. CHD and stroke were defined using the WHO Multinational Monitoring of Trends and Determinants in Cardiovascular Diseases (MONICA) criteria. The agreement between MetS definitions was estimated by κ statistics. Odds ratios (ORs) and their 95% CIs were obtained using logistic regression.

Results The prevalence of MetS was 51.6% (58.2% in men and 48.4% in women) by revised NCEP definition and 40.4% (42.7% in men and 39.3% in women) IDF definition. The agreement was 79.2% ($\kappa = 0.762$) in men and 94.9% ($\kappa = 0.950$) in women between revised NCEP and IDF definitions. The ORs for CHD were 1.50 (95% CI: 1.16-1.94) ($p = 0.002$) by revised NCEP definition and 1.75 (95% CI: 1.37-2.25) ($p < 0.0001$). The ORs for stroke were 1.64 (95% CI: 1.24-2.17) ($p = 0.001$) and 1.71 (95% CI: 1.301-2.24) ($p < 0.0001$) by the corresponding definitions.

Conclusions The revised NECP definition identified more Mets subjects than IDF definition in Taiyuan. Their agreement between those definitions is very high in women.

17

Genetic Variants in the Renin-angiotensin System and Blood Pressure in Chinese Population

Lu XF, Li HF, Gu DF

Department of Evidence Based Medicine and Population Genetics, Cardiovascular Institute and Fu Wai Hospital, Chinese Academy of Medical Sciences and Peking Union Medical College, Beijing, China

Objective The renin-angiotensin system (RAS) has a central role in controlling BP and sodium homeostasis. The objective of this analysis was to examine the association between genetic variants of RAS candidate genes [angiotensinogen (AGT), renin (REN), renin-binding protein (RENBP), angiotensin converting enzyme (ACE), angiotensin II type 1 receptor (AGTR1), and angiotensin II type 1 receptor 2 (AGTR2)] and systolic (SBP), diastolic (DBP), and mean arterial (MAP) pressure.

Methods The current study was conducted in a large, homogeneous sample of Han Chinese families who took part in the Genetic Epidemiology Network of Salt Sensitivity (GenSalt). A total of 3142 persons from 636 families from six field-centres in rural north China were recruited. A standard questionnaire was administered by trained staff to collect information on family structure, demographic characteristics, personal and family medical history, and lifestyle risk factors. Three morning BP measurements were obtained according to a standard protocol by trained and certified observers using a random-zero sphygmomanomete. Body weight and height were measured twice in light indoor clothing without shoes.

Sixty-seven SNPs in six candidate genes were chosen for genotyping based on linkage disequilibrium (LD) structure in the Chinese population, or based on previously reported associations with BP. Additive associations between SNP genotypes and BP level were assessed using a mixed linear regression model. Age, gender, body mass index (BMI), BP measurement room temperature, and study site were adjusted in multivariable analyses. To adjust for multiple comparisons, the false discovery rate (FDR) q-value was calculated for all SNPs.

Results Of the sixty-seven genotyped SNPs, 6 monomorphic SNPs, 2 SNPs with missing marker data, and 1 SNP that significantly deviated from HWE were excluded from the analysis. RENBP SNP rs4898373 located on the X-chromosome was significantly associated with SBP, DBP and MAP ($P < 0.001$, respectively, all false discovery rates < 0.05). Compared to those with the T allele, men with C allele appeared to have lower SBP (115.09 ± 2.10 vs. 122.69 ± 0.45 mmHg), DBP (69.82 ± 1.42 vs. 75.18 ± 0.30 mmHg) and MAP (84.86 ± 1.48 vs. 91.03 ± 0.33 mmHg).

Conclusions In summary, these data support a role for the RENBP gene in BP regulation. Future studies aimed at replicating these novel findings are warranted.

18

Heart Rate Influence on Incidence of Cardiovascular Disease among Adults in China

Mao QX, Huang JF, Gu DF

Department of Evidence Based Medicine, Cardiovascular Institute and Fu Wai Hospital, Chinese Academy of Medical Sciences and Peking Union Medical College, Beijing, China

Objective To examine heart rate influence on the incidence of cardiovascular disease in Chinese adults

Methods A population-based sample of 169 871 Chinese adults aged ≥40 years at 1991 baseline was followed up in 1999-2000 with a response rate of 93.4% (158 666). Data on demographic characteristics, blood pressure, heart rate and other related variables were collected at baseline. Cox proportional hazard regression model was used to analyze the data. Cardiovascular disease was defined as diagnosed as acute myocardial infarction or stroke or died due to cardiovascular disease (ICD-9:390.0-398.9, 401.0-429.9 and 430.0-438.9). Heart rate was entered as both a continuous and a categorical variable.

Results After 8.3 years of follow-up, the incidence rate of cardiovascular disease was 804.6 per 100 000 person-years (men: 942.3 per 100 000 person-years and women: 671.5 per 100 000 person-years).

For men, compared with the participants with heart rate of 60-74 b.p.m, hazard ratios of cardiovascular disease for those with heart rate of < 60 b.p.m, 75-89 b.p.m and ≥90 b.p.m were 1.06 (95% confidence interval [CI], 0.76-1.49), 1.12 (95% CI, 1.04-1.20) and 1.33 (95% CI, 1.19-1.48), respectively, after adjusted for baseline systolic blood pressure, age, cigarette smoking, alcohol consumption, body mass index (BMI), physical activity, education, geographic region (north vs. south), and urbanization (urban vs. rural). For women, compared with participants with heart rate of 60-74 b.p.m, only those with heart rate of ≥90 b.p.m had higher risk of cardiovascular disease, with the multivariate-adjusted hazard ratio: 1.28 (95% CI, 1.13-1.44). While the hazard ratios of per 10 b.p.m increased in heart rate, were 1.10 (95% CI, 1.06-1.13) for men and 1.08 (95% CI, 1.04-1.12) for women, respectively, after adjusted for baseline systolic blood pressure, age, cigarette smoking, alcohol consumption, body mass index (BMI), physical activity, education, geographic region (north vs. south), and urbanization (urban vs. rural). After excluding participants who developed cardiovascular disease within the first 1 years of follow-up, compared with the participants with heart rate of 60-74 b.p.m, those with higher heart rate still had a higher risk of cardiovascular disease both in men and women. For men, compared with the participants with heart rate of 60-74 b.p.m, the multivariate-adjusted hazards of the cardiovascular disease for those with heart rate of 75-89 b.p.m and ≥90 b.p.m were 1.09 (95% CI, 1.02-1.17) and 1.28 (95% CI, 1.14-1.43), respectively. For women, compared with the participants with heart rate of 60-74 b.p.m, the multivariate-adjusted hazard of the cardiovascular disease for those with ≥90 b.p.m was: 1.27 (95% CI, 1.12-1.44).

Conclusions High heart rate was associated with high incidence of cardiovascular disease in Chinese adults, especially for men. This suggests that controlling the heart rate <90 b.p.m by all means reduce the incidence of cardiovascular disease in Chinese adults.

19

Heart Rate and Cardiovascular Mortality in Chinese Adults

Mao QX, Huang JF, Gu DF
Department of Evidence Based Medicine, Cardiovascular Institute and Fu Wai Hospital, Chinese Academy of Medical Sciences and Peking Union Medical College, Beijing, China

Objective To study the relationship between heart rate and cardiovascular disease mortality in a large population-based prospective cohort study of Chinese adults.

Methods Blood pressure, heart rate and other variables were measured in China National Hypertension Survey in 1991 for aged at 15 and over. Of them, 169 871 Chinese men and women aged 40 years or older in 1991 were followed up using standard protocols in 1999-2000 with a response rate of 93.4% (158 666). Data were analyzed by Cox proportional hazard regression model. Heart rate was analyzed both as a continuous and as a categorical variable. Cardiovascular death was determined according to the underlying cause of death ICD-9 (390.0-398.9, 401.0-429.9 and 430.0-438.9).

Results Over a mean of 8.3 years of follow-up, the mortality of heart disease was 305.3 per 100 000 person-years, and the mortality of cerebrovascular disease was 261.5 per 100 000 person-years.

For men, compared with participants with heart rate of 60-74 b.p.m, the hazard ratios of cardiovascular death for participants with heart rate of <60, 75-89 and ≥90 b.p.m were 1.07, (95% confidence interval [CI], 0.72-1.60), 1.14 (95% CI, 1.05-1.24) and 1.37 (95% CI, 1.21-1.55), respectively, after adjusted for baseline systolic blood pressure, age, cigarette smoking, alcohol consumption, body mass index (BMI), and other variables. For women, participants with heart rate of ≥90 b.p.m had a higher risk of cardiovascular death than those with heart rate of 60-74 b.p.m, with the multivariate-adjusted hazard ratio: 1.26 (95% CI, 1.10-1.45). The hazard ratios of per 10 b.p.m increased in heart rate were 1.10 (95% CI, 1.06-1.14) for men and 1.08 (95% CI, 1.04-1.13) for women, respectively, after adjusted for baseline systolic blood pressure, age, cigarette smoking, alcohol consumption, body mass index (BMI), and other variables. After excluding participants who died during the first 1 years of follow-up, compared with the participants with heart rate of 60-74 b.p.m, those with higher heart rate still had a higher risk of cardiovascular death both in men and women.

Conclusions High heart rate was associated with high cardiovascular disease mortality in Chinese adults, especially in men. The results indicate that heart rate is one of precursors predicting the long-term cardiovascular death in Chinese adults.

20

Cigarette Smoking, Blood Pressure and Risk of Cardiovascular Disease in Chinese Adults

Sun DL, Cao J, Chen JC, Lu XF, Li JX, Wu XG, Gu DF
Cardiovascular Institute and Fu Wai Hospital, CAMS and PUMC, Beijing 100037, China

Objective Aim to identify the joint effects of cigarette smoking and blood pressure (BP) on the risk of CVD incidence in Chinese adults.

Methods Overall, 83, 533 men and 86, 338 women aged 40 years or older at their baseline examination in 1991 were eligible to participate in the follow-up study in 1999-2000. Cox proportional hazards models were used to study the associations between both smoking and BP and CVD incidence by stratified analyses. To evaluate biological interaction between high BP and smoking on CVD incidence, we used the method of the additive interaction according to Rothman. Statistical analyses were conducted using SAS statistical software (version 9.0; SAS Institute Inc).

Results During an average of 8.3 years follow-up, we recorded a total of 11, 785 CVD events. Compared with those with SBP < 120 or DBP < 80 mmHg, a linear relationship between SBP or DBP and CVD incidence among nonsmokers, former smokers, and current smokers (all $P < 0.05$ for linear trend) was found, with higher slope of CVD risk against the increased BP among current smokers, compared with among nonsmokers and former smokers. Both former and current smokers were associated with the increased risk of CVD among men and women. We found a significant additive interaction of high SBP (≥140 mmHg) and current smoking for the risk of CVD after adjusting for other risk factors among men and women. The relative excess risk due to interaction (RERI), attributable proportion due to interaction (AP), and synergy index (SI) were 1.03 (95% CI 0.53, 2.03), 31% (95% CI 13%, 38%), and 1.78 (95% CI 1.44, 2.21), respectively. The relationships persisted in relation to diastolic BP in combination with current smoking in men and women.

Conclusions There was a statistically significant additive interaction between high SBP or DBP and current smoking on the risk of CVD, after adjusting for other risk factors.

21

Blood Pressure, Body Mass Index and Risk of Cardiovascular Disease in Chinese Men and Women

Wang HW, Cao J, Wu XG, Gu DF
Department of Evidence Based Medicine, Cardiovascular Institute and Fu Wai Hospital, Chinese Academy of Medical Sciences and Peking Union Medical College, Beijing 100037, China

Objective It is still uncertain whether increased blood pressure (BP) has a stronger effect on the risk of cardiovascular disease (CVD) in lean persons than in obese persons, we tested it using the data set collected from a large cohort of Chinese adults.
Methods Systolic and diastolic BP, body mass index (BMI) and other variables were measured in 169, 871 Chinese men and women ≥40 years of age in 1991 using standard protocols. Follow-up evaluation was conducted in 1999-2000, with a response rate of 93.4%. According to the definition of obesity from Working Group on Obesity in China, participants in the present study were divided into 4 BMI levels including underweight (< 18.5 kg/m^2), normal (18.5-23.9 kg/m^2), overweight (24-27.9 kg/m^2), and obese (≥28 kg/m^2). Data were analyzed with Cox proportional hazards models.
Results After adjusted for age, sex, cigarette smoking, alcohol consumption, high school education, physical inactivity, geographic region, and urbanization, we found that the effects of systolic or diastolic BP on risk of CVD generally increased with the increasing BMI levels (underweight, normal, overweight, and obese). For example, HRs and 95% CI per 10 mmHg increase in systolic BP within corresponding BMI levels were 1.11 (1.08-1.14), 1.19 (1.17-1.21), 1.25 (1.21-1.28) and 1.30 (1.22-1.39), respectively. Statistically significant interactions ($P < 0.0001$) were observed between systolic BP, diastolic BP and BMI in relation to CVD. In baseline hypertensive participants we found both obese men and women had higher risk of CVD than normal-weight persons. The multivariate-adjusted relative risks (95% CI) were 1.23 (1.03-1.47) and 1.20 (1.02-1.40), respectively for incidence of CVD.
Conclusions The present study indicates that there is a general increase in the magnitude of the association between BP and CVD with increasing BMI. Hypertension is not a less serious risk factor in obese than in lean or normal-weight persons in Chinese adults.

22

Hypertension Control in Communities (HCC): Preliminary Result of Blood Pressure Management among Hypertensive

Wang ZW[1], Wang X[1], Zhang LF[1], Wang W[1], Chen WW[1], Zhu ML[1], Hu SS[1], Lei ZL[2], Kong LZ[2], Liu LS[1]
1. The National center of Cardiovascular Disease, Beijing 100037;
2. Bureau of disease control, Ministry of Health of China, Beijing 100044;

Objective To determine the effect of community-based standardized blood pressure management on the control of hypertension.
Methods A protocol of community-based standardized blood pressure management was developed based on the current Chinese guideline for prevention, treatment of hypertension. The grass-roots doctors from community health service centers across China were trained using this protocol and required to manage hypertensive patients according to the protocol; patients were treaded with therapy life style change or/and medication, and followed up based on risk stratification. The control rate of hypertension was evaluated after 1 year. Effect of intervention (EI) was estimated as rate (mean) in 1 year minus it in baseline.
Results By the end of 2008, a total of 29 411 hypertensive patients (47.2% for male, mean age 61.4 ± 10.9 years) with full information have been managed for one year according to the protocol. Among all patients, 8.9% were classified to low risk, 50.8% as moderate risk and 40.3% as high and very high risk in baseline. After standardized management, the EI of smoking, drinking and systolic/diastolic blood pressure was-7.1% ($P < 0.05$), -7.3% ($P < 0.05$), and-14.8/-8.3 mmHg ($P < 0.05$), respectively. However, EI of overweight/obesity was 0.3% ($P > 0.05$). For all patients, the control rate rose to 74.7%, EI was 53.1%, and each sub-group, including age, risk stratification, had a significant increase. The longer the management was, the higher the control rate was. The results of multivariate logistic regression

showed that older age, male and higher blood level were adverse factors for the control and management of hypertension.
Conclusions Our study showed that standardized management could significantly improve the control of hypertension in communities in China.

23

Surveys on Arrhythmias among Hospitalized Patients in Major Parts of China

Wang ZW[1], Wang X[2], Cheng KP[1], Chen Z[1], Li X[1], Chen WW[1], Fu W[3], Zhu ML[1], Zhang S[2]
[1]National Center of Cardiovascular Disease, Fu Wai Hospital, CAMS and PUMC, Beijing 100037, China;
[2]Center of Arrhythmia Diagnosis and Treatment, Fu Wai Hospital, CAMS and PUMC, Beijing 100037, China

Objective To understand the epidemiological distribution of different kind of arrhythmia among hospitalized patients in major parts of China.
Methods Hospital records of patients who aged? 18 years and were with diagnosis of arrhythmia, were collected from 22 provincial-level hospitals across China with the standard protocol and questionnaire, for patients hospitalized at the period from January 1, 2007 to June 30, 2007. 6 122 cases of arrhythmia were eligible for analysis.
Results The proportion of patients with diagnosis of arrhythmia among the patients in department of cardiology was 26.8%. Among patients with arrhythmia, the frequency of atrial fibrillation was the highest (35.0%); frequency of paroxysmal superventricular tachycardia (PSVT), sick sinus syndrome (SSS), premature ventricular beat (PVB) was 28.0%, 11.9% and 11.6%, respectively. Frequencies of SSS, ventricular tachycardia, and PSVT were higher among female patients of arrhythmia. Most of arrhythmias increased with age, with the highest proportion of PSVT (60.4%) for the young patients and AF (44.7%) for the elder patients, respectively. Patients with arrhythmia, 38% were accompanied with hypertension, 24.7% with coronary artery disease, and 10.2% with cardiac valve disease.
Conclusions Among the hospitalized patients, atrial fibrillation was the major type of arrhythmia, especially in elder patients. Most of the patients with arrhythmia were accompanied with hypertension.

24

Hypertension Control in Communities (HCC): Protocol and description of baseline characteristics

Wang ZW[1], Wang W, Wang X[1], Chen WW[1], Zhu ML[1], Hu SS[1], Lei ZL[2], Kong LZ[2], Liu LS[1]
1. The National center of Cardiovascular Disease, Beijing 100037;
2. Bureau of disease control, Ministry of Health of China, Beijing 100044.

Objective The project of Hypertension Control in Communities (HCC) aimed to determine the effect of community-based standardized management on control of hypertension.
Methods The protocol of community-based standardized hypertension management was developed by expert board with being oriented by guidelines. Community health service centers across China were selected to implement the protocol. After trained with the protocol, the grass-roots doctors from selected centers were asked to manage hypertensives in their communities according to the protocol. The control of hypertension was evaluated after 1 year the program preformed.
Results By the end of 2008, the program contained 110 610 patients with eligible baseline data for analysis. 47.7% were male patients. In baseline, the mean level of systolic/diastolic blood pressure (BP) was 145.5 ± 17.3/88.3 ± 10.7 mmHg, about 31.5% patients ate highly salted food, and 17.1% and 18.5% were with drinking and smoking habit, respectively, the levels of all variables were higher in male than in female ($P < 0.05$). Among the patients, grade I, grade II, and grade III hypertension was 47.1%, 22.4% and 8.1%, respectively; low-, moderate-, and high-risk group were 9.4%, 53.9% and 36.7%, respectively. At baseline, 75.7% were under treatment and 22.5% were controlled (< 140/90 mmHg).
Conclusions The baseline characteristic of HCC subjects was described in this article. It showed standardized management was needed to further improve the control of hypertension.

25

Prevalence and Trend of Metabolic Syndrome in Middle-aged Chinese Population

Wang ZW, Wang X, Li X, Chen Z, Zhao LC, Li Y, Wu YF
National Center of Cardiovascular Disease, Cardiovascular Institute and Fu Wai Hospital, Chinese Academy of Medical Science, Beijing 100037, China
Department of Epidemiology and Biostatistics, Peking University School of Public Health, Beijing 100083, China

Objective To analyze the current prevalence of metabolic syndrome (MS) and its trend in the past 5 years in China in middle-aged population.
Methods In 2004-2005, cross-sectional sampling surveys were conducted in 13 populations from southern and northern parts including urban and rural areas in China, with internationally standardized criteria and measurement. 1000-2000 participants from each population with the same percentage of man and women, were examined. Out of them, there were 13 732 participants aged 35-59 years. Comparison was made for 10 populations with comparable data in 1998 to observe the trend in the period of 1998 to 2004. MS was defined according to Chinese Medical Association Diabetes Branch definition set in 2004.
Results The prevalence of MS was 12.1%. The age-adjusted prevalence was higher in men (13.9%) than in women (8.5%), higher in residents from the northern (15.0%) than the southern (6.8%) and from urban (11.3%) than rural (10.1%). Among the participants with MS, 60.4% were with obesity, high blood pressure or with dyslipidemia. Comparing with data in 1998, the age-adjusted prevalence rates of MS in 2004-2005 had a significantly increase (10.0% vs. 7.2%, $P<0.05$), and the increase level was higher in men than in women, and in residents of the northern part than in the southern ($P<0.05$). Regardless the geographic region and urbanization, the mean levels of triglyceride, body mass index and waist circumference were higher in participants in survey in 2004-2005 than in 1998.
Conclusions The prevalence of MS was increasing in middle aged Chinese population during years of 1998 to 2004. Lifestyle therapeutic changes for obesity, high blood pressure and dyslipidemia should be emphasized to control MS.

26

Efficacy and Safety of Statin

Wuhanbilige
Fu Wai-Oxford Collaborative Centre for Cardiovascular Health, Cardiovascular Institute and Fu Wai Hospital, CAMS and PUMC, Beijing 100037, China

Coronary heart disease (CHD) is believed to be the major cause of disability and death in developed and developing countries. Previous results and observations indicated that Statins is an effective way of treatment to reduce the risk of CHD by lowering the low-density lipoprotein cholesterol (LDL-C) better than other medicines. Publication of several large-scale clinical trials in past 10 years has provided direct evidences which lead to popular use of statins in the clinic. Recently, a prospective meta-analysis data from 90056 participants in the 14 randomized LDL-C lowering clinical tails was published in the Lancet by the Cholesterol Treatment Trialists' (CTT) Collaboration[1]. In this report we will discuss the efficacy and safety of Statins by analyzing the main results from the meta-analysis and clarify the misunderstandings about it in the clinical practice.
CTT meta-analysis result showed that: During a mean of 5 years, there were 8, 186 deaths, 14, 348 individuals had major vascular events and 5, 103 developed cancer. According to the meta-analysis, over all in these 14 selected trials, the weighted average difference in LDL cholesterol at 1 year was 1.09 mmol/L (0.35-1.77 mmol/L). By reducing per mmol/L LDL cholesterol, Statins caused a 12% proportional reduction ($p<0.0001$) in all-cause mortality, which attributed mainly from 19% proportional reduction in CHD deaths ($p<0.0001$), however, the reduction of non-coronary vascular mortality ($p=0.2$) and non-vascular mortality ($p=0.1$) are both non-significant. These benefits were significant within the first year, but were greater in subsequent years. Taking all 5 years together, the overall reduction of major vascular incidences is about one fifth per mmol/L LDL cholesterol reduction, which translated into 48 fewer participants having major vascular events per 1000 among those with pre-existing CHD at baseline, compared with 25 per 1000 among participants with no such history. For the safety indications, the meta-analysis noted that, no evidence of increased risk of cancer in statin therapy by lowering LDL cholesterol for 1.0 mmol/L, and the therapy induced also extremely low rate of Myopathy (0.01%, SE0.01). Information on episodes of raised liver enzymes was not

sought for this meta-analysis. In summary, the potential hazard of these statin regimens seemed to be extremely small in relation to its clear benefits; hence, statin treatment can last for long time safely.

Previous large-scale randomized trials showed that, statin can significantly reduce the mortality and morbidity of cardiovascular disease in high risk populations by lowering the level of LDL-C. In these reports, Statin therapy can safely reduce the 5-year incidence of non-fatal myocardial infarction (MI) and CHD death by about one quarter per mmol/L reduction in LDL cholesterol[2-7]. These findings clearly showed the importance of statin in the secondary prevention after MI. Despite all those positive results reported by these large-scale, randomized trials, the clinical use of statin in the secondary prevention is not so popular until now, usually because of patients' lack of knowledge about Blood cholesterol and doctors' worry about negative effects after using higher concentration. Hence, we should try our best to knowledge patient's mind with importantce of LDL-C lowering treatment and knowledge doctor's minds with correct understanding of efficacy and safety of statin; finally to benefit people by turning the result of evidence based medicine to clinical practices.

27

Relationship between Smoking and Hypertension in Residents in Jiangsu Province, China

Xiang QY, Pan XQ, Lu SR, Wu M

Center for Disease Control and Prevention, Jiangsu province, No. 172, Jiangsu Lu, Nanjing, China

Objective To assess association of smoking with systolic blood pressure (SBP), diastolic blood pressure (DBP), and the rank of blood pressure level.

Methods 4480 subjects were included in this study by random sampling. Information on age, gender, smoking, drinking, dietary habit and physical activity was obtained by questionnaire. Body weight, height, waistline, blood pressure and other variables were measured for all subjects. We analyzed data from 4318 individuals with completed questionnaires.

Results The average SBP and DBP in men and smoking group were significant higher than in women and nonsmoking, separately. There were a significant positive correlation between the amount of tobacco use and SBP (Pearson correlation coefficient $r = 0.067$, $p = 0.004$), DBP ($r = 0.075$, $p = 0.001$), and rank of blood pressure ($r = 0.053$, $p = 0.022$), respectively. When age, sex, BMI, waistline were adjusted, the results of logistic analysis indicated that odds ratio (OR) of hypertension was 2.08 (95% CI was 1.13-4.26) in smoking group compared with the nonsmoking. Moreover, the OR for smoking individuals was increased as the amount of tobacco consumed.

Conclusions Smoking positively associated with SPB, DBP and the rank of blood pressure. Smoking significantly increased the risk of hypertension.

28

Four Blood Pressure Measures Predicting Risk of Cardiovascular Disease among Chinese Adults

Yu DH, Huang JF, Chen JC, Cao J, Li JX, Gu DF

Department of Evidence-Based Medicine Cardiovascular Institute and Fu Wai Hospital of the Chinese Academy of Medical Science and Peking Union Medical College 167 Beilishi Rd Beijing 100037, PR China

Objective To identify which is the best predictor among four blood pressure (BP) measures, SBP, DBP, pulse pressure (PP), or mean arterial pressure (MAP)? How about the quantitative association between BP levels and risk of CVD?

Methods We conducted a prospective cohort study in a nationally representative sample of 169, 871 Chinese men and women aged ≥40 years. Data on SBP and DBP and other variables were obtained at a baseline examination in 1991 with a standard protocol. Follow-up evaluation was conducted in 1999-2000, with a response rate of 93.4%. We calculated the MAP as 1/3 (SBP) + 2/3 (DBP). Cox proportional hazards models were used to examine the multivariate adjusted relationship of BP with the incidence of CVD. To explore further the association of BP with CVD and to allow a detailed examination of the association between BP and CVD risk across a wide range of BP values without a priori assumptions about the shape of the dose-response curve. We determined the incidence and hazard ratios of CVD for quintile of SBP (<108, 108 to 118, 119 to 128, 129 to 140, >140 mmHg), (<67, 67-73, 74 to 79, 80 to 87, >87 mmHg), PP (<36, 36 to 42, 43 to 49, 50 to 59, >59 mmHg), and MAP (<82, 82 to 88, 89 to 94, 95 to 104, >104 mmHg).

Results The incidence of CVD is 2919. 6/100, 000 person-years, 1853. 8/100, 000 person-years, 2205. 8/100, 000 person-years, and 2140. 2/100, 000 person-years for SBP > 140 mmHg, DBP > 87 mmHg, PP > 59 mmHg, MAP > 104 mmHg, respectively. Contrasted with SBP < 108 mmHg, DBP < 67 mmHg, PP < 36 mmHg, MAP < 82 mmHg classification, the relative risk (RR) of CVD is 1. 54, 1. 32, 1. 18, 1. 54 for SBP129-140 mmHg, DBP 80-87 mmHg, PP 50-59 mmHg, MAP 95-104 mmHg as well as 2. 74, 2. 26, 2. 24 and 2. 54 for SBP > 140 mmHg, DBP > 87 mmHg, PP > 59 mmHg, MAP > 104 mmHg, respectively. Compared with SBP < 108 mmHg, DBP < 67 mmHg, PP < 36 mmHg, MAP < 82 mmHg, the PAR of CVD is 9. 1%, 6. 1%, 8. 8%, and 11. 0% for SBP129-140 mmHg, DBP 80-87 mmHg, PP 50-59 mmHg, MAP 95-104 mmHg as well as 25. 7%, 20. 0%, 20. 5% and 24. 1% for SBP > 140 mmHg, DBP > 87 mmHg, PP > 59 mmHg, MAP > 104 mmHg, respectively. Moreover, 1 standard deviation increase of 4 BP measures (22 mmHg for SBP, 12 mmHg for DBP, 16 mmHg for PP, and 14 mmHg for MAP) leads to the increase of risk for CVD as 1. 45-, 1. 46-, 1. 28-and 1. 49 fold, respectively.

Conclusions SBP is an important predictor for CVD as well as MAP. Lifestyle therapeutic modifications should be emphasized in the prevention and control of hypertension, especially for prehypertensive individuals.

29

Prevalence of Arterial Stiffness and Risk Factors for Ankle-brachial Pulse Wave Velocity in Han ethnical group in Xinjiang, China

Hu YH, Ma YT

Cardiology Dept. of the First Affiliated Hospital of Xinjiang Medical University, China

Objective To investigate the prevalence of arterial stiffness and study the risk factors for the ankle-brachial pulse wave velocity (baPWV) in Han ethnic, Xinjiang, China.

Methods The baPWV was examined from Han population who live around Urumqi, Kelamayi, Yili by arterial stiffness early detection equipment VP-1000 (Colin Company of Japan). Data on age, gender, body height, fasting blood glucose, triglyceride, total cholesterol and other biochemical indicators were collected. Disease status like hypertension, coronary heart disease, diabetes mellitus and stroke was also obtained. Subjects were divided into baPWV < 1400 cm/s and baPWV ≥1400 cm/s group. baPWV ≥1400 cm/s was considered as the arterial stiffness increase.

Results 43. 27% of Han community residents in Xinjiang had the increased arterial stiffness. The prevalence of increased arterial stiffness was increased with age, and was higher in men than in women. Logistic regression showed that age (OR: 1. 31, 95% CI: 1. 16-1. 52), systolic blood pressure (OR: 2. 03, 95% CI: 1. 73-2. 38), diastolic blood pressure (OR: 1. 55, 95% CI: 1. 28-1. 88), total cholesterol (OR: 1. 30, 95% CI: 1. 10-1. 52) were the risk for arterial stiffness.

Conclusions The prevalence of increased arterial stiffness is high in Han community residents in Xinjiang at the age of 35-60 years. Age, systolic and diastolic blood pressure, total cholesterol is associated with baPWV, an indicator of arterial stiffness in Han ethnical group, in Xinjiang.

30

Atherosclerosis Measured by Non-invasive Method in Zhaosu Hazakh in Xinxiang

Liu C, Ma YT, Ma X, Yang YN

Cardiology Dept. of the First Affiliated Hospital of Xinjiang Medical University

Objective To describe the distribution of atherosclerosis of Hazakh ethnicity in Xinjiang, China and to evaluate the relationship between atherosclerosis (AS) and the risk factors of cardiovascular (CVD) in Hazakh ethnicity.

Methods 1274 volunteers included 469 male and 805 female from Zhaosu city of YiLi hazakh autonomous prefecture in Xinxiang were enrolled in the study. All participants underwent physical checkup and interview for collecting data on lifestyle such as smoking, systolic blood pressure (SBP), diastolic blood pressure (DBP), duration of diabetes, body mass index (BMI), total cholesterol (TC), triglyceride (TG), low density lipoprotein cholesterol (LDL-C), high density lipoprotein cholesterol (HDL-C). The intima-media thickness (IMT) of carotid arteries, pulse pressure (PP), ankle-brachial index (ABI), and brachial-ankle pulse wave velocity (b-a PWV) were measured by non-invasive method. The relationship between atherosclerosis and the risk factors of cardiovascular disease in Hazakh nationality was analyzed.

Results AS prevalence was 42. 6% , 48. 6% , 38. 2% in general group and in male and female group, respectively. The prevalence was higher in male group ($p < 0.05$). AS prevalence was elevated with the increase of age ($p < 0.05$). The hypertension, DM, hyperlipidemia prevalence and the rate of awareness and under control were 43. 3% 63. 7% , 44. 9% ;52% , 59. 6% , 49. 1% ;59. 5% , 25. 8% , 6. 4% in Hazakh nationality in Zhousu, Xinxiang. Compared with non-atherosclerosis group, hypertension, age, low density lipoprotein cholesterol level, hyperlipidemia, adiposity, hypercholesterolemia were higher in the atherosclerosis group ($p < 0.05$). But, no differences were found in smoking, hypertriglyceridemia, family history, drinking habits between two groups. AS prevalence was 40. 1% for individuals with one CVD risk, and the prevalence rate was 85. 7% for those with 3 CVD risks.

Conclusions AS prevalence of Hazakh nationality in Zhaosu, Xinxiang is 42. 6% by the non-invasive method. Hypertension and age are independent risk factors of atherosclerosis for hazakh nationality in Xinjiang. AS were associated with the increased number of CVD risks.

31

Prevalence of Cardiovascular Disease Risk Factors among the Kazakh, Uygur Mongolia and Han population in Xinjiang, China

Li NF, Wang HM, Ling Z, Wang XL, Ya ZF, Zhang DL, Yang WJ, Chen QY
The Center of Hypertension of the People's Hospital of Xinjiang Uygur Autonomous Region; The Institute of Hypertension of Xinjiang; Urumqi, Xinjiang 830001, China

Objective Effective prevention of cardiovascular disease (CVD) requires early detection and modification of risk factors in susceptible subjects. The prevalence and component of CVD risk factors varies with different ethnicity. There are less studies of CVD epidemiology conducted in ethnic populations including Kazakh, Uygur, Mongolia in Xinjiang. Aim of this study is to investigate the prevalence of CVD risk factors among Kazakh, Uygur, Mongolia and Han population in Xinjiang.

Methods A cross-sectional study was conducted in Xinjiang ($n = 11197$, including 5046 males and 6151 females aged more than 30 years) during 2006 to 2008. A set of questionnaires was completed and the demographic data, blood pressure, body mass index, fasting and postprandial blood were obtained. Serum lipid, fasting plasma glucose and 2-hour postprandial glucose levels were determined.

Results The age-standardized prevalence of dyslipidemia, hypertension, diabetes, current smoking, and overweight was 62. 61% , 43. 43% , 11. 54% , 23. 37% and 62. 8% , respectively. Dyslipidemia, overweight and smoking prevalence was higher in men than in women (all $P < 0.001$). Hypertension, dyslipidemia and overweight were more common in Kazakh (54. 21% , 68. 83% , 65. 57% , respectively), Uygur (39. 96% , 71. 40% , 70. 44% , respectively), Mongolia (53. 4% , 73. 93% , 57. 43% , respectively) population than in Han (31. 59% , 47. 7% , 54. 36% , respectively), respectively (all $P < 0.001$). Diabetes was more common in Uygur (18. 14%) than in Kazakh (7. 74%) and in Han (8. 44%), respectively (all $P < 0.001$). Smoking was more common in Mongolia (33. 38%), Han (37. 29%), than in Kazakh (16. 21%), Uygur (16. 72%), respectively (all $P < 0.001$). After adjusting for gender, age, smoking and drinking, covariate variance analysis showed that compared with Han, the mean levels of SBP, DBP, BMI, FBG, LDL-c were significantly higher but HDL-c was lower in Kazakh, Uygur and Mongolia population (all $P < 0.001$). Overall, 88. 6% , 63. 2% , and 31. 0% of Xinjiang population had ≥ 1, ≥ 2, and ≥ 3 modifiable CVD risk factors (dyslipidemia, hypertension, diabetes, cigarette smoking, and overweight), respectively.

Conclusions The prevalence of dyslipidemia, hypertension, diabetes, smoking, and overweight is common and varies with ethnicity in Xinjiang. Ethnic-specific and cost-effective strategies to prevent CVD risk factors are needed in Xinjiang, China.

32

Serum Uric Acid is associated with Common Cardiovascular Risk Factors in Uygur Population

Wang HM, Hong J, Zhou L, Yan ZT, Yao XG, Li NF
The Center of Hypertension of the People's Hospital of Xinjiang Uygur Autonomous Region; the Institute of Hypertension of Xinjiang; Urumqi, Xinjiang 830001, China

Objective The prevalence of hypertension was low in Uygur ethnical population which has high prevalence of cardiovascular risk factors including hypertension, overweight/obesity, dyslipidemia, diabetes (DM), impaired fasting glucose (IFG), impaired glucose tolerance (IGT) and insulin resistance (IR). The study was to investigate the relationship between serum uric acid (UA) and these risk factors in Uygur, China.
Methods A cross-sectional study was conducted in Uygur (892 males, 1323 females) aged from 20 to 108 years. The demographic data, systolic blood pressure (SBP), diastolic blood pressure (DBP), body mass index (BMI), fasting and postprandial blood were obtained. Serum uric acid (UA), total cholesterol (TC), high-density lipoprotein cholesterol (HDL-c), low-density lipoprotein cholesterol (LDL-c), triglyceride (TG), fasting blood glucose (FBG), 2-hour postprandial glucose (2HPG) and fasting insulin (FINS) were determined. Relationship between UA and cardiovascular risk factors were compared among different groups of UA.
Results The prevalence of hyperuricemia was 3.1% in the present population. The mean of BMI, SBP, DBP, TC, HDL-c, LDL-c, TG, FBG, FINS and HOMA-IR and the prevalence of hypertension, IR, hyperglycemia, overweight/obesity, hypercholesteremia, hyper-LDL-c and hypertriglyceridemia increased with UA but the prevalence of hypo-HDL-c decreased ($P < 0.05$). Adjusted for confounding factors, Logistic regression analysis confirmed the odds ratios for hypertension, hyperglycemia, IR, overweight/obesity, hypercholesteremia, hyper-LDL-c, hypertriglyceridemia increased significantly with UA, however, it decreased with UA for Hypo-HDL-c. After adjusting for confounding factors, covariate variance analysis showed that compared with the normal controls, the serum UA was significantly higher in hypertension, overweight/obesity, hyperglycemia and IR, hypercholesteremia and hypertriglyceridemia and hyper-LDL-c groups, respectively. However, the serum UA in hypo-HDL-c group was significantly lower than that of normal group ($P < 0.05$).
Conclusions Elevated UA level is associated with hypertension, overweight/obesity, hypercholesteremia, LDL-c, hypertriglyceridemia, hyperglycemia and IR in Uygur. Further studies are needed to clarify why UA is positively correlated to HDL-c. An ethnic-specific UA-based prevention strategy is needed for reducing these risk factors to control CVD more efficiently in Uygur.

33

Metabolic Syndrome and Carotid Atherosclerosis in a Group of Community Population

Zou XX, Li Y, Zhang HG, Chen Z, Wang H, Zhao LC, Gu DF
Fu Wai Hospital, Peking Union Medical College & Chinese Academy of Medical Sciences, Beijing 100037, China

Objective To explore the relationships of metabolic syndromes (MS) and carotid atherosclerosis in a middle aged community population in China and to estimate the predictive role of MS diagnosed by different definitions.
Methods Data were collected from the National Project of "The 11th Five Year Plan". There were 685 subjects (313 men, 372 women), aged 45-64, free of cardiovascular disease, stroke or cancer, recruited in this cross-sectional study. Data on life style, disease history, and physical examination were obtained with the same protocol. Color Doppler Ultrasonic Diagnostic System was used for the measurement of carotid intima-media thickness and plaque. MS was diagnosed by the criteria of IDF, NCEP ATP Ⅲ and The Guidelines of Dyslipidemia Control for Chinese Adult ("Guideline"), which was published in 2007.
Results 1. The prevalence of MS was 40.6%, 30.1% and 33.0% according to the criteria of IDF, NCEP ATP Ⅲ and "Guideline" respectively. The Kappa value was 0.77, 0.82 and 0.72, respectively between each pair of three criteria. 2. The mean ± sd of intima-media thickness in common carotid artery (CCA-IMT) was 0.76 ± 0.14mm, 0.77 ± 0.14mm, 0.77 ± 0.14mm; the prevalence of atherosclerotic plaques was 46.0%, 52.1% and 48.7% respectively in MS groups diagnosed with the criteria of IDF、NCEP ATP Ⅲ and "Guideline" respectively. The differences was still significant ($P < 0.001$) after adjustment for age, gender, LDL-C, current smoking and drinking habit. 3. Multiple linear regression analyses showed that classification of MS with each of the criteria was significantly correlated with CCA-IMT; the regression coefficient was 0.04 (95% CI: 0.02-0.07) for IDF, 0.056 (95% CI: 0.03-0.08) for NCEP ATP Ⅲ; and 0.040 (95% CI: 0.02-0.06) for

"Guideline" after adjustment for age, gender, LDL-C, smoking and drinking habit. 4. Logistic regression analyses showed that each classification of MS increased the prevalence of carotid atherosclerotic plaques. The Odds Ratio (OR) was 1.50 (95% CI: 1.06-2.11) for IDF, 1.77 (95% CI: 1.22-2.57) for NCEP ATP Ⅲ, 1.64 (95% CI: 1.16-2.33) for "Guideline" after adjustment for age, gender, LDL-C, smoking, and drinking habit respectively, compared with the group without MS.

Conclusions The results indicate that MS increases the risk of atherosclerosis independently in general population.

34

Left Atrial Maze Procedure for Chronic Atrial Fibrillation associated with Rheumatic Valve Disease: a follow-up of 7 years

Li L, Xu ZY, Zhang BR
Changhai hospital, Second military medical university, PLA, Shanghai 200433

Objective To assess the long-term electrophysiologic and heart function outcome in patients with chronic atrial fibrillation (AF) associated with rheumatic heart disease who underwent concomitant maze procedure.

Methods From 1998 to 2001, 15 patients underwent left atrial maze procedure combined with valve surgery. Epicardial mapping electrograms was performed during operation. In a postoperative follow-up of 84.2 ± 8.9 months 12-lead electrocardiograms, holter monitoring and echocardiograms were recorded.

Results: Epicardial mapping electrograms during surgery showed that slow conduction was most often located in the middle of posterior left atrial wall (26.4%). Double potentials and fragmented potentials mostly occurred at posterior left atrial wall (41.3% and 19.4% respectively). Epicardial two-atrium mapping after recovery of heartbeat showed that 75% of patients had two-atrium sinus rhythm and 25% atrail flutter. There were no perioperative complications. At 3 months after maze procedure 67% of all patients were free of AF without any antiarrhythmic medication, 80% at 1 year, and 92.8% at the end of follow-up. Sinus node and atrioventricular node function were normal in 84.6% of the patients who maintained sinus rhythm. Permanent pacemakers were implanted in 2 patients at 3 and 5 years after operation due to sinus arrest more than 3 seconds. Echocardiographic examination showed that left atrial volume (LAV), left atrial dimension (LAD), end-diastolic left ventricular dimension (LVEDd), and end-diastolic left ventricular volume (LVEDV) were significantly smaller than those of postoperation. (LAV 69.06 ± 21.23 cm3 VS 105.51 ± 33.79 cm3, $P < 0.05$; LAD 2.56 ± 0.5 cm VS 3.67 ± 1.10 cm, $P < 0.05$; LVEDd 4.12 ± 0.24 cm VS 4.63 ± 0.49 cm, $P < 0.05$; LVEDV 82.61 ± 15.50 cm3 VS. 103.80 ± 24.48 cm3, $P < 0.05$). Cardiac output (CO) markedly decreased comparing to that of postoperation (4.60 ± 1.35 L/min VS. 5.66 ± 0.05 L/min $P < 0.05$). During the follow-up period the mean ejection fraction was 66.6 ± 7.10% and the mean left ventricular fractional shortenings was 36.9 ± 6.4%. Eighty-seven percent had documented, and 93% had right atrial function. The rehospitalization rate was 29.8%.

Conclusions Left atrial maze procedure combined with valve operation is a safe and effective treatment for eliminating AF associated with rheumatic valve disease. During long-term follow-up period 90.8% of patients maintained sinus rhythm, 89% had left atrial function.

35

How to Predict the Public Health Impact of Statins?

Boissel JP, Kahoul R
Dept. de Pharmacologie Clinique, Faculte RTH Laennec rue Guillaume Paradin, France

The public health impact (PHI) of a treatment/prevention strategy is the number of spared event (NSE) when the intervention is applied to a population for a given period of time. Among the population, the people to whom the strategy is applied constitute the intervention target population (ITP). In order to compute the NSE and to delineate the ITP, we need: a precisely defined therapeutic objective (TO), the intervention effect model (EM), the risk distribution in the population and an external constraint. The EM is obtained from a meta-analysis of all the available randomized clinical trials (RCT) with the intervention. From the EM a relation that links the absolute benefit with the intervention to subject's characteristics, especially his/her risk of presenting the event (the TO), is derived which will be used to compute the NSE. One needs further the rate of event distribution in the population. It was obtained from the French Virtual Representative Population (VRP). The EM could be linear or curvilinear. In both case, it could present a natural threshold, i. e. when subjects with risk lower than this threshold will fare worse with the intervention than without. In the other cases, there is no natural threshold, which means that for very low risk subjects there is benefit which is quite tiny and not worth the cost and/or burden of intervention.

For the statin case, prevention of death of any cause was selected as the TO. We collected 91 RCT comparing a statin to a placebo or nothing. The statin EM against total death occurred to be linear with a [0, 0] intercept. This means that the meta-analysis common relative risk (RR), actually 0.90 ($p < 0.001$), could be used instead of a more complicated EM. There was no natural threshold. Note that the RCT strength of evidence was correlated with the common RR estimate. The external constraint was the resources that the community accepts to pay for the intervention. The other parameter was the cost of each statin. Given this cost, a marketed statin was the most efficient. However, for a 1 M French VRP between 45 and 65 years of age, the number of spared deaths over 1 year was 753 with a ITP of 628855, and 100M. With the least efficient statin and the same resources the figures were 33 and 280622 respectively. This approach could be applied to any type of treatment/prevention strategy provided that enough data on efficacy are available and risk distribution in the population is known or could be approximate.

Nursing

1

The modern overall nursing model needs standardized healthy education

Zhai JW, Zhang YF, Zhao R
Cardiovascular Institute and Fu Wai Hospital, Beijing 100037

Objective To investigate the contribution of effective, standardize healthy education in improving the coronary artery disease patient's satisfaction, in order to enhance the healthy education's significance and quantity in clinical practice.
Methods From 2003, the year of quantity control year, patients are chosen from the four ward of Fu Wai hospital, in the forms of one-on-one, divided groups, collective education based on patient's need to give them concrete designed, specific, effective and integrity healthy education. Simultaneously, hand out healthy education materials, on which both the name of people giving education and educated patients are write down. The most important thing different from past is we calculate the patient assessment and evaluate the effective of education. Feedback and supplementary are given in time. This work are charge by specific person, overall planning, unceasing improve the ways of work, always refresh the content, attain the goal of planning and effective. The standardized healthy education has received a very good result.
Results After the implementation of healthy education, the patient satisfaction has greatly improved($P < 0.05$), the patient satisfactory about healthy education rise form 89.07% to 99.01%, the patient satisfactory about nursing service rise from 91.07 % to 98.30%, the patient satisfactory about nursing technology rise from 90.82% to 97.63%.
Conclusions Strengthen the healthy education is more suitable for the modern nursing model, and has great significance in promoting nursing quantity and satisfy the patients' need of healthy. In clinical practice, nurses should promote the quantity of healthy education, guarantee the efficiency of healthy education. Finally attain the goal of meet the patients' healthy need, improve their quantity of live. Nurses should take advantage of this platform, emphasize the communication between nurses and patients, enhancing their confidence in nurse, and improve their impressions about nurses, make nurse's ability are approbated, through healthy education, reduce the contradiction between nurses and patients, enhance the patients satisfactory during hospitalization.

2

Nursing of Severe Acute Left Heart Failure after Cardiovascular Operations by Reducing the Heart Preload using Continuous Veno-venous Hemofiltration Combine with Mild Hypothermia

Wu YY, Zhang HT, Wang JX
Intensive Care Unit, Department of Vascular Surgery, Cardiovascular Institute and Fu Wai Hospital, Beijing 100037

Objective Discuss the nursing experience of improving the condition of acute left heart failure after cardiovascular operations by using continuous veno-venous hemofiltration (CVVH) and mild hypothermia.
Methods By means of CVVH system, indwelling dual-lumen catheter through femoral vein and putting CVVH pipeline into container filled with mixture of ice and water, control the central temperatures of six patients between 34℃ and 35℃, meanwhile warm up the ending. Calm the pa-

tients and assist their breath by ventilator.

Results The cardiac function of six patients is significantly improved and all of their monitoring indexes are stable. During the period of using CVVH, the phenomenon of anticoagulation deficiency and serious bleeding complications did not occur. Five of the patients discharged from hospital after completely cured and one died of the rupture of residual aortic dissection.

Conclusions This paper present the method of reducing the heart preload and curing acute left heart failure by using continuous veno-venous hemofiltration and mild hypothermia, which apply the basic principle of traditional therapy. Clean out the moisture and solute continuously, slowly and isotonic, keep the balance of liquid, excrete the added liquid and output keep more than the input, make the patient at the state of ultrafiltration and reduce the load and the work of heart; Did not occur the adverse reaction of increasing of oxygen consumption and heart work by chilling, which win the time and condition for repairing of functional injured myocardial cells. The method is simple in cooling, good in effect, and it can avoid the disadvantages that the effect of regional hypothermia simple in limb peripheral is not good, there are many adverse reactions and so on.

3

Post-operative Care of Heart Transplantation with Extracorporeal Membrane Oxygenation

Wu R, Shi L, Wei YY, Liu JL
Cardiovascular Institute and Fu Wai Hospital, Beijing 100037

Objective To summarize nursing care experience about ten patients using ECMO in the post-operative period of heart transplantation.

Methods We performed 131 orthotopic heart transplantations from Jun. 2004 to Dec. 2008. Ten patients required the use of veno-artery ECMO support in the post-operative period of heart transplantation for acute graft failure or acute heart failure. All patients were monitored by electrocardiography, hemodynamics, body temperature, urine volume, activated coagulation time, liver & renal function, free hemoglobin & colloid osmotic pressure.

Results Nine survivals discharged with NYHA I, one patient died. The ECMO time was 40-824 h. After bedside UCG evaluating heart function recovery, ECMO could be weaned off uneventfully after 100h, long-term follow-up results were good.

Conclusions Intensive care of heart & lung function during ECMO, reasonable adjusting respirator index, intensive lung & respiratory tract care, nutrition support, preventing arrhythmia, bleeding & embolism, infection, bedsores & other complications, may decrease mortality of severe patients in the post-operative period of heart transplantation.

4

Replacement of a Permanent Artificial Pacemaker Clinical Analysis

Li W, Wu LR, Fang Y, Liu XD, Li P, Liang JF, Lei MM, Li AM, Chen Y, Lang Y
Department of Cardiology, Guiyang Medical College Affiliated Hospital, Guiyang 550004

Objective To analyze reasons of the replacement of a permanent artificial heart pacemaker electrodes and evaluation of the parameters of the old features.

Methods A total of pacemaker replacement of 59 cases of cases, 36 males and 23 females, aged 70 ± 8 (29-87) years, Ⅲ degree atrioventricular block in 27 cases, 32 cases of sick sinus syndrome ; Single chamber pacemaker 36 cases, 23 cases of dual-chamber pacemaker, pacemaker average time 86 ± 11 (48-142) months. A total of 10 cases electrode replacement; the replacement of the process of Ⅲ degree atrioventricular block in patients with temporary pacemakers are preset to protect them.

Results The reasons for pacemaker replacement natural pacemaker battery depletion of 46 cases meeting, battery depletion of 13 cases in advance; Lead replacement of reasons: 6 with single-chamber pacemakers for the double, pacing threshold too high, too low impedance electrodes, the diaphragm and contraction of the pocket of infection in 1 case. When the replacement of ventricular pacemaker, atrial pacing threshold [(1.1 ±0.4) V, (1.2 ±0.5) V] with the first threshold at the time of implantation [(0.5 ±0.2) V, (0.6 ±0.3) V], compared to significantly higher ($P<0.01$). Replacement of ventricular, atrial electrode impedance [(640.7 ± 171.5) Ω, (637.2 ± 143.6) Ω], R-wave, P wave amplitude [(11.0 ±3.4) mV, (3.8 ± 1.8) mV] when the first implant [(596.3 ± 169.5) Ω, (623.7 ± 135.1) Ω], [(10.3 ±3.8)

mV, (3.7 ± 1.7) mV] compared the difference was not statistically significant (all $P > 0.05$).
Conclusions The main reasons for the replacement of pacemaker battery depletion of natural, early battery depletion and failure to follow-up of it; pacemaker electrode replacement can continue to use the most; Ⅲ degree atrioventricular block in patients with implantation in replacement of the provisional starting when pacing device to protect them.

5

CNS Outcomes After Cardiac Surgery: A 20 Year Update

Murkin JM
Dirctor of cardiac Anesthesiology Research
Professor of Anesthesiology
University of Western Ontario London, Ontario, Canada

The current understanding of the etiology of adverse central nervous (CNS) events following cardiac surgery involves several identifiable, evidence-based mechanisms: atherosclerotic emboli, microgaseous and microgaseous and microparticulate emboli, and hypoperfusion Secondary factors including patient co-morbidities and inherent genetic suscepibilities, as well as systemic inflammatory processes and a suboptimal metabolic milieu may interact to potentiate the extent of injury. More than two decades ago clinical physiology studies were focused on understanding the relationship beween cerebralblood flow (CBF) and cerebral oxygen metabolism during cardiopulmonary bypass (CPB) This result in the generation of hypotheses relating the delivery of cerebral emboli as beingproportional to CBF, and emphasized the role of cerebral emboli in the genesis of CNS injury.
Specifically, alpha-stat PH management was hypothesized to result in a lower incidence of CNS injury due to lowered cerebral embolic delivery and avoidence of intracerebral steal. Subsequently there have been several independent prospective randomized clinical trials demonstrating improved neurological and neuropsychological outcomes associated with alpha-stat management in adult patients undergoing moderately hypothermic CPB. Pulsatile perfusion has also been shown to improve averrall clinical outcomes and remains a topic of interest. With appropiate management atreteges during CPB, current studies have demonstrated no significant difference Iin the Iincedence of cognitive dysfunction whether or not CPB is employed during coronary revascularization. There is some confilicting envidence whether or not the incidence of late cognitive dysfunction is similar beween surgical patients and those undergoing medical management or nor-surgical revascularization using percutaneous coronary intervention with the suggestion that late cognitive decline is due to issues that will be further considered in this discussion of perioperative cognitive dysfuntion are:
i) The influlence of phenotype and inflammatory processes
ii) The role of cardiopulmonary bypass versus beating heart surgery
iii) The ralative impact of microemboli versus hypoperfusion
iv) Susceptibility of subpopulation eg diabetics
v) The influence of surgucal intervention versus medical management
vi) The long term impact of cogntive dysfuntion.

6

A New Look for An Old Drug: Vitamin D in Prevention of Cardiovascular Disease-Prepared for International Heart Forum Beijing 2009

Wang L
Division of Preventive Medicine, Department of Medicine
Brigham and Women's Hospital, Harvard Medical School, 900 Commonwealth Ave 3rd Floor Boston, MA 02215, USA

Vitamin D deficiency was well recognized in the early 20th century for its severe clinical outcomes related to bone health. Synthesis of vitamin D3 in the skin through sun exposure is the major source of vitamin D for humans. Only a small amount of vitamin D comes from dietary intake. Vitamin D is metabolized through two sequential hydroxylation steps to form 25-hydroxy vitamin D (25 (OH) D, calcidiol) and 1, 25-dihydroxy vitamin D (1, 25 (OH) 2D, calcitriol). 25 (OH) D is the major circulating form of vitamin D, and has been used as the standard clinical assessment for vitamin D status. Whereas 1, 25 (OH) 2D is the most active metabolite. Recent advances in research have linked vitamin D status to many non-skeletal health conditions, including cardiovascular disease (CVD). Vitamin D functions as a negative endocrine regulator of the renin-angiotensin system, improves insulin secretion and insulin sensitivity, inhibits vascular smooth muscle cell proliferation and angiogenesis, and modulates inflammatory processes. These effects of vitamin D may potentially improve cardiovascular risk factor profile and reduce CVD event risk. Ecological studies and cross-sectional studies have linked deficient or insufficient vitamin D status to higher prevalence of CVD in different populations. Retrospective case-control studies found lower levels of circulating 25 (OH) D in patients of myocardial infarction, stroke, peripheral vascular disease, and heart failure compared to healthy controls. Evidences from prospective studies are accumulating in support of an inverse association between baseline circulating 25 (OH) D level and subsequent risk of CVD. Use of vitamin D supplement has been associated with a reduced cardiovascular mortality or CVD event rate in patients with chronic kidney disease as well as in general population. An alarming epidemic of vitamin D deficiency/insufficiency worldwide and availability of low-risk, high-efficacy intervention strategy underscore the public health importance to elucidate the role of vitamin D inadequacy in the development of CVD. Future studies of vitamin D and risk of CVD, particularly large-scale, randomized trials with adequate doses of vitamin D supplement and CVD ascertained as the primary endpoint, are critically needed to evaluate any potential benefit of vitamin D supplementation in the prevention of CVD.

INDEX

A

B

C

D

M

N

P

Q

R

S

T

V

W

X

Y

Z

An invaluable aid in understanding and treating heart disease

CARDIOLOGY

International Journal of Cardiovascular Medicine, Surgery, Pathology and Pharmacology

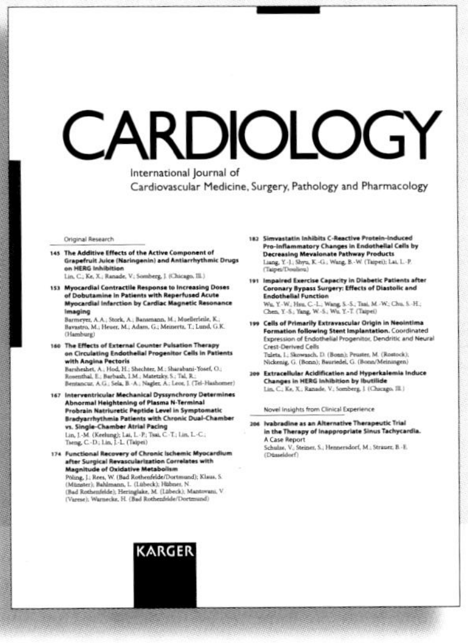

Cardiology features first reports on original clinical, preclinical and fundamental research as well as instructive case reports and topical comprehensive reviews in selected areas of cardiovascular disease. Investigators from all over the world contribute to keep readers regularly informed of current strategies in the prevention, recognition and treatment of heart disease. Their articles not only describe but offer critical appraisals of new developments in non-invasive and invasive diagnostic methods and in pharmacologic, nutritional and mechanical/surgical therapies. Following the recent incorporation of the journal *HeartDrug*, *Cardiology* will increase its coverage of issues relating to cardiovascular clinical pharmacology and drug trials. Special sections in a variety of subspecialty areas reinforce the journal's value as a complete record of recent progress for all cardiologists, internists, cardiac surgeons, clinical physiologists, pharmacologists and professionals in other areas of medicine interested in current activity in cardiovascular diseases.

Selected contributions

Cell Therapy of Acute Myocardial Infarction: Open Questions: **Dimmeler, S.; Zeiher, A.M.** (Frankfurt)

The Impact of Statin Treatment on Presentation Mode and Early Outcomes in Acute Coronary Syndromes: **Cuculi, F.; Radovanovic, D.; Eberli, F.R.; Stauffer, J.C.; Bertel, O.; Erne, P.** (Luzern) **on behalf of the AMIS Plus Investigators**

Clinical and Hemodynamic Effects of Bosentan Dose Optimization in Symptomatic Heart Failure Patients with Severe Systolic Dysfunction, Associated with Secondary Pulmonary Hypertension – A Multi-Center Randomized Study: **Kaluski, E.** (Newark, N.J.); **Cotter, G.** (Durham, N.C.); **Leitman, M.** (Tel Aviv); **Milo-Cotter, O.** (Durham, N.C.); **Krakover, R.** (Tel Aviv); **Kobrin, I.; Moriconi, T.; Rainisio, M.** (Allschwil); **Caspi, A.** (Jerusalem); **Reizin, L.** (Beer Sheva); **Zimlichman, R.; Vered, Z.** (Tel Aviv)

State of the Art Percutaneous Intervention for the Treatment of Valvular Heart Disease: A Review of the Current Technologies and Ongoing Research in the Field of Percutaneous Valve Replacement and Repair: **Babaliaros, V.; Block, P.** (Atlanta, Ga.)

Low-Molecular-Weight Heparins in Conjunction with Thrombolysis for ST-Elevation Acute Myocardial Infarction. A Critical Review of the Literature: **Rubboli, A.** (Bologna); **Ottani, F.** (Forlì); **Capecchi, A.; Brancaleoni, R.** (Bologna); **Galvani, M.** (Forlì); **Swahn, E.** (Linköping)

Weight Lifting and Aortic Dissection: More Evidence for a Connection: **Hatzaras, I.; Tranquilli, M.; Coady, M.; Barrett, P.M.; Bible, J.; Elefteriades, J.A.** (New Haven, Conn.)

Chronic Development of Ischaemic Mitral Regurgitation during Post-Infarction Remodelling: **Nixdorff, U.; Klinghammer, L.** (Erlangen-Nuremberg); **Wüstefeld, G.; Mohr-Kahaly, S.; von Bardeleben, R.S.** (Mainz)

Tracking Coronary Calcification and Atherosclerotic Lesions in Patients with Stable Angina Pectoris Undergoing Nifedipine Therapy: **Motro, M.** (Tel Aviv); **Kirwan, B.-A.; de Brouwer, S.** (Nyon); **Poole-Wilson, P.A.** (London); **Shemesh, J.** (Tel Aviv) **on behalf of the Action CC side-arm study**

More information at
www.karger.com/crd

- Pay-per-View and Subscriber Access to Full Text
- Full Table of Contents
- Full Editorial Board
- Free Abstracts and Selected Articles
- Online Sample Issue
- Submission/Guidelines for Authors
- Subscription Details
- Free Alert Service
- Online Library Recommendation

Cardiology
2009: Volumes 112, 113, 114
4 issues per volume
Language: English
ISSN 0008–6312 (print)
ISSN 1421–9751 (online)

Listed in bibliographic services, including *Current Contents®/Life Sciences, MEDLINE, Biological Abstracts, EMBASE/Excerpta Medica.*

KARGER